Non-Motor Parkinson's Disease

Non-Motor Parkinson's Disease

Edited by

Néstor Gálvez-Jiménez
Florida International University

Amos D. Korczyn
Tel-Aviv University

Ramón Lugo-Sanchez
Cleveland Clinic

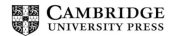

CAMBRIDGE
UNIVERSITY PRESS

CAMBRIDGE
UNIVERSITY PRESS

University Printing House, Cambridge CB2 8BS, United Kingdom

One Liberty Plaza, 20th Floor, New York, NY 10006, USA

477 Williamstown Road, Port Melbourne, VIC 3207, Australia

314–321, 3rd Floor, Plot 3, Splendor Forum, Jasola District Centre, New Delhi – 110025, India

103 Penang Road, #05–06/07, Visioncrest Commercial, Singapore 238467

Cambridge University Press is part of the University of Cambridge.

It furthers the University's mission by disseminating knowledge in the pursuit of education, learning, and research at the highest international levels of excellence.

www.cambridge.org
Information on this title: www.cambridge.org/9781316510650
DOI: 10.1017/9781009039291

© Cambridge University Press 2022

First published 2022

Printed in the United Kingdom by TJ Books Limited, Padstow Cornwall

A catalogue record for this publication is available from the British Library.

Library of Congress Cataloging-in-Publication Data
Names: Gálvez-Jiménez, Néstor, author. | Korczyn, Amos D., 1940– author. | Lugo-Sanchez, Ramón, author.
Title: Non-motor Parkinson's disease / edited by Néstor Gálvez-Jiménez, Florida International University, Amos Korczyn, Tel-Aviv University, Ramón Lugo-Sanchez, Cleveland Clinic.
Description: Cambridge, United Kingdom ; New York, NY : Cambridge University Press, 2021. | Includes bibliographical references and index.
Identifiers: LCCN 2021026816 (print) | LCCN 2021026817 (ebook) | ISBN 9781316510650 (hardback) | ISBN 9781009039291 (ebook)
Subjects: LCSH: Parkinson's disease.
Classification: LCC RC382 .G35 2021 (print) | LCC RC382 (ebook) | DDC 616.8/33–dc23
LC record available at https://lccn.loc.gov/2021026816
LC ebook record available at https://lccn.loc.gov/2021026817

ISBN 978-1-316-51065-0 Hardback

....

Contents

Contents

Contributors

Roy N. Alcalay, MD, MSc,
Department of Neurology, College of Physicians
and Surgeons, Columbia University, New York;
and Taub Institute for Research on Alzheimer's
Disease and the Aging Brain, Columbia
University, New York.

Tim Anderson,
New Zealand Brain Research Institute,
Christchurch, New Zealand.

Camila Aquino, MD, MSc, PhD,
Department of Clinical Neurosciences,
Hotchkiss Brain Institute,
University of Calgary,
Calgary, Alberta, Canada.

Esther Azizi MD,
Department of Dermatology, Sackler Faculty of
Medicine,Tel Aviv University, Israel.

Ovidiu-Alexandru Bajenaru, Deceased.
From the Department of Neurology,
Bucharest University, Romania

Kailash P. Bhatia,
Prof. KP Bhatia, FRCP Professor of Clinical
Neurology Department of Clinical and
Movement Neurosciences UCL, Institute of
Neurology, NHNN, Queen Square London
WC1N 3BG, UK.

Bianca Brim,
Department for Neurology, University Clinic
Tulln, Karl Landsteiner University of Health
Sciences, site Tulln, Austria.

Gila Bronner,
Sex Therapy Clinic,
Lis Maternity and Women's Hospital, and
Movement Disorders Unit,
Tel-Aviv Medical Center, Tel-Aviv,
Israel

Adolfo M. Bronstein,
Department of Brain Sciences, Imperial College
London, London, UK.

David J Brooks MD DSc,
FRCP (UK) FMedSci (UK)Professor of
NeurologyPET Center, Aarhus University
Denmark.

K. Ray Chaudhuri MD FRCP DSc,
King's College London, Department of
Neurosciences, Institute of Psychiatry,
Psychology & Neuroscience, De Crespigny Park,
London; and Parkinson's Foundation Centre of
Excellence, King's College Hospital, Denmark
Hill, London.

Ștefania Diaconu,
County Emergency Clinic Hospital, Faculty of
Medicine, Transilvania University Brașov,
Romania.

Atbin Djamshidian MD PhD,
Department of Neurology, Medical University of
Innsbruck, Innsbruck, Austria.

Richard L. Doty, PhD, FAAN,
Professor and Director Smell and Taste
Center Perelman School of Medicine
University of Pennsylvania' 5 Ravdin
Pavilion 3400 Spruce Street Philadelphia,
PA 19104.

Cristian Falup-Pecurariu,
County Emergency Clinic Hospital, Faculty of
Medicine, Transilvania University Brașov,
Romania.

Chloe Farrell,
National Parkinson Foundation International
Centre of Excellence, King's College London
and King's College Hospital, London,
UK.

Hubert H. Fernandez MD,
Department of Neurology and Center for
Neurological Restoration
Neurological Institute Cleveland Clinic,
Cleveland, OH, USA

Thomas Foki,
Department for Neurology,
University Clinic Tulln, Karl Landsteiner
University of Health Sciences, site Tulln, Austria.

Michael J. Frank MD Prof,
Department of Neuroscience, Brown University,
Providence, RI, USA.

Joseph H. Friedman MD Prof,
Department of Neurology, Butler Hospital,
Warren Alpert Medical School of Brown
University, USA.

Nestor Galvez-Jimenez,
Department of Neurology, Cleveland Clinic
Florida, Weston, FL, USA.

Ziv Gan-Or, MD, PhD,
The Neuro (Montreal Neurological Institute-
Hospital), McGill University, Montréal, Canada;
Department of Neurology and Neurosurgery,
McGill University, Montréal, Canada; and
Department of Human Genetics, McGill
University, Montréal, Canada.

Ganesh Gopalakrishna,
Banner Alzheimer's Institute
University of Arizona College of Medicine
Phoenix, AZ.

Tanya Gurevich,
Movement Disorders Unit and Parkinson's
Foundation Centre of Excellence, Neurological
Institute, Tel-Aviv Medical Center, Sackler
Faculty of Medicine and Sagol School of
Neuroscience, Tel Aviv Aviv University, Tel Aviv,
Israel.

Kasia Gustaw Rothenberg MD, PhD,
Geriatric Psychiatrist/Neuropsychiatrist Center
for Brain Health Neurological Institute Cleveland
Clinic.

Christopher Hawkes MD FRCP FAAN,
Department of Neurology
Nuffield Health Brentwood Hospital, UK.

Helmut Heinsen,
Department of Radiology, Hospital das Clinicas
HCFMUSP, University of São Paulo School of
Medicine, São Paulo, Brazil; and Morphological
Brain Research Unit, Department of Psychiatry,
University of Würzburg, Würzburg, Germany.

Rivka Inzelberg MD,
Department of Neurology and Neurosurgery,
Sackler Faculty of Medicine, and Sagol
School of Neuroscience, Tel Aviv University,
Israel.

Wolfgang H. Jost, MD,
Parkinson-Klinik Ortenau, Kreuzbergstr. 12–16,
77709 Wolfach, Germany.

Diego Kaski,
Department of Clinical and Motor Neurosciences,
University College London, London, UK.

Lisa Klingelhoefer, MD, PD habil,
Department of Neurology, Technical University
Dresden, Dresden, Germany.

Amos D. Korczyn,
Tel Aviv University, Tel-Aviv, Israel.

Valentina Leta MD,
King's College London, Department of
Neurosciences, Institute of Psychiatry,
Psychology & Neuroscience, De Crespigny Park,
London; and Parkinson's Foundation Centre of
Excellence, King's College Hospital, Denmark
Hill, London.

Ramon Lugo-Sanchez,
Department of Neurology, Cleveland Clinic
Florida, Weston, FL, USA.

Michael MacAskill,
New Zealand Brain Research Institute,
Christchurch, New Zealand.

Adam Margolius MD,
Department of Neurology and Center for
Neurological Restoration Neurological
Institute Cleveland Clinic, Cleveland,
OH, USA.

Shira McMahan,
Cleveland Clinic Martin health system Outpatient
Neuro.

Eoin Mulroy,
Department of Clinical and Movement Neurosciences National Hospital for Neurology and Neurosurgery Queen Square London United Kingdom.

Maria-Lucia Muntean,
Paracelsus Elena Hospital, Center for Parkinson's Disease and Movement Disorders Kassel, Germany.

Guillaume Pagnier MS,
Department of Neuroscience, Brown University, Providence, RI, USA.

Birgit Riemer,
Department for Neurology, University Clinic Tulln, Karl Landsteiner University of Health Sciences, site Tulln, Austria.

Carmen Rodriguez-Blazquez,
National Center of Epidemiology and CIBERNED, Carlos III Institute of Health, Madrid, Spain.

Damon Salzman, MD,
Cleveland Clinic Florida Department of Neurology2950 Cleveland Clinic BoulevardWeston, FL 33331.

Anna Sauerbier, Department of Neurology,
University Hospital Cologne, Cologne, Germany; and National Parkinson Foundation International Centre of Excellence, King's College London and King's College Hospital, London, UK.

Konstantin Senkevich, MD, PhD,
The Neuro (Montreal Neurological Institute-Hospital) University, Montréal, Canada; and Department of Neurology and Neurosurgery, McGill University, Montréal, Canada.

Aasef Shaikh,
Neurological Institute, University Hospitals, Cleveland, Ohio, USA.

Umar Shuaib MD,
Department of Neurology and Center for Neurological Restoration Neurological Institute Cleveland Clinic, Cleveland, OH, USA.

Walter Struhal,
Department for Neurology, University Clinic Tulln, Karl Landsteiner University of Health Sciences, site Tulln, Austria.

Shakeel Tabish MD,
Cleveland clinic Florida.

Lea Tenenholz Grinberg,
University of California, San Francisco, Memory and Aging Center, Weill Institute for Neurosciences; Departments of Neurology and Pathology, San Francisco; LIM-22, Department of Pathology, University of São Paulo School of Medicine, São Paulo, Brazil; and University of California, Global Brain Health Institute, San Francisco.

Po-Heng Tsai,
Banner Alzheimer's Institute University of Arizona College of Medicine Phoenix, AZ.

Daniele Urso,
National Parkinson Foundation International Centre of Excellence, King's College London and King's College Hospital, London, UK.

Daniel van Wamelen MD PhD,
King's College London, Department of Neurosciences, Institute of Psychiatry, Psychology & Neuroscience, De Crespigny Park, London; Parkinson's Foundation Centre of Excellence, King's College Hospital, Denmark Hill, London; and Radboud University Medical Centre; Donders Institute for Brain, Cognition and Behaviour; Department of Neurology, Nijmegen, Netherlands.

Introduction

The non-motor manifestations of Parkinson's disease have been known since the description of the disease by James Parkinson in 1817. In his "Essay of the Shaking Palsy", he clearly stated *"sleep becomes much disturbed … the bowels, which had been all along torpid, in most cases demand stimulating medicines of very considerable power … sometimes the expulsion of feces requiring mechanical aid"* [1]. However, for years the emphasis has been on the motor features which define the disease, largely by the availability of dopaminergic and other agents which alleviate the bradykinesia and rigidity, and partly also the tremor. In fact, these drugs added new non-motor manifestations.

As seen in this book, the spectrum of non-motor features is extremely large and spans practically all body organs and functions [2]. Awareness of these can help in their prevention or treatment. In this volume we have included chapters dedicated to all of them.

It should be recognized that non-motor features of Parkinson's disease occur in all stages of the disease, may precede the appearance of the classical motor symptoms [3] and thus are challenging the diagnosis of the cause of these phenomena. Some, such as hyposmia or anosmia, may in fact serve as biomarkers, alerting the clinician to the evolving disease and allowing early initiation of neuroprotective therapy [4].

Once diagnosed with Parkinson's disease, it may become clear why patients have reported constipation, pains, loss of smell sense, erectile difficulties, depression, and sleep problems, particularly REM sleep behavior disorder (RSBD) for several years [5], in many preceding the onset of the motor symptoms. These manifestations are important for several reasons. They indicate that the neuropathology of Parkinson's disease is not limited to the nigrostriatal system or dopamine itself, and emphasize the need to develop specific therapies. For example, although depression is very common in Parkinson's disease, and in many cases affective manifestations may precede by several years the motor symptoms, we do not know what the underlying pathophysiology is and it is unclear whether there should be a specific treatment in these cases [6].

The existence of these pre-motor manifestations shows the heterogeneous phenotypic expression of the disease, which will continue in the more advanced stages. In addition, they may help in the early diagnosis of the disease. We still do not know the exact sensitivities and specificities for each of them, however RSBD and hyposmia have proven to have a stronger correlation as predictors of the disease than others [7]. As such, there are increasing attempts to develop and validate clinical biomarkers which can diagnose Parkinson's disease at an early stage. This will be particularly relevant once a disease-modifying therapy is developed, as ideally these should be used early for a diagnosis, if we are to change the natural history of the disease.

A special case is cognitive impairment. As the frequency of dementia increases gradually over the years in patients with Parkinson's disease, many will become demented, placing a huge burden on the patients themselves, caregivers and healthcare services. The cognitive decline may begin at any time in the neurodegenerative process, before or after the onset of motor symptoms. Patients in whom the onset of the cognitive impairment begins prior to the motor symptoms have been termed Dementia with Lewy bodies, but there is nothing known about the underlying mechanisms that cause the early α-synucleinopathy deposition in the cortex and particularly in the limbic system [8].

Thus there is still a long way to go in deciphering the underlying mechanisms of Parkinson's disease and finding interventions to alleviate the associated suffering. We hope that this volume will help in addressing these issues.

Néstor Gálvez-Jiménez MD, MSc, MHA, Amos D. Korczyn MD, MSc, Ramón Lugo-Sanchez MD

1. Parkinson J. An essay on the shaking palsy. J Neuropsychiatry Clin Neurosci 2002; **14**(2): 223–236.

2. Schapira AH, Chaudhuri KR, Jenner P. Non-motor features of Parkinson disease. Nat Rev Neurosci 2017; **18**(7): 435.

3. Korczyn AD, Gurevich T. Parkinson's disease: before the motor symptoms and beyond. J Neurolog Sci 2010; **289**(1–2): 2–6.

4. Doty RL. Olfaction in Parkinson's disease and related disorders. Neurobiol Dis 2012; **46**(3): 527–552.

5. Boeve BF, Silber MH, Ferman TJ. REM sleep behavior disorder in Parkinson's disease and dementia with Lewy bodies. J Geriatr Psychiatry Neurol 2004; **17**(3): 146–157.

6. Korczyn AD, Hassin-Baer S. Can the disease course in Parkinson's disease be slowed? BMC Med 2015; **13**(1): 1–6.

7. Roos DS, Twisk JW, Raijmakers PG, Doty RL, Berendse HW. Hyposmia as a marker of (non-) motor disease severity in Parkinson's disease. J Neural Transm 2019; **126**(11): 1471–1478.

8. Jellinger KA, Korczyn AD. Are dementia with Lewy bodies and Parkinson's disease dementia the same disease? BMC Med 2018; **16**(1): 1–6.

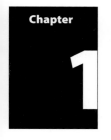
Parkinson's Disease: An Overview of the Non-Motor Symptomatology

Daniel van Wamelen, Valentina Leta, K. Ray Chaudhuri

Introduction

Non-motor symptoms (NMS) are a crucial component of Parkinson's disease (PD) and the burden of the range of NMS that occurs in PD is one of the main determinants of quality of life [1]. In 1817, Dr. James Parkinson already described several NMS in his "shaking palsy," the condition that would later be named after him, including pain, constipation, and sleep disturbances [2]. Nonetheless, after a long period of inertia, over the last 20 to 25 years, the interest in NMS has increased and evidence suggests that the overall burden of NMS dominates and can influence the risk of developing motor parkinsonism in the premotor stage of PD while being a driving factor for quality of life [3]. The identification of NMS in PD has been greatly aided by the development of specific tools, such as the NMS questionnaire (NMSQ) in 2006 [4] and the NMS Scale (NMSS) in 2007 [5]. The NMSS, which was based on the previously validated NMSQ, addresses a wide range of NMS in PD which are grouped into nine domains, measured over the period of the last month and quantified by severity and frequency (NMS symptomatic burden) [5]. Recently, a new version of the NMSS, the Movement Disorder Society Non-Motor Scale (MDS-NMS), has been published which will further aid in the identification and quantification of NMS burden of PD [6].

In this chapter, we will describe the phenomenology of NMS in PD, including non-motor fluctuations (NMF), and how to measure these symptoms.

Non-Motor Burden

Non-motor symptoms are present in every stage of the disease, from prodromal (Table 1.1) to palliative, with a tangible impact on quality of life. This has been demonstrated in several studies, where NMS burden has been found to be positively associated with health-related quality of life measures [7]. NMS, and in particular depression, have a higher impact on quality of life compared to motor symptoms and motor complications as exemplified by higher R^2 values in uni- and multivariate analyses [5]. Patients' non-motor burden also impacts on caregiver quality of life [8].

Holistic Non-Motor Measurements

Over the years, several tools have been developed to measure non-motor burden, and specific NMS, in PD. As specific NMS are the topic of other chapters, here we will focus on the measurement of general non-motor burden. Several dedicated scales are available, the most widely used include the Non-Motor Symptoms Scale (NMSS), the MDS-UPDRS Part I, and the recently validated Movement Disorder Society Non-Motor Scale (MDS-NMS) (Table 1.2).

The NMSS has nine non-motor domains and shows a strong correlation with the NMSQ, underlining the link between patient-reported and physician-gathered outcomes related to NMS in PD [5]. The other common tool to assess

Table 1.1 Prodromal non-motor symptoms in Parkinson's disease

Sleep disorders
Rapid eye movement behavior disorder/events Excessive daytime somnolence
Neuropsychiatric
(Episodic) major depression Abnormal color vision/visual perception Cognitive impairment
Other
Hyposmia/anosmia Constipation Fatigue Erectile dysfunction Neurogenic orthostatic hypotension Pain

Table 1.2 Holistic scales used to assess and quantify non-motor symptoms in Parkinson's disease

Scale	Non-motor symptoms covered	Main features

Non-Motor Symptoms Scale	• Orthostatic hypotension (two items)
	• Sleep/fatigue (four items)
	• Mood/cognition (six items)
	• Perceptual problems (three items)
	• Attention/memory (three items)
	• Gastrointestinal symptoms (three items)
	• Urinary symptoms (three items)
	• Sexual dysfunction (two items)
	• Miscellaneous (four items)
	   o Pain
	   o Hyposmia
	   o Weight change
	   o Hyperhidrosis
		Rater-completed
		30 items
		10–15 minutes

Movement Disorders Society Unified Parkinson's Disease Rating Scale Part I	• Cognitive impairment • Hallucinations and illusions • Depressed mood • Anxiety • Apathy • Dopamine dysregulation syndrome • Sleep problems • Excessive daytime sleepiness • Pain • Urinary problems • Constipation • Orthostatic hypotension • Fatigue • Sialorrhea • Dysphagia	Six items rater-completed Eight items patient-completed 10 minutes

Movement Disorders Society Non-Motor Scale	• Depression (five items)
	• Anxiety (four items)
	• Apathy (three items)
	• Psychosis (four items)
	• Impulse control disorders (four items)
	• Cognition (six items)
	• Orthostatic hypotension (two items)
	• Urinary symptoms (three items)
	• Sexual symptoms (two items)
	• Gastrointestinal symptoms (four items)
	• Sleep and wakefulness (six items)
	• Miscellaneous
	   o Weight change
	   o Hyposmia
	   o Mental fatigue
	   o Physical fatigue
	   o Hyperhidrosis
	• Non-motor fluctuations (eight items)
		Rater-completed
		52 items
		15–40 minutes

NMS in PD is the MDS-UPDRS Part I, although substantial differences exist between the two tools, NMSS being a rater-based standalone instrument to comprehensively assess the NMS, while the non-motor assessment in MDS-UPDRS (Part I) is a mixture of self-rated and rater-based items contained in a comprehensive PD scale that also addresses motor symptoms [9]. There is overlap between the two scales and in the updated version of the NMSS, the MDS-NMS, additional emphasis has been put on depression, cognition, impulse control disorders (ICD), pain, and non-motor fluctuations [6].

Digitalized Measurements for Non-Motor Symptoms

An interesting field that is currently developing in PD is the digital capture and follow-up of NMS, in line with similar developments in other neurological diseases to provide objective outcome measures instead of relying on classical scales and questionnaires. Although findings are mostly preliminary and need further validation, several measures and surrogate markers for NMS in PD have been developed. Examples include the association of cognitive performance with circadian rest-activity patterns as measured by actigraphy [10], and the use of wrist-worn wearable sensors to measure impulse control disorder and sleep disorders in PD [11]. Moreover, it has been suggested that wearable sensor severity measures of bradykinesia are associated with constipation severity in PD patients [12], and the iPrognosis project is aiming to measure e.g. gastric and colonic motility as objective measures for delayed gastric emptying and constipation in PD (www.i-prognosis.eu).

Prevalence and Burden

Non-motor symptoms are already present in, and even define, the prodromal phase of the disease when motor symptoms have not yet emerged. Such prodromal NMS consist of hyposmia, fatigue, constipation, and rapid eye movement sleep behavior disorder (RBD) as the most common, but not only NMS (Table 1.1) [13]. Interestingly, a recent study by Schrag et al. showed that these NMS, starting in the prodromal phase before motor symptoms, tend to occur in specific clusters: a) a neuropsychiatric cluster with anxiety, depression, apathy, stress, and sleep disorders; b) an axial motor phenotype associated mainly with dysphagia; and c) a motor phenotype with additional non-motor features [14]. Also other studies have shown the differential association of NMS with specific motor phenotypes, such as motor-predominant, intermediate, and diffuse malignant subtypes of PD [15] (Table 1.3).

When looking at the burden of NMS, it is necessary to distinguish between patients with early-on and later-on NMS during the motor in-life manifestation of the disease, as with increasing disease progression not only do motor symptoms get worse but also NMS. From the available literature, it becomes clear that the presence of NMS appears to be spread more or less equivalently across the motor stages, where 93.7% of patients with a disease duration of less than 2 years are affected compared to 93.9% of patients with disease duration of over 10 years [16]; some studies have even higher prevalence, of up to 99.1% [17]. In terms of burden (as measured by the UPDRS), there is almost a 50% increase over a period of 5 years after diagnosis compared to the burden around time of diagnosis [18–20]. Similarly, mean NMS Questionnaire (NMSQ) scores increased from 5.3 to 8.2 after 4 years [21] with no correlation to motor scores. However, some studies have shown stable burden or only mild progression [22].

The Influence of Gender

In addition to the already mentioned motor profiles that tend to associate with specific NMS, gender also plays an important role in NMS burden. For example, Picillo et al. showed that men have a greater number of NMS compared to women, with specifically sialorrhea and nocturia being more prevalent [23]. Other studies have shown similar findings, with the additional identification of depressive symptoms, anxiety, and RBD as more prevalent in male patients, and apathy in female patients [24]. On the other hand, female PD patients are more likely to develop non-motor fluctuations [25].

Non-Motor Symptoms in the Palliative Phase of Parkinson's Disease

Like motor symptoms, NMS are prevalent among patients with advanced PD, and NMS burden has been reported to have a similar impact as metastatic cancer [26]. Moreover, in the palliative stage, patients have an average of 10.7 physical symptoms [27, 28], with pain, fatigue, daytime somnolence, and mobility problems observed in over 80% of PD patients, and constipation, loss of bladder control, swallowing difficulties, sialorrhea, breathing and sleep problems in over half. Also, anxiety and depression were reported to be very prevalent in 70% and 60% of patients, respectively [28].

Non-Motor Symptoms in Animal Models of Parkinson's Disease

Experimental models of the disease that feature at least some of the key NMS are of great interest, and crucial for the development of NMS-targeted

Table 1.3 Studies identifying subgroups within Parkinson's disease based on cluster analysis and including non-motor symptoms

Authors and year	Population	Identified subtypes
Graham and Sagar, 1990	176 unselected PD patients (83 F, 93 M; mean age 63.2 (SD 10.2) years; mean disease duration 7.5 (SD 6.4) years)	1. Motor only 2. Motor and cognitive 3. Rapid progression
Dujardin et al., 2004	50 drug-naïve PD patients (24 F, 26 M; median age 66 years; median disease duration 1 year)	1. Preserved cognition and mild motor dysfunction 2. Cognitive dysfunction and more severe motor deficits
Lewis et al., 2005	120 unselected PD patients (43 F, 77 M; mean age 64.4 (SD 9.3) years; mean disease duration 7.8 (5.4) years)	1. Younger disease onset 2. Tremor-dominant 3. Non-tremor-dominant, significant cognitive impairment, and mild depression 4. Rapid progression without cognitive impairment
Post et al., 2008	131 de novo PD patients (F 60, M 71; mean age 66.7 (SD 10.4) years; mean disease duration 20 (SD 11.2) months)	1. Younger onset group 2. Intermediate older onset group 3. Oldest onset group
Reijnders et al., 2009	173 unselected PD patients	1. Rapid disease progression 2. Young onset 3. Non-tremor-dominant with psychopathology 4. Tremor-dominant subtype
Van Rooden et al., 2011	344 PD patients of a Dutch cohort (118 F, 226 M; mean age 60.8 (SD 11.3) years; mean disease duration 9.9 (SD 6.2) years) 357 PD patients of a Spanish cohort (164 F, 193 M; mean age 66.2 (SD 11.2) years; mean disease duration 7.7 (SD 5.8) years)	1. Mild severity in all clinical domains 2. Severe motor complications 3. Intermediate severity in non-dopaminergic domains without prominent motor complications 4. Moderate motor complications, higher age and age at onset, long duration of Levodopa use, and female gender
Erro et al., 2013	100 de novo PD patients (41 F, 59 M; mean age 59.7 (SD 8.3) years; mean disease duration 13.4 (SD 5.6) months)	1. Benign pure motor 2. Benign mixed motor and non-motor 3. Non-motor-dominant 4. Motor-dominant
Kim et al., 2014	180 unselected PD patients (106 F, 74 M; mean age 62.6 (SD 10.2) years; mean disease duration 7.2 (SD 5.7) years)	1. Mood, sleep/fatigue, attention/memory, urinary symptoms, and miscellaneous symptoms 2. Perceptual problems, gastrointestinal issues, and cardiovascular symptoms
Pont-Sunyer et al., 2015	109 drug-naïve PD patients (40 F, 69 M; mean age 66.6 (SD 9.3) years; median disease duration 1 (IQR 0–2) month)	1. RBD-like and constipation cluster 2. Mood-related cluster 3. Cognition-related cluster 4. Sensory cluster
Lawton et al., 2015	769 unselected PD patients (261 F, 508 M; mean age at onset 64.8 (SD 9.7) years; mean disease duration 1.3 (SD 0.96) years)	1. Mild motor and non-motor disease 2. Poor posture and cognition 3. Severe tremor 4. Poor psychological well-being, RBD, and sleep 5. Severe motor and non-motor disease with poor psychological well-being
Fereshtehnejad et al., 2015	113 unselected PD patients (40 F, 73 M; mean age 66.7 (SD 8.9) years; mean disease duration 5.7 (SD 4.2) years)	1. Mainly motor/slow progression 2. Intermediate 3. Diffuse/malignant
Ma et al., 2015	1510 unselected PD patients (596 F, 914 M; mean age 66.7 (SD 10.5) years; mean disease duration 63.9 (SD 51.9) months)	1. Non-tremor-dominant 2. Rapid disease progression with late onset 3. Benign pure motor characteristics without non-motor disturbances

Table 1.3 (cont.)

Authors and year	Population	Identified subtypes
		4. Tremor-dominant with slow disease progression
Tsujikawa et al., 2015	70 unselected PD patients (44 F, 26 M; mean age 69.5 (SD 8.7) years; mean disease duration 1.9 (SD 2.4) years)	1. Markedly low MIBG uptakes at baseline 2. Normal or mildly low MIBG uptakes at baseline, female-dominant, young onset, slow motor progression and preserved cognitive function
Szeto et al., 2015	209 PD patients in the early motor stages (65 F, 144 M; mean age 66.7 (SD 8.9) years; mean disease duration 5.9 (SD 4.9) years)	1. Younger disease onset 2. Tremor-dominant 3. Non-tremor-dominant with higher prevalence of freezing of gait and NMS (MCI, hallucinations, daytime somnolence, and RBD) 4. Rapid disease progression
Dujardin et al., 2015	156 unselected PD patients	1. Cognitively intact patients with high level of performance in all cognitive domains 2. Cognitively intact slightly slower than those in cluster 1 3. Deficits in executive functions 4. Severe deficits in all cognitive domains, particularly executive functions 5. Severe deficits in all cognitive domains, particularly working memory and recall in verbal episodic memory
Uribe et al., 2016	• 88 non-demented PD patients • (37 F, 51 M; mean age 64.1 (SD 10.6) years; mean disease duration 8.0 (SD 5.7) years)	1. Parieto-temporal pattern of atrophy with worse cognitive performance 2. Occipital and frontal cortical atrophy and younger disease onset 3. No detectable cortical atrophy
van Balkom et al., 2016	• 226 unselected PD patients • (81 F, 145 M; mean age 63.4 (SD 10.2) years; median disease duration 3.0 (range 0–20) years)	1. Young age, mildly affected 2. Old age with severe motor and non-motor symptoms 3. Mild motor symptoms, below-average executive functioning, and affective symptoms 4. Severe motor symptoms, affective symptoms, and below-average verbal memory
Petrovic et al., 2016	• 360 unselected PD patients • (126 F, 234 M; mean age 63.5 (SD 10.3) years; median disease duration 7.2 (SD 5.1) years)	1. No or few neuropsychiatric symptoms 2. Mild to moderate depression, anxiety, and apathy 3. High agitation, disinhibition, and irritability scores
Souza et al., 2016	100 unselected PD patients	Three general distinct cognitive profiles which represented a continuum from mild to severe cognitive impairment, without distinguishing specific cognitive profiles
Fereshtehnejad et al., 2017	• 422 de novo PD patients • (146 F, 276 M; mean age 61.1 (SD 9.7) years; median disease duration 6.5 (SD 6.5) months)	1. Mild motor-predominant 2. Intermediate 3. Diffuse malignant (motor and non-motor) more profound dopaminergic deficit, increased atrophy in PD brain networks, a more AD-like CSF profile, and faster progression of motor and cognitive deficits
Mu et al., 2017	951 unselected PD patients from two independent international cohorts (360 F, 591 M; mean age 66.2 (SD 11.2) years; mean disease duration 8.0 (SD 5.8) years)	1. Mild 2. Non-motor-dominant 3. Motor-dominant 4. Severe
Kawabata et al., 2018	44 PD patients with cognitive impairment	1. PD with amnestic cognitive deficits 2. PD with non-amnestic cognitive deficits

Table 1.3 (cont.)

Authors and year	Population	Identified subtypes
Lawton et al., 2018	2545 unselected PD patients from two independent cohorts	1. Fast motor progression with symmetrical motor disease, poor olfaction, cognition, and postural hypotension 2. Mild motor and non-motor disease with intermediate motor progression 3. Severe motor disease, poor psychological well-being, and poor sleep with an intermediate motor progression 4. Slow motor progression with tremor-dominant and unilateral disease

Abbreviations: AD, Alzheimer disease; CSF, cerebrospinal fluid; F, female; M male; MIBG, metaiodobenzylguanidine; PD, Parkinson's disease; RBD, REM sleep behavior disorder; SD, standard deviation.

Table 1.4 Examples of non-motor symptoms in common animal models of Parkinson's disease

Animal model	Non-motor symptoms	Reference
α-Synuclein-overexpressing mice	• Olfaction disorder • Autonomic signs • Constipation • Sleep (circadian dysfunction) • Cognition	[29]
LRRK2-overexpressing mice	• Gastrointestinal dysfunction • Olfactory dysfunction	[30]
GBA-deficient mice	• Memory/attention dysfunction • Cognitive dysfunction	[31]
Parkin knockout mice	• Anxiety • Cognition	[32]
VMAT2-deficient mice	• Olfactory discrimination • Delayed gastric emptying • Sleep disturbances • Altered sleep latency • Anxiety-like behavior • Depressive behavior	[33]
6-OHDA-lesioned rodents	• Sleep/wakefulness, circadian rhythms, RBD	[34]
MPTP-treated primates	• sleep–wake cycle • REM sleep/RBD	[34]

treatment in PD. Although the assessment of many of the potential NMS in animal models is limited to the inherent nature of the models, it has so far been observed that key NMS in PD, such as reduced olfactory discrimination, gastrointestinal and autonomic dysfunction, cognitive decline, and anxiety and depressive-like behavior are present [29–34]. An exhaustive overview of NMS in animal models is beyond the purpose of this chapter. In Table 1.4, we show examples of NMS observed in common animal models of PD. These studies illustrate that NMS are present in many of the commonly used models to study PD, but in their number and detail studies aiming to explore

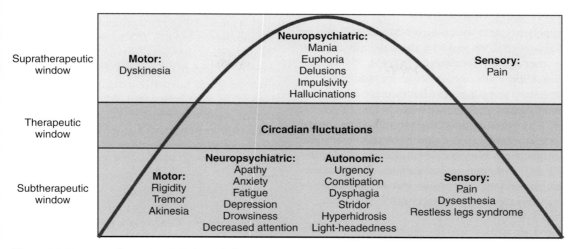

Figure 1.1 Non-motor fluctuations in Parkinson's disease.

them lag far behind the dopaminergic-driven motor studies and interventions to ameliorate these. A further complicating matter is that in all these animal models, a PD-like condition was induced through interference with dopaminergic neurotransmission or lesioning of the *substantia nigra*. Even though many NMS are partially responsive to dopamine replacement therapy, others are clearly non-dopaminergic in origin, resulting from the degeneration of non-dopaminergic nuclei [35].

Non-Motor Fluctuations

The concept of fluctuations in PD, in response to dopaminergic medication, is well recognized, yet often these fluctuations are linked to motor rather than non-motor function. The first structured concept of non-motor fluctuations (NMF) was described in 1998 by Quinn, who noticed that several key NMS showed fluctuations in line with motor fluctuations. These fluctuations, including Off-related pain, beginning and end-of-dose pain, and peak-dose pain, clearly underline the close link of this key NMS with motor fluctuations [36]. Interestingly, he also noted that over two-thirds of PD patients treated with levodopa preparations experienced mood fluctuations, i.e. changes in depressive feelings, anxiety and panic, irritability, and apathy, mostly occurring during Off-periods, while symptoms such as euphoria and hypersexuality were more common during the On-period [36].

The prevalence of NMF is high among patients with motor fluctuations and prevalence rates for NMF in general range between 17% and 100% in these patients [25, 37–43]. Although NMF often present alongside motor fluctuations in most, they rarely occur independently or in the absence of motor fluctuations [44, 45]. Indeed, NMF are considered a heterogeneous and complex group of fluctuations, which include neuropsychiatric, autonomic, and sensory symptom fluctuations [40, 46] (Figure 1.1). Moreover, NMF appear to cause a greater degree of disability and distress than motor fluctuations, at least in some patients [37, 39, 40, 47, 48].

Neuropsychiatric Fluctuations

The most common NMF in PD patients consist of neuropsychiatric fluctuations and are present in approximately half of patients with neuropsychiatric NMS [45], and especially anxiety and mood fluctuations appear to have the most pronounced impact on quality of life [40]. Many of these neuropsychiatric symptoms are mainly present during Off-periods (82%) [49]. Other common NMF include changes in motivation, cognition, and apathy [50–53]. The latter symptom is mainly present during Off-periods and is replaced by excessive motivation and impulse control disorder during On-periods [54]. Hallucinations, on the other hand, which are often considered as classic hyperdopaminergic symptoms, can occur both during On- and Off-state [55].

Autonomic Fluctuations

In patients who experience NMF, it was shown that between 29% and 94% also have a fluctuation in autonomic symptoms [42–45]. Symptoms coinciding with motor state include dyspnea, excessive sweating, cardiovascular symptoms, constipation, and urinary urgency [36, 39, 42, 43, 56]. The evidence that these symptoms are indeed fluctuating comes from the observation that some of them improve with dopaminergic medication [57–59], although some authors demonstrated that autonomic symptoms showed only minor changes in symptom severity [40].

Sensory and Pain Fluctuations

Pain in PD is a common feature, especially in the motor Off-state [39, 42, 43]. Pathologically, pain may be related to a muscular component with increased rigidity and dystonia during motor Off-state, but can also be attributed to dysfunction in sensory striatal cortical afferents due to dopamine depletion [60–62]. Part of pain-related symptoms can be improved with dopaminergic medication [63], in particular, leg motor restlessness which occurs in up to 54% of patients with NMF [39]. Less common NMF, such as sensory symptoms, occur in about 25% of patients with NMF [44].

Dopamine-Induced Non-Motor Symptoms

While most of NMS are an intrinsic component of PD, some of them may be regarded as induced by dopaminergic medication intake. As the disease progresses and the patient requires higher doses of dopaminergic medication, however, it becomes difficult to distinguish the contribution of one or the other component to the development of some NMS, particularly neuropsychiatric disorders, autonomic dysfunction, and sleep-related disturbances [64].

Neuropsychiatric disorders secondary to dopaminergic medication encompass hallucinations, psychosis as well as impulse control disorders (ICDs), and ICD-related disorders [64]. Behavioral changes, including pathological gambling, binge eating, hypersexuality, and compulsive buying, are typical clinical manifestations of ICDs which occur in 20% of PD population [65]. As it may lead to serious financial, legal, and health-related problems for both patients and carers, early detection and treatment represent a key aspect of PD management [66]. Although commonly reported in PD patients on dopaminergic medication, especially dopamine agonists, symptoms suggestive of ICDs have also been observed in de novo PD patients [67] and post deep brain stimulation [68]. Additional risk factors for the development of ICD are male gender, young age at PD onset, history of ICD or other psychopathologies, and genetic predisposition [68]. As well as ICD, ICD-related disorders, including dopamine dysregulation syndrome (DDS), punding, hobbyism, walkabout and hoarding, may have a major impact on quality of life and patient's functioning [66]. Prevention of ICD is relevant, as treatment is limited to reduction of dopaminergic medication (with risk of withdrawal syndrome) and cognitive behavioral therapy. Evidence on other pharmacological approaches, including use of antipsychotics, serotonin reuptake inhibitors, opioid antagonists, and GABA inhibitors, is controversial [66].

Among the other common and disabling treatment-related symptoms are autonomic conditions secondary to dopaminergic medication intake including nausea and orthostatic hypotension [64]. Usually, these drug-induced NMS may be prevented by slowly titrating dopaminergic medication dose and managed by non-pharmacological approaches when they occur; occasionally, use of peripheral-dopamine antagonists and fludrocortisone, midodrine, or droxidopa may be required for nausea and orthostatic hypotension respectively [69].

Finally, excessive daytime sleepiness and even narcoleptic attacks are commonly seen in medicated PD patients [64]. These NMS may have serious safety implications, including road traffic accidents [70]. As excessive daytime sleepiness has been linked to reductions in hypothalamic dopamine D3 receptor availability [71], the use of drugs with high D3 receptor affinity should be avoided in this particular subgroup of PD patients.

Non-Motor Biomarkers and Evidence for Non-Dopaminergic Causes of Non-Motor Symptoms

In order to develop effective disease-modifying treatments for PD, an early and accurate diagnosis

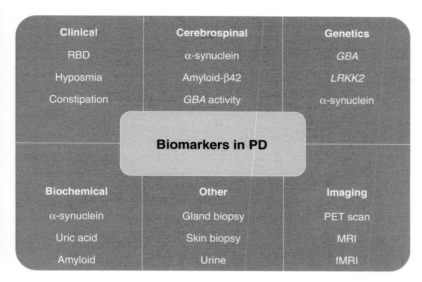

Clinical	Cerebrospinal	Genetics
RBD	α-synuclein	GBA
Hyposmia	Amyloid-β42	LRKK2
Constipation	GBA activity	α-synuclein

Biomarkers in PD

Biochemical	Other	Imaging
α-synuclein	Gland biopsy	PET scan
Uric acid	Skin biopsy	MRI
Amyloid	Urine	fMRI

Figure 1.2 Examples of biomarkers in Parkinson's disease. RBD, rapid eye movement behavior disorders; *GBA*, glucocerebridase; *LRKK2*, leucine-rich repeat kinase 2; PET, positron emission tomography; MRI, magnetic resonance imaging; fMRI, functional magnetic resonance imaging; PD, Parkinson's disease.

and prognostic monitoring is crucial, but current challenges are posed by the variable symptom onset and progression [72]. Many types of biomarkers have been proposed to assist in this problem, and have been extensively reviewed elsewhere, including cerebrospinal fluid and serum biomarkers [73], positron emission tomography (PET) [74], and magnetic resonance imaging (MRI) [75] (Figure 1.2).

In addition to the clear role of PET/SPECT in the visualization of the dopaminergic system in PD (Dopamine Transporter (DaT) imaging), this technique can also be used to enable the study of non-dopaminergic systems. Changes in serotonergic, noradrenergic, and cholinergic neurotransmission can be detected and were associated with NMS, including dementia, depressive symptoms, and sleep disorders [74]. Although primarily used as a supportive technique in the diagnosis of PD, DaT imaging can also provide some insights into dopaminergic NMS. Currently, there is evidence for over ten dopaminergic NMS, which include attention deficits [76], anxiety [77], urinary problems [78], REM sleep behavior disorder [79], olfaction [80], restless legs syndrome [81], and weight changes [82].

Also, resting state functional MRI (fMRI) is increasingly being used to study NMS in PD and several reviews are available on this topic [83, 84]. The best studied NMS using fMRI is cognitive decline and several studies have suggested that cognitive network alterations might predict the development of cognitive deficits in PD patients, although the interpretation of the current data is largely hampered by the lack of longitudinal studies [83]. Other NMS that are associated with changes in fMRI include REM sleep behavior disorder, associated with a decreased functional connectivity of the ponto-striato-cortical pathway [85], and hyposmia, whose severity was linked to decreased functional connectivity within the limbic/paralimbic systems and between the amygdala and parietal/occipital areas [86, 87]. Moreover, functional connectivity alterations within the prefrontal-limbic network have been shown in PD patients with depression, fatigue, hallucinations, and pain [83]. Although fMRI looks promising as a tool to link structural and connectivity disorders to NMS in PD, fMRI studies on specific NMS remain few and do not allow identification of specific and useful markers to anticipate the onset of these symptoms, or to monitor the effect of dedicated treatments.

In terms of biomarkers, especially the serum and cerebrospinal fluid (CSF) have been extensively studied in order to identify PD-specific footprints. A comprehensive review is not within the scope of this chapter, but has been recently published by Sarkar et al. [88]. Examples include increased levels of serum amyloid P component and transferrin, and decreased levels of apolipoprotein A-1 and coagulation factor V in PD patients compared to healthy control subjects. These changes may contribute to protein aggregation, oxidative stress, mitochondrial function, and neuroinflammation [88]. Depression, as one of the most common NMS in PD, on the other hand, has been associated with lipid and glucose metabolic changes [89]. CSF, often considered to be more reliable than serum markers due to its intimate relationship with the brain, shows other changes that appear to be promising biomarkers. Here, a reduction in the pathological hallmark protein of PD, α-synuclein, has been shown to be linked to the development of dementia, especially when combined with β-synuclein levels [90]. The usefulness of CSF markers for other NMS remains underexplored as well as the potential applications of α-synuclein deposits detection in peripheral tissues [91–93].

Treatment

Treatment for Specific Non-Motor Symptoms

The evidence base for the treatment of NMS in PD has substantially grown over the years, and several treatments are considered efficacious for a range of NMS. The best evidence is available for the treatment of depressive symptoms, where Pramipexole, Nortriptyline, Desipramine, Venlafaxine, and cognitive behavioral therapy have been shown to be efficacious or likely efficacious [94]. Also, cognitive decline has been the focus of many interventional studies. Here, the acetylcholinesterase inhibitor Rivastigmine is the only efficacious therapy, even though many other interventions, including Memantine, Galantamine, cognitive rehabilitation, and transcranial magnetic stimulation have been investigated [94, 95]. An overview of all efficacious and likely efficacious medication for NMS in PD is provided in Table 1.5.

Non-Motor Fluctuations

Similar to motor symptoms, NMF can, at least in part, respond to changes in dopaminergic medication [96]. Therefore, the primary goal in treating NMF is to aim for continuous dopaminergic therapy, with e.g. the use of prolonged release

Table 1.5 Efficacious and likely efficacious treatments for non-motor symptoms in Parkinson's disease

Symptom	Treatment	Efficacy
Depressive symptoms and depression	Pramipexole	Efficacious
	Venlafaxine	Efficacious
	Nortriptyline	Efficacious
	Desipramine	Likely efficacious
	Cognitive behavioral therapy	Likely efficacious
Apathy	Rivastigmine	Efficacious
Dementia	Rivastigmine	Efficacious
Psychosis	Clozapine	Efficacious
	Pimavanserin	Efficacious
Insomnia	Rotigotine	Likely efficacious
	Continuous positive airway pressure therapy (CPAP)	Likely efficacious
Excessive daytime sleepiness	CPAP	Likely efficacious
Fatigue	Rasagiline	Efficacious
Orthostatic hypotension	Droxidopa	Efficacious (short term)
Sexual dysfunction	Sildenafil	Efficacious
Constipation	Macrogol	Likely efficacious
	Lubiprostone	Likely efficacious
	Probiotics	Efficacious
Nausea	Domperidone	Likely efficacious
Sialorrhea	Glycopyrrolate	Efficacious
	Botulinum toxin A or B to salivary glands	Efficacious

Table 1.5 based on Seppi et al. [94]. Efficacious: Supported by data from at least one high-quality (score ≥75%) randomized controlled trial without conflicting level I data; Likely efficacious: Supported by data from any level I trial without conflicting level I data.

dopaminergic preparations. The latter is exemplified by the Rotigotine transdermal patch, which in a recent post-hoc analysis of the RECOVER trial showed improvements in pain, sleep/fatigue, and mood/apathy [97]. According to the recently published Movement Disorder Society update on treatment for NMS of PD, patients with pain-dominant NMF may also benefit from Rotigotine [94]. Not only for NMF, but also for NMS in advanced PD in general, non-oral therapies provide a powerful option to address these symptoms. In both EuroInf studies, subcutaneous Apomorphine infusion and intrajejunal levodopa infusion (IJLI) improved NMS burden, but with a spectrum of improvement unique to each therapy. Apomorphine mainly improved mood/cognition, perceptual problems, attention/memory, and the miscellaneous domains of the NMSS, where IJLI mainly improved sleep/fatigue, and gastrointestinal NMSS domains [98]. Also, deep brain stimulation was able to improve NMS, but the profile of improvement was distinct from the infusion therapies, with additional effects on urinary and sexual dysfunction domains, although the effect on the other domains was less pronounced compared to the infusion therapies [99]. In fact, night-time sleep disturbances have been suggested as the only NMS within the criteria for the eligibility of device-aided therapy [100].

Conclusions

The non-motor aspect of PD is complex, both in terms of pathophysiology and clinical phenotypes. Even so, it is becoming increasingly clear that proper identification of NMS through dedicated instruments, such as the NMSS, MDS-UPDRS Part I, and the recently validated MDS-NMS, aids in addressing these symptoms which have a tangible impact on quality of life in PD patients. Identification of NMS, and the developing potential for biomarkers to track their progression, will contribute toward the currently underexplored therapeutic potential for treatment of NMS in PD.

References

1. Politis M, Wu K, Molloy S, et al. Parkinson's disease symptoms: the patient's perspective. Mov Disord 2010; 25: 1646–1651.

2. Parkinson J. An essay on the shaking palsy. 1817. J Neuropsychiatry Clin Neurosci 2002; 14: 223–236; discussion 222.

3. Titova N, Padmakumar C, Lewis SJG, Chaudhuri KR. Parkinson's: a syndrome rather than a disease? J Neural Transm 2017; 124: 907–914.

4. Chaudhuri KR, Martinez-Martin P, Schapira AH, et al. International multicenter pilot study of the first comprehensive self-completed nonmotor symptoms questionnaire for Parkinson's disease: the NMSQuest study. Mov Disord 2006; 21: 916–923.

5. Chaudhuri KR, Martinez-Martin P, Brown RG, et al. The metric properties of a novel non-motor symptoms scale for Parkinson's disease: results from an international pilot study. Mov Disord 2007; 22: 1901–1911.

6. Martinez-Martin P, Schrag A, Weintraub D, et al. Pilot Study of the International Parkinson and Movement Disorder Society-sponsored Non-motor Rating Scale (MDS-NMS). Mov Disord Clin Pract 2019; 6: 227–234.

7. Zis P, Martinez-Martin P, Sauerbier A, et al. Non-motor symptoms burden in treated and untreated early Parkinson's disease patients: argument for non-motor subtypes. Eur J Neurol 2015; 22: 1145–1150.

8. Carod-Artal FJ, Mesquita HM, Ziomkowski S, Martinez-Martin P. Burden and health-related quality of life among caregivers of Brazilian Parkinson's disease patients. Parkinsonism Relat Disord 2013; 19: 943–948.

9. Goetz CG, Tilley BC, Shaftman SR, et al. Movement Disorder Society-sponsored revision of the Unified Parkinson's Disease Rating Scale (MDS-UPDRS): scale presentation and clinimetric testing results. Mov Disord 2008; 23: 2129–2170.

10. Wu JQ, Li P, Stavitsky Gilbert K, et al. Circadian rest-activity rhythms predict cognitive function in early Parkinson's disease independently of sleep. Mov Disord Clin Pract 2018; 5: 614–619.

11. Klingelhoefer L, Rizos A, Sauerbier A, et al. Night-time sleep in Parkinson's disease – the potential use of Parkinson's KinetiGraph: a prospective comparative study. Eur J Neurol 2016; 23: 1275–1288.

12. van Wamelen DJ, Hota S, Podlewska A, et al. Non-motor correlates of wrist-worn wearable sensor use in Parkinson's disease: an exploratory analysis. NPJ Parkinsons Dis 2019; 5: 22.

13. Titova N, Chaudhuri KR. Non-motor Parkinson disease: new concepts and personalised management. Med J Aust 2018; 208: 404–409.

14. Schrag A, Zhelev SS, Hotham S, et al. Heterogeneity in progression of prodromal features in Parkinson's disease. Parkinsonism Relat Disord 2019; 64: 275–279.

15. Fereshtehnejad SM, Zeighami Y, Dagher A, Postuma RB. Clinical criteria for subtyping Parkinson's disease: biomarkers and longitudinal progression. Brain 2017; **140**: 1959–1976.

16. Guo X, Song W, Chen K, et al. Disease duration-related differences in non-motor symptoms: a study of 616 Chinese Parkinson's disease patients. J Neurol Sci 2013; **330**: 32–37.

17. Ou R, Yang J, Cao B, et al. Progression of non-motor symptoms in Parkinson's disease among different age populations: a two-year follow-up study. J Neurol Sci 2016; **360**: 72–77.

18. Simuni T, Caspell-Garcia C, Coffey CS, et al. Baseline prevalence and longitudinal evolution of non-motor symptoms in early Parkinson's disease: the PPMI cohort. J Neurol Neurosurg Psychiatry 2018; **89**: 78–88.

19. Aleksovski D, Miljkovic D, Bravi D, Antonini A. Disease progression in Parkinson subtypes: the PPMI dataset. Neurol Sci 2018; **39**: 1971–1976.

20. Holden SK, Finseth T, Sillau SH, Berman BD. Progression of MDS-UPDRS scores over five years in de novo Parkinson disease from the Parkinson's progression markers initiative cohort. Mov Disord Clin Pract 2018; **5**: 47–53.

21. Erro R, Picillo M, Vitale C, et al. The non-motor side of the honeymoon period of Parkinson's disease and its relationship with quality of life: a 4-year longitudinal study. Eur J Neurol 2016; **23**: 1673–1679.

22. Antonini A, Barone P, Marconi R, et al. The progression of non-motor symptoms in Parkinson's disease and their contribution to motor disability and quality of life. J Neurol 2012; **259**: 2621–2631.

23. Picillo M, Erro R, Amboni M, et al. Gender differences in non-motor symptoms in early Parkinson's disease: a 2-year follow-up study on previously untreated patients. Parkinsonism Relat Disord 2014; **20**: 850–854.

24. Picillo M, Amboni M, Erro R, et al. Gender differences in non-motor symptoms in early, drug naive Parkinson's disease. J Neurol 2013; **260**: 2849–2855.

25. Picillo M, Palladino R, Moccia M, et al. Gender and non-motor fluctuations in Parkinson's disease: a prospective study. Parkinsonism Relat Disord 2016; **27**: 89–92.

26. Miyasaki JM, Long J, Mancini D, et al. Palliative care for advanced Parkinson disease: an interdisciplinary clinic and new scale, the ESAS-PD. Parkinsonism Relat Disord 2012; **18** Suppl 3: S6–9.

27. Higginson IJ, Gao W, Saleem TZ, et al. Symptoms and quality of life in late-stage Parkinson syndromes: a longitudinal community study of predictive factors. PLoS One 2012; **7**: e46327.

28. Saleem TZ, Higginson IJ, Chaudhuri KR, et al. Symptom prevalence, severity and palliative care needs assessment using the Palliative Outcome Scale: a cross-sectional study of patients with Parkinson's disease and related neurological conditions. Palliat Med 2013; **27**: 722–731.

29. Chesselet MF, Richter F, Zhu C, et al. A progressive mouse model of Parkinson's disease: the Thy1-aSyn ("Line 61") mice. Neurotherapeutics 2012; **9**: 297–314.

30. Bichler Z, Lim HC, Zeng L, Tan EK. Non-motor and motor features in LRRK2 transgenic mice. PLoS One 2013; **8**: e70249.

31. Sardi SP, Clarke J, Kinnecom C, et al. CNS expression of glucocerebrosidase corrects alpha-synuclein pathology and memory in a mouse model of Gaucher-related synucleinopathy. Proc Natl Acad Sci USA 2011; **108**: 12101–12106.

32. Zhu XR, Maskri L, Herold C, et al. Non-motor behavioural impairments in parkin-deficient mice. Eur J Neurosci 2007; **26**: 1902–1911.

33. Taylor TN, Caudle WM, Shepherd KR, et al. Nonmotor symptoms of Parkinson's disease revealed in an animal model with reduced monoamine storage capacity. J Neurosci 2009; **29**: 8103–8113.

34. Duty S, Jenner P. Animal models of Parkinson's disease: a source of novel treatments and clues to the cause of the disease. Br J Pharmacol 2011; **164**: 1357–1391.

35. Jellinger KA. Neuropathobiology of non-motor symptoms in Parkinson disease. J Neural Transm 2015; **122**: 1429–1440.

36. Quinn NP. Classification of fluctuations in patients with Parkinson's disease. Neurology 1998; **51**: S25–29.

37. Rodriguez-Violante M, Ospina-Garcia N, Davila-Avila NM, et al. Motor and non-motor wearing-off and its impact in the quality of life of patients with Parkinson's disease. Arq Neuropsiquiatr 2018; **76**: 517–521.

38. Rahmani M, Benabdeljlil M, Bellakhdar F, et al. Deep brain stimulation in Moroccan patients with Parkinson's disease: the experience of the Neurology Department of Rabat. Front Neurol 2018; **9**: 532.

39. Witjas T, Kaphan E, Azulay JP, et al. Nonmotor fluctuations in Parkinson's disease: frequent and disabling. Neurology 2002; **59**: 408–413.

40. Storch A, Schneider CB, Wolz M, et al. Nonmotor fluctuations in Parkinson disease: severity and correlation with motor complications. Neurology 2013; **80**: 800–809.

41. Lohle M, Hermann W, Hausbrand D, et al. Putaminal dopamine turnover in de novo Parkinson's disease predicts later neuropsychiatric fluctuations but not other major health outcomes. J Parkinsons Dis 2019; **9**(4): 1–12.

42. Hillen ME, Sage JI. Nonmotor fluctuations in patients with Parkinson's disease. Neurology 1996; **47**: 1180–1183.

43. Gunal DI, Nurichalichi K, Tuncer N, et al. The clinical profile of nonmotor fluctuations in Parkinson's disease patients. Can J Neurol Sci 2002; **29**: 61–64.

44. Brun L, Lefaucheur R, Fetter D, et al. Non-motor fluctuations in Parkinson's disease: prevalence, characteristics and management in a large cohort of parkinsonian outpatients. Clin Neurol Neurosurg 2014; **127**: 93–96.

45. Seki M, Takahashi K, Uematsu D, et al. Clinical features and varieties of non-motor fluctuations in Parkinson's disease: a Japanese multicenter study. Parkinsonism Relat Disord 2013; **19**: 104–108.

46. Storch A, Rosqvist K, Ebersbach G, Odin P. Disease stage dependency of motor and non-motor fluctuations in Parkinson's disease. J Neural Transm 2019; **126**: 841–851.

47. Rieu I, Houeto JL, Pereira B, et al. Impact of mood and behavioral disorders on quality of life in Parkinson's disease. J Parkinsons Dis 2016; **6**: 267–277.

48. Muller B, Assmus J, Herlofson K, et al. Importance of motor vs. non-motor symptoms for health-related quality of life in early Parkinson's disease. Parkinsonism Relat Disord 2013; **19**: 1027–1032.

49. Martinez-Fernandez R, Schmitt E, Martinez-Martin P, Krack P. The hidden sister of motor fluctuations in Parkinson's disease: a review on nonmotor fluctuations. Mov Disord 2016; **31**: 1080–1094.

50. Nissenbaum H, Quinn NP, Brown RG, et al. Mood swings associated with the 'on-off' phenomenon in Parkinson's disease. Psychol Med 1987; **17**: 899–904.

51. Racette BA, Hartlein JM, Hershey T, et al. Clinical features and comorbidity of mood fluctuations in Parkinson's disease. J Neuropsychiatry Clin Neurosci 2002; **14**: 438–442.

52. Richard IH, Justus AW, Kurlan R. Relationship between mood and motor fluctuations in Parkinson's disease. J Neuropsychiatry Clin Neurosci 2001; **13**: 35–41.

53. Friedenberg DL, Cummings JL. Parkinson's disease, depression, and the on-off phenomenon. Psychosomatics 1989; **30**: 94–99.

54. Sierra M, Carnicella S, Strafella AP, et al. Apathy and impulse control disorders: yin & yang of dopamine dependent behaviors. J Parkinsons Dis 2015; **5**: 625–636.

55. Pagonabarraga J, Martinez-Horta S, Fernandez de Bobadilla R, et al. Minor hallucinations occur in drug-naive Parkinson's disease patients, even from the premotor phase. Mov Disord 2016; **31**: 45–52.

56. Stacy M, Bowron A, Guttman M, et al. Identification of motor and nonmotor wearing-off in Parkinson's disease: comparison of a patient questionnaire versus a clinician assessment. Mov Disord 2005; **20**: 726–733.

57. Goetz CG, Lutge W, Tanner CM. Autonomic dysfunction in Parkinson's disease. Neurology 1986; **36**: 73–75.

58. Pursiainen V, Korpelainen JT, Haapaniemi TH, et al. Blood pressure and heart rate in parkinsonian patients with and without wearing-off. Eur J Neurol 2007; **14**: 373–378.

59. Leta V, van Wamelen DJ, Rukavina K, et al. Sweating and other thermoregulatory abnormalities in Parkinson's disease: a review. Mov Disord 2019; **2**: 39.

60. Juri C, Rodriguez-Oroz M, Obeso JA. The pathophysiological basis of sensory disturbances in Parkinson's disease. J Neurol Sci 2010; **289**: 60–65.

61. Tinazzi M, Recchia S, Simonetto S, et al. Muscular pain in Parkinson's disease and nociceptive processing assessed with CO_2 laser-evoked potentials. Mov Disord 2010; **25**: 213–220.

62. Rukavina K, Leta V, Sportelli C, et al. Pain in Parkinson's disease: new concepts in pathogenesis and treatment. Curr Opin Neurol 2019; **32**: 579–588.

63. Ford B. Pain in Parkinson's disease. Mov Disord 2010; 25 Suppl1: S98–103.

64. Park A, Stacy M. Dopamine-induced nonmotor symptoms of Parkinson's disease. Parkinsons Dis 2011; **2011**: 485063.

65. Weintraub D, Claassen DO. Impulse control and related disorders in Parkinson's disease. Int Rev Neurobiol 2017; **133**: 679–717.

66. Gatto EM, Aldinio V. Impulse control disorders in Parkinson's disease. A brief and comprehensive review. Front Neurol 2019; **10**: 351.

67. Smith KM, Xie SX, Weintraub D. Incident impulse control disorder symptoms and dopamine transporter imaging in Parkinson disease. J Neurol Neurosurg Psychiatry 2016; **87**: 864–870.

68. Eisinger RS, Ramirez-Zamora A, Carbunaru S, et al. Medications, deep brain stimulation, and other factors influencing impulse control disorders in Parkinson's disease. Front Neurol 2019; **10**: 86.

69. Palma JA, Kaufmann H. Treatment of autonomic dysfunction in Parkinson disease and other synucleinopathies. Mov Disord 2018; **33**: 372–390.

70. Frucht S, Rogers JD, Greene PE, et al. Falling asleep at the wheel: motor vehicle mishaps in persons taking pramipexole and ropinirole. Neurology 1999; **52**: 1908–1910.

71. Pagano G, Molloy S, Bain PG, et al. Sleep problems and hypothalamic dopamine D3 receptor availability in Parkinson disease. Neurology 2016; **87**: 2451–2456.

72. Schapira AHV, Chaudhuri KR, Jenner P. Non-motor features of Parkinson disease. Nat Rev Neurosci 2017; **18**: 509.

73. Parnetti L, Gaetani L, Eusebi P, et al. CSF and blood biomarkers for Parkinson's disease. Lancet Neurol 2019; **18**(6): 573–586.

74. Brooks DJ, Pavese N. Imaging biomarkers in Parkinson's disease. Prog Neurobiol 2011; **95**: 614–628.

75. Ryman SG, Poston KL. MRI biomarkers of motor and non-motor symptoms in Parkinson's disease. Parkinsonism Relat Disord 2019; **73**: 85–93.

76. Rinne JO, Portin R, Ruottinen H, et al. Cognitive impairment and the brain dopaminergic system in Parkinson disease: [18 F]fluorodopa positron emission tomographic study. Arch Neurol 2000; **57**: 470–475.

77. Weintraub D. Dopamine and impulse control disorders in Parkinson's disease. Ann Neurol 2008; **64**: S93–S100.

78. Sakakibara R, Shinotoh H, Uchiyama T, et al. SPECT imaging of the dopamine transporter with [(123)I]-beta-CIT reveals marked decline of nigrostriatal dopaminergic function in Parkinson's disease with urinary dysfunction. J Neurol Sci 2001; **187**: 55–59.

79. Eisensehr I, Linke R, Tatsch K, et al. Increased muscle activity during rapid eye movement sleep correlates with decrease of striatal presynaptic dopamine transporters. IPT and IBZM SPECT imaging in subclinical and clinically manifest idiopathic REM sleep behavior disorder, Parkinson's disease, and controls. Sleep 2003; **26**: 507–512.

80. Bohnen NI, Gedela S, Kuwabara H, et al. Selective hyposmia and nigrostriatal dopaminergic denervation in Parkinson's disease. J Neurol 2007; **254**: 84–90.

81. Moccia M, Erro R, Picillo M, et al. A four-year longitudinal study on restless legs syndrome in Parkinson disease. Sleep 2016; **39**: 405–412.

82. Lee JJ, Oh JS, Ham JH, et al. Association of body mass index and the depletion of nigrostriatal dopamine in Parkinson's disease. Neurobiol Aging 2016; **38**: 197–204.

83. Filippi M, Sarasso E, Agosta F. Resting-state functional MRI in Parkinsonian syndromes. Mov Disord Clin Pract 2019; **6**: 104–117.

84. Wolters AF, van de Weijer SCF, Leentjens AFG, et al. Resting-state fMRI in Parkinson's disease patients with cognitive impairment: a meta-analysis. Parkinsonism Relat Disord 2019; **62**: 16–27.

85. Gallea C, Ewenczyk C, Degos B, et al. Pedunculopontine network dysfunction in Parkinson's disease with postural control and sleep disorders. Mov Disord 2017; **32**: 693–704.

86. Su M, Wang S, Fang W, et al. Alterations in the limbic/paralimbic cortices of Parkinson's disease patients with hyposmia under resting-state functional MRI by regional homogeneity and functional connectivity analysis. Parkinsonism Relat Disord 2015; **21**: 698–703.

87. Yoneyama N, Watanabe H, Kawabata K, et al. Severe hyposmia and aberrant functional connectivity in cognitively normal Parkinson's disease. PloS One 2018; **13**: e0190072.

88. Sarkar A, Rawat N, Sachan N, Singh MP. Unequivocal biomarker for Parkinson's disease: a hunt that remains a pester. Neurotox Res 2019; **36**: 627–644.

89. Dong MX, Feng X, Xu XM, et al. Integrated analysis reveals altered lipid and glucose metabolism and identifies NOTCH2 as a biomarker for Parkinson's disease related depression. Front Mol Neurosci 2018; **11**: 257.

90. Oeckl P, Metzger F, Nagl M, et al. Alpha-, beta-, and gamma-synuclein quantification in cerebrospinal fluid by multiple reaction monitoring reveals increased concentrations in Alzheimer's and Creutzfeldt-Jakob disease but no alteration in synucleinopathies. Mol Cell Proteomics 2016; **15**: 3126–3138.

91. Donadio V, Incensi A, Leta V, et al. Skin nerve α-synuclein deposits: a biomarker for idiopathic Parkinson disease. Neurology 2014; **82**: 1362–1369.

92. Borghammer P. Is constipation in Parkinson's disease caused by gut or brain pathology? Parkinsonism Relat Disord 2018; **55**: 6–7.

93. Beach TG, Adler CH, Dugger BN, et al. Submandibular gland biopsy for the diagnosis of Parkinson disease. J Neuropathol Exp Neurol 2013; **72**: 130–136.

94. Seppi K, K. Ray Chaudhuri, Coelho M, et al. Update on treatments for nonmotor symptoms of Parkinson's disease: an evidence-based medicine review. Mov Disord 2019; **34**: 180–198.

95. Goldman JG, Guerra CM. Treatment of nonmotor symptoms associated with Parkinson disease. Neurol Clin 2020; **38**(2): 269–292.

96. Stacy MA, Murck H, Kroenke K. Responsiveness of motor and nonmotor symptoms of Parkinson disease to dopaminergic therapy. Prog Neuropsychopharmacol Biol Psychiatry 2010; **34**: 57–61.

97. Kassubek J, Chaudhuri KR, Zesiewicz T, et al. Rotigotine transdermal system and evaluation of pain in patients with Parkinson's disease: a post hoc analysis of the RECOVER study. BMC Neurol 2014; **14**: 42.

98. Martinez-Martin P, Reddy P, Katzenschlager R, et al. EuroInf: a multicenter comparative observational study of apomorphine and levodopa infusion in Parkinson's disease. Mov Disord 2015; **30**: 510–516.

99. Dafsari HS, Martinez-Martin P, Rizos A, et al. EuroInf 2: Subthalamic stimulation, apomorphine, and levodopa infusion in Parkinson's disease. Mov Disord 2019; **34**: 353–365.

100. Antonini A, Stoessl AJ, Kleinman LS, et al. Developing consensus among movement disorder specialists on clinical indicators for identification and management of advanced Parkinson's disease: a multi-country Delphi-panel approach. Curr Med Res Opin 2018; **34**: 2063–2073.

Chapter 2

Evaluation of the Patient with Parkinson's Disease in the Early Stages: Non-Motor Phase

Anna Sauerbier, Daniele Urso, Chloe Farrell, K. Ray Chaudhuri, Carmen Rodriguez-Blazquez

Introduction

Value-based healthcare is a key aspect of modern approaches of delivery of medical care. Outcome measures are therefore a major aspect of addressing the importance of healthcare delivery and the objectives it aims to achieve. Besides motor symptoms, non-motor symptoms (NMS) in Parkinson's disease (PD) drive quality of life across all stages of the disease, as well as societal costs. Objective measurement is possible using validated tools, both patient self-rated and healthcare professional-administered. Mixed motor and non-motor objective assessments are therefore recommended in order to achieve an adequate evaluation and management tailored to the patients' specific needs [1]. Furthermore, the availability of assessment instruments for detecting and measuring NMS has allowed understanding of their importance, prevalence, presentation, progression, and impact on the patients' daily life, and the evaluation of the effect of interventions in PD patients [2].

In this book chapter, we will summarize some of the key assessment tools for NMS, being the core symptoms during the early phase of PD [3]. First, we will review tools addressing NMS holistically and second, we will review tools addressing specific NMS (Table 2.1).

Holistic Assessment Tools for Non-Motor Symptoms in Parkinson's Disease

Non-Motor Symptoms Questionnaire

The NMS Questionnaire (NMSQuest) is a screening instrument for the detection of NMS in patients with PD and was the first validated tool in 2006 that specifically assesses NMS in PD in a holistic manner. The NMSQuest is a self-administered questionnaire and is answered in a "yes" and "no" fashion that can be easily completed by the patient or carer within 5–7 minutes. It includes 30 items composed of nine different NMS domains: digestive (seven items); urinary (two items); apathy/attention/memory (three items);

Table 2.1 Overview of the Parkinson's disease-specific non-motor tools addressed in this chapter

Parkinson's disease specific assessment tools for non-motor symptoms
Holistic assessment tools
Non-Motor Symptoms Questionnaire (NMSQuest)
Non-Motor Symptoms Scale (NMSS)
Movement Disorder Society Non-Motor Rating Scale (MDS-NMS)
Movement Disorder Society-Sponsored Revision of the Unified Parkinson's Disease Rating Scale (MDS-UPDRS)
Specific assessment tools
King's Parkinson's Disease Pain Scale (KPPS)
SCales for Outcomes in PArkinson's disease – Sleep (SCOPA-Sleep)
Parkinson's Disease Sleep Scale (PDSS) and revised PDSS-2
SCOPA-Autonomic (SCOPA-AUT)
Parkinson Fatigue Scale-16 item (PFS-16)
Parkinson Anxiety Scale (PAS)
Apathy Scale (AS)
Parkinson Fatigue Scale (PFS)
Parkinson Psychosis Questionnaire (PPQ)
Ardouin Scale of Behavior in Parkinson's Disease (ASBPD)
Scales for Outcome in Parkinson's Disease-Psychiatric Complications (SCOPA-PC)
Scale for Evaluation of Neuropsychiatric Disorders in Parkinson's Disease (SEND-PD)
Questionnaire for Impulsive-Compulsive Disorders in PD (QUIP) and QUIP-Rating Scale (QUIP-RS)

hallucinations/delusions (two items); depression/anxiety (two items); sexual function (two items); cardiovascular (two items); sleep disorders (five items); and miscellaneous (pain, weight change, swelling, sweating, diplopia) (five items) [4].

The total score (range: 0–30) is easily obtained from the sum of the "yes" responses, revealing the number of NMS experienced by the patient over the last month. Chaudhuri and colleagues proposed a grading classification of NMS burden based on the NMSQuest total score; 0 = no NMS; 1–5 NMS = mild burden; 6–9 NMS = moderate burden; 10–13 NMS = severe burden; and >13 NMS = very severe burden [5].

As a result of its design and content, the NMSQuest can be applied in other neurological disorders and has been already used in motor neuron disease (MND) and restless legs syndrome (RLS), for example [6, 7]. The NMSQuest has been translated into a number of different languages including Chinese (Mandarin), Dutch, French, German, Greek, Italian, Japanese, Malay, Spanish, Swedish, and is owned by the Movement Disorders Society (MDS) thus requires their permission for use.

The NMSQuest provides the clinician and specialist nurse, even at a primary care level, with a tool to easily screen for NMS in a simple manner which might help to refer patients to multidisciplinary care and can measure the effect of therapeutic interventions [8]. Grading of NMS using the NMSQuest is considered a quality standard for assessment of PD as also reflected in the NICE guidelines (2017) for PD [9].

Non-Motor Symptoms Scale

The Non-Motor Symptoms Scale (NMSS) for Parkinson's disease (PD) was developed by the MDS Non-Motor-PD study group in order to comprehensively assess a wide spectrum of NMS in PD patients across all stages of the disease [10]. The 30-item scale includes nine different NMS domains: cardiovascular (two items), sleep/fatigue (four items), mood/cognition (six items), perceptual problems/hallucinations (three items), attention/memory (three items) gastrointestinal tract (three items), urinary (three items), sexual function (two items), and miscellaneous (four items). Each item is scored for severity (0 = not present to 3 = severe) and frequency (1 = rarely to 4 = daily) and then multiplied to obtain the item

total score (0–12). By adding all corresponding item scores, the score for each domain is calculated. The NMSS total score is obtained from the sum of the nine domain scores and ranges between 0 and 360, with higher scores indicating a more severe NMS burden. Similar to the NMSQuest, based on the NMSS total score a NMS burden grading has been categorized as follows: 0 = no NMS; 1–20 = mild burden; 21–40 = moderate burden; 41–70 = severe burden, and ≥71 = very severe burden [11]. The NMSS is administered by a trained healthcare professional through direct questioning/interviewing of the patient and/or their carer and typically takes 10–15 minutes to complete. The NMSS has been internationally validated and is available in a number of different languages, including French, German, Italian, Norwegian, Spanish, Swedish, and Japanese [12–14]. More recently, the MDS has supported an update of the above described NMSS considering the strengths and weaknesses that have been noticed over the years. The primary clinimetric validation of the English version of the so-called Movement Disorder Society Non-Motor Rating Scale (MDS-NMS) has just been published [15]. Similar to the NMSS, the MDS-NMS is also health-professional completed, it includes 52 items grouped into 13 different non-motor domains: depression (five items), anxiety (four items), apathy (three items), psychosis (four items), impulse control and related disorders (four items), cognition (six items), orthostatic hypotension (two items), urinary (three items), sexual (two items), gastrointestinal (four items), sleep and wakefulness (six items), pain (four items), and other (five items; unintentional weight loss, decreased smell, physical fatigue, mental fatigue, and excessive sweating). Each item is scored by severity (0 = not present to 4 = severe) and frequency (0 = never to 4 =majority of time) and then multiplied to obtain the item total score (0–16). Total scale score range is 0 to 832 points.

Based on the NMSS, the new MDS-NMS has been specifically improved with domains assessing cognition and other neuropsychiatric symptoms and a new domain to address impulse control and related disorders. Furthermore, a new subscale evaluating non-motor fluctuations has been added, an aspect that was not sufficiently captured with the NMSS. The estimated time to complete the MDS-NMS varies between 15 and

40 minutes according to the non-motor burden and health status of the respective patient.

In the research setting, the NMSS and now the new MDS-NMS serve as both primary and secondary outcome measures in clinical trials [1] which provide the scientific community with invaluable information on tracking disease progression, disease subgroups, and responses to existing and novel therapies [15].

The Movement Disorder Society-Sponsored Revision of the Unified Parkinson's Disease Rating Scale

The great importance of the accurate detection and evaluation of NMS in PD was recognized by the MDS who in 2008 sponsored a revision of the original Unified Parkinson's Disease Rating Scale (UPDRS) [16] initially designed [17]. The so-called MDS–UPDRS evaluates the severity of the main motor and non-motor manifestations in PD combining clinician-reported and patient-reported outcomes. The scale is composed of four sections: Part I, Non-Motor Aspects of Experiences of Daily Living (13 items); Part II, Motor Aspects of Experiences of Daily Living (13 items); Part III, Motor Examination (33 items); and Part IV, Motor Complications (six items). It takes approximately 30 minutes to complete the MDS-UPDRS.

Each item scores from 0 (normal) to 4 (severe), and the total score for each part is obtained from the sum of the item scores [16]. The total scale score range is 0 to 260, with higher scores indicating a more severe burden.

In more detail, the MDS-UPDRS Part I, the section of the MDS-UPDRS designed to evaluate NMS, includes 13 items, six rater-based, evaluated through interview, and seven through a self-completed patient questionnaire, each one evaluating the severity of a NMS relevant in PD. The MDS-UPDRS has been made available in numerous languages including Arabic, Chinese (traditional and simplified), Czech, Dutch, Estonian, French, German, Greek, Hebrew, Hindi, Hungarian, Italian, Japanese, Korean, Polish, Portuguese, Russian, Slovak, Spanish, Thai, and Turkish.

Gallagher and colleagues [18] analyzed the convergent validity of the MDS-UPDRS Part I and suggested that the MDS-UPDRS Part I, despite its brevity, appropriately reflects the burden of NMS in PD patients and is indicative of performance on an extensive battery of established scales, making the MDS–UPDRS Part I an easy and practical tool to assess the burden of NMS in PD.

The MDS-UPDRS is nowadays among the standardized clinical assessment tools most widely used in PD, having been cross-culturally adapted to many countries [19], and having proven good reliability and intra- and inter-observer validity [20–22]. As a limitation, one needs to acknowledge that completion time of the MDS-UPDRS is relatively long and, similar to the NMSS, needs specific training to be administered [2].

Specific Assessment Tools for Individual Non-Motor Symptoms in Parkinson's Disease

For years, different rating scales have been developed to assess specific NMS in PD patients. In this section, we will review those PD-specific instruments that have been deemed as recommended by the MDS and that have been used in studies with newly diagnosed or early-stage PD patients.

Pain

Several rating scales have been used in clinical research and practice for assessing pain in PD, such as the McGill Pain Questionnaire [23], the Brief Pain Inventory [24], and the Neuropathic Pain Symptoms Inventory [25]. However, there is only one PD-specific rating scale that has been classified as recommended for assessing pain by the MDS Task Force [26], the King's PD Pain Scale (KPPS) [27]. There are also items on pain in the main comprehensive instruments for assessing NMS in PD, the NMSS (one item on pain), the MDS-NMS (one domain that includes different types of pain), and the MDS-UPDRS (one item on painful OFF-state dystonia). These scales have been presented earlier in this chapter.

The KPPS is composed of 14 items assessing musculoskeletal, chronic, fluctuation-related, nocturnal, orofacial, swelling, and radicular pain in the past month. Items are scored for severity (0 to 3) and frequency (0 to 4) and then multiplied to obtain the item total score. Total scale score range is 0 to 168 points, with higher scores indicating more pain. It is administered by a clinician through interview and it takes around 10 minutes to be completed. The KPPS has a complete validation study, with good acceptability, reliability, and validity. It has been used in clinical trials [28, 29], and has been demonstrated to be sensitive to changes due to treatment [30]. Among its weaknesses, the need for training of clinicians to recognize the nosological categories of pain included in the scale, the absence of information on the interpretability of scores, and the lack of versions adapted to and validated in languages other than English should be cited [26].

Sleep

Main PD-specific rating scales for assessing sleep disturbances include the SCales for Outcomes in PArkinson's disease – Sleep (SCOPA-Sleep) and the Parkinson's Disease Sleep Scale (PDSS) and its revised version (PDSS-2) [31–33]. Multidomain scales such as the NMSQuest, the NMSS, and the MDS-UPDRS include items that evaluate sleep disorders, and the MDS-NMS includes a six-item domain assessing sleep and wakefulness. These scales, together with other widely used generic instruments for evaluation of sleep disorders in PD, have been previously reviewed by the MDS and other authors [34, 35].

The SCOPA-Sleep was the first instrument specifically developed to assess sleep problems in PD. It is a self-completed scale, using the previous month as its time frame, composed of 12 items grouped in two domains: night-time sleep (five items) and daytime sleepiness (six items), scored from 0 (not at all) to 3 (very much). Higher scores in both domains reflect more severe sleep disorders. Cut-off points have been identified: 6/7 for nocturnal sleep to differentiate good sleepers from poor sleepers, and 4/5 for daytime sleepiness, to separate excessive daytime sleepiness from normal scores. The scale also contains a single question rating sleep quality on a seven-point scale (from slept very well to slept very badly) which is not included in the total scale score. The scale shows good reliability and validity in the validation studies, it is easy to complete (5–10 minutes), and seems to be sensitive to changes due to treatment [36, 37]. SCOPA-Sleep has been originally developed in Dutch, but it has been translated and validated in several languages, including English, Spanish, German, and Korean. Due to its properties, it is recommended and owned by the MDS [35]. Its limitations include the need for further studies on its responsiveness and interpretability and the lack of specific items addressing some sleep-related disturbances, such as RLS and REM behavior disorder (RBD).

The PDSS is a PD-specific, 15-item self-rated scale that mainly evaluates night-time sleep problems over the previous week, with only one item pertaining to daytime sleepiness. Each item is rated in a visual analog scale (VAS) from 0 (severe and always present) to 10 (not present). Item scores are summed, with a maximum total score of 150 indicative of absence of sleep problems. The PDSS has satisfactory psychometric properties and is easy to use; thus it is recommended for screening and measuring severity of sleep disturbances in PD [34, 35]. It has been proven to be responsive to changes due to treatment and it has been translated into several languages [38]. The scale has been used to characterize sleep problems and their physiological correlates in untreated PD patients [39–42]. However, patients could require explanation on how to score the VAS, and the scale does not include information from the caregiver. It does not screen for specific sleep disorders in PD, such as sleep apnea, RBD, or RLS and the only item on daytime somnolence is not enough to assess it.

The PDSS-2 was designed to overcome two of the shortcomings of the PDSS: the scoring system has been replaced by a Likert-type one (from 0, never, to 4, very frequent), and all the 15 items are focused on nocturnal sleep [33]. Maximum total score is 60, reflecting higher sleep problems severity. Cut-off values have been determined: ≥15 points have been determined to distinguish between good and bad sleepers, and ≥18 to define clinically relevant PD-specific sleep disturbances [43, 44]. Its time frame is the last week, and is easily self-responded, taking around 10 minutes to be completed. The PDSS-2 has satisfactory reliability and validity, it seems to be responsive to changes, and it has versions in several languages. A roommate-based version in Spanish has been also tested [45, 46]. In drug-naïve PD patients, the RBD as assessed with the PDSS-2 was associated with cognitive dysfunction, anxiety, and other sleep disturbances [47]. However, there is a need for further studies on its responsiveness.

Autonomic Dysfunction

The rating scales for assessing dysautonomia have been reviewed by two MDS Task Forces [48, 49].

There are several instruments for assessing autonomic symptoms, such as the Drooling Rating Scale (DRS), Sialorrhea Clinical Scale for PD (SCS-PD), and the Composite Autonomic Symptom Scale (COMPASS). The main global, PD-specific measure for autonomic dysfunction is the SCOPA-Autonomic (SCOPA-AUT), although the NMSQuest, the NMSS, the MDS-UPDRS, and the MDS-NMS contain items or domains focused on autonomic symptoms [50].

The SCOPA-AUT is a self-completed instrument composed of 25 items assessing the following domains: gastrointestinal (seven items), urinary (six items), cardiovascular (three items), thermoregulatory (four items), pupillomotor (one item), and sexual (two items for men and two items for women). The response options for each item range from 0 (never) to 3 (often), with higher total scores reflecting worse autonomic functioning. It is easy to apply (around 10 minutes), and has good psychometric properties using both Classical Test Theory and Item Response Theory, although its association with objective physiological autonomic measures is not clear [51]. Using the SCOPA-AUT, researchers have found there are autonomic symptoms in early stages of PD, although mild, and they can be an early marker of cognitive impairment in de novo PD patients [52, 53]. The SCOPA-AUT has been translated and validated in several languages. It is a recommended scale by the MDS, but several limitations must be accounted for: its sensitivity for screening orthostatic symptoms is low and its responsiveness has not been determined.

Fatigue

Fatigue is a prominent NMS in PD patients, even in early stages, and thus, it has been addressed in a high number of studies using a wide variety of rating scales. The MDS Task Force on fatigue recommended the use of the instruments Fatigue Severity Scale (FSS) for both screening and severity rating; the Functional Assessment of Chronic Illness Therapy-Fatigue (FACIT), and the Parkinson Fatigue Scale-16 item (PFS-16) for screening; and the Multidimensional Fatigue Inventory (MFI) for severity [54]. Between the multidimensional instruments, the MDS-UPDRS and the NMSS contain one item on fatigue, and the MDS-NMS includes one item on physical fatigue and one item on mental fatigue.

The PFS-16 is the only PD-specific instrument available for assessing fatigue. It is focused on physical, but not on cognitive or emotional, aspects of fatigue, and includes items on the impact of fatigue in activities of daily living [55]. The item response options range from 1 (strongly disagree) to 5 (strongly agree), and the final score can be calculated as the mean of item responses, using a binary approach (options agree and strongly agree score as 1 and the rest as 0), or summing the 16 items' scores. The time frame is the last 2 weeks, and it takes around 15 minutes to be administered. It has versions validated in several languages, with satisfactory psychometric properties, although the binary scoring showed lower measurement precision [56]. The PFS-16 is useful to detect fatigue and assess changes due to treatment in early PD patients [57]. The main criticism is this scale may not adequately reflect clinically significant non-physical aspects of fatigue [54].

Neuropsychiatric Symptoms

Several MDS Task Force committees have reviewed the available rating scales for the main neuropsychiatric symptoms in PD, that can be present even in early stages: anxiety, depression, apathy, fatigue, psychosis, and impulsive and compulsive behaviors [54, 58–61].

For anxiety, none of the revised scales, all generic, reached the category of recommended. For this reason, a new PD-specific scale, the Parkinson Anxiety Scale (PAS) was developed [62]. The PAS includes 12 items, grouped into subscales for persistent and episodic anxiety and avoidance behaviors. Items are scored from 0 (not or never) to 4 (severe or almost always), with a maximum total score of 48 points, suggestive of severe anxiety. A cut-off ≥14 points for anxiety has been suggested. It is a brief and easy-to-apply scale, with clinician- and patient-rated versions and good psychometric properties. In an Italian study, 58.4% of early PD patients showed anxiety symptoms using the PAS [60, 63]. The disadvantages of the PAS include the lack of information on its responsiveness and its adequateness for patients with dementia.

The main multidimensional scales for NMS in PD also include questions for assessing anxiety: the NMSQuest, the NMSS, and the MDS-UPDRS each have one item, while the MDS-NMS has a four-item domain, focused on general anxiety, panic attacks, and worries about being in public and in social situations [15].

For depression, three generic rating scales reached the classification recommended by the MDS Task Force: the Hamilton Depression Scale (Ham-D), the Montgomery-Asberg Depression Rating Scale (MADRS), and the Beck Depression Inventory-II (BDI-II). No PD-specific rating scale for depression exists, but the MDS Task Force does not recommend developing new scales [59]. Multidimensional PD rating scales also contain items for assessing depression: one in NMSQuest, NMSS, and MDS-UPDRS and a domain in the MDS-NMS [59]. In this instrument, the five items that compose the domain are addressed to assess the emotional component of depression: sadness, difficulty experiencing pleasure, hopelessness, negative thoughts, and feelings that life is not worth living.

Apathy is also a component of the main multidimensional rating scales for PD: the NMSQuest, the NMSS, and the MDS-UPDRS, with one item on apathy in each one; and the MDS-NMS with a domain composed of three items. The MDS Task Force on apathy categorized one PD-specific rating scale as recommended, the Apathy Scale (AS) [64, 65]. This scale consists of 14 items, scored from 0 (a lot) to 3 (not at all) for items 1–8, and from 0 (not at all) to 3 (a lot) for items 9–14. Maximum total score, indicative of severe apathy, is 42 points. The cut-off value for the presence of apathy is ≥14 points. The AS is rapid, simple, and suitable for screening and has demonstrated good reliability, validity, and sensitivity to change. It has been specifically validated in early-stage PD patients, and some studies have shown that apathy is present in up to 26% of these patients [66, 67]. However, there are concerns about its adequateness for PD patients with dementia.

For psychosis, the MDS Task Force recommended the following generic rating scales: the Neuropsychiatric Inventory (NPI), the Schedule for Assessment of Positive Symptoms (SAPS), the Positive and Negative Syndrome Scale (PANSS), and the Brief Psychiatric Rating Scale (BPRS) [58]. Before this review, some PD-specific scales for assessing psychosis have been developed and validated: the Parkinson Psychosis Questionnaire (PPQ), the Ardouin Scale of Behavior in Parkinson's Disease (ASBPD), and the Scales for

Outcomes in Parkinson's Disease-Psychiatric Complications (SCOPA-PC) [69–71].

Parkinson's disease-related psychosis is captured in other validated multidomain scales such as the MDS-UPDRS, the NMSS, and the MDS-NMS, with a domain composed by four items. The Scale for Evaluation of Neuropsychiatric Disorders in Parkinson's Disease (SEND-PD) is another PD-specific instrument that evaluates the presence and severity of psychotic symptoms, mood/apathy, and impulse control disorders (ICD) [72].

The MDS Task Force reviewed the instruments for assessing impulsive and compulsive behaviors, recommending the Questionnaire for Impulsive-Compulsive Disorders in PD (QUIP) for screening, the QUIP-Rating Scale (QUIP-RS) for screening and severity rating, the Self-Assessment Scale For Dopamine Dependent Behaviors in Parkinson's Disease (Ardouin short screen), recommended for severity assessment, and the Scale for Outcomes in Parkinson's Disease–Psychiatric Complications (SCOPA-PC), recommended only for the assessment of hypersexuality and gambling/shopping [61].

Conclusion

The assessment of NMS in a holistic manner using a burden-based strategy or a more detailed individual NMS-based assessment is feasible in a clinical setting with the available validated tools as addressed in this chapter [1]. Some symptoms may remain unnoticed by the patient (sleep disorders, for example) or undeclared (as sexual problems), and rating scales and questionnaires can be essential for adequately assessing the patient and for monitoring and adjusting treatment to the patient's specific needs [73]. It is indeed important that objective measurements are incorporated into clinical practice as well as clinical studies and form part of evidence-based management guidelines as well as audit process. To achieve this, selection of the most appropriate instrument for each specific application is required and should be guided by information on its psychometric properties and its main characteristics, such as length or measured construct. The MDS section on rating scales and reviews can help researchers and clinicians to select the most appropriate instrument. The construction of new instruments, the study of the psychometric attributes of some of them, and the exploration of new forms of administration (item banks, wearables) are future developments in this field.

References

1. Martinez-Martin P, Chaudhuri K. Ray. Comprehensive grading of Parkinson's disease using motor and non-motor assessments: addressing a key unmet need. Expert Rev Neurother 2018; **18**(1): 41–50.

2. Martinez-Martin P, et al. Measurement of nonmotor symptoms in clinical practice. Int Rev Neurobiol 2017; **133**: 291–345.

3. Schapira AHV, Chaudhuri KR, Jenner P. Non-motor features of Parkinson disease. Nat Rev Neurosci 2017; **18**(8): 509.

4. Chaudhuri KR, et al. International multicenter pilot study of the first comprehensive self-completed nonmotor symptoms questionnaire for Parkinson's disease: the NMSQuest study. Mov Disord 2006; **21**(7): 916–923.

5. Chaudhuri KR, et al. The burden of non-motor symptoms in Parkinson's disease using a self-completed non-motor questionnaire: a simple grading system. Parkinsonism Relat Disord 2015; **21**(3): 287–291.

6. Gunther R, et al. Non-motor symptoms in patients suffering from motor neuron diseases. Front Neurol 2016; **7**: 117.

7. Sauerbier A, et al. Restless legs syndrome – the under-recognised non-motor burden: a questionnaire-based cohort study. Postgrad Med 2019; **131**(7): 473–478.

8. Dafsari HS, et al. Beneficial effects of bilateral subthalamic stimulation on non-motor symptoms in Parkinson's disease. Brain Stimul 2016; **9**(1): 78–85.

9. NICE. *Parkinson's Disease in Adults*. NICE Guidelines. 2017: 23.

10. Chaudhuri KR, et al. The metric properties of a novel non-motor symptoms scale for Parkinson's disease: results from an international pilot study. Mov Disord 2007; **22**(13): 1901–1911.

11. K. Ray Chaudhuri, et al. A proposal for a comprehensive grading of Parkinson's disease severity combining motor and non-motor assessments: meeting an unmet need. PloS One 2013; **8**(2): e57221–e57221.

12. Storch A, et al. Non-motor Symptoms Questionnaire and Scale for Parkinson's disease. Cross-cultural adaptation into the German language. Nervenarzt 2010; **81**(8): 980–985.

13. Cova I, et al. Validation of the Italian version of the Non-Motor Symptoms Scale for Parkinson's disease. Parkinsonism Relat Disord 2017; **34**: 38–42.

14. Sauerbier A, et al. A global survey of the use and linguistic translation of the NMSQuest and NMSScale: implication for non-motor studies in Parkinson's disease. Mov Disord 2017; **32**.

15. Chaudhuri KR, et al. The movement disorder society nonmotor rating scale: Initial validation study. Mov Disord 2020; **35**(1): 116–133.

16. Goetz CG, et al. Movement Disorder Society-sponsored revision of the Unified Parkinson's Disease Rating Scale (MDS-UPDRS): process, format, and clinimetric testing plan. Mov Disord 2007; **22**(1): 41–47.

17. Fahn S, Elton R, U.D. Committee. The Unified Parkinson's Disease Rating Scale. In: Fahn S, Marsden CD, Calne DB, Goldstein M (eds). *Recent Developments in Parkinson's Disease*, 2nd ed. Macmillan Healthcare Information; 1987, 153–163, 293–304.

18. Gallagher DA, et al. Validation of the MDS-UPDRS Part I for nonmotor symptoms in Parkinson's disease. Mov Disord 2012; **27**(1): 79–83.

19. Goetz CG, et al. IPMDS-sponsored scale translation program: process, format, and clinimetric testing plan for the MDS-UPDRS and UDysRS. Mov Disord Clin Pract 2014; **1**(2): 97–101.

20. Goetz CG, et al. Movement Disorder Society-sponsored revision of the Unified Parkinson's Disease Rating Scale (MDS-UPDRS): scale presentation and clinimetric testing results. Mov Disord 2008; **23**(15): 2129–2170.

21. Martinez-Martin P, et al. Expanded and independent validation of the Movement Disorder Society-Unified Parkinson's Disease Rating Scale (MDS-UPDRS). J Neurol 2013; **260**(1): 228–236.

22. Antonini A, et al. Validation of the Italian version of the Movement Disorder Society–Unified Parkinson's Disease Rating Scale. Neurol Sci 2013; **34**(5): 683–687.

23. Melzack R. The McGill Pain Questionnaire: major properties and scoring methods. Pain 1975; **1**(3): 277–299.

24. Cleeland C. Measurement of pain by subjective report. In: Chapman CR, Loeser JD, (eds.). *Issues in Pain Measurement*, 1st ed. Raven; 1989, 391–403.

25. Bouhassira D, et al. Development and validation of the Neuropathic Pain Symptom Inventory. Pain 2004; **108**(3): 248–257.

26. Perez-Lloret S, et al. Rating scales for pain in Parkinson's disease: critique and recommendations. Mov Disord Clin Pract 2016; **3**(6): 527–537.

27. Chaudhuri KR, et al. King's Parkinson's disease pain scale, the first scale for pain in PD: An international validation. Mov Disord 2015; **30**(12): 1623–1631.

28. Trenkwalder C, et al. Prolonged release oxycodone-naloxone for treatment of severe restless legs syndrome after failure of previous treatment: a double-blind, randomised, placebo-controlled trial with an open-label extension. Lancet Neurol 2013; **12**(12): 1141–1150.

29. Rascol O, et al. A randomized controlled exploratory pilot study to evaluate the effect of rotigotine transdermal patch on Parkinson's disease-associated chronic pain. J Clin Pharmacol 2016; **56**(7): 852–861.

30. Silverdale MA, et al. A detailed clinical study of pain in 1957 participants with early/moderate Parkinson's disease. Parkinsonism Relat Disord 2018; **56**: 27–32.

31. Marinus J, et al. A short scale for the assessment of motor impairments and disabilities in Parkinson's disease: the SPES/SCOPA. J Neurol Neurosurg Psychiatry 2004; **75**(3): 388–395.

32. Chaudhuri KR, et al. The Parkinson's disease sleep scale: a new instrument for assessing sleep and nocturnal disability in Parkinson's disease. J Neurol Neurosurg Psychiatry 2002; **73**(6): 629–635.

33. Trenkwalder C, et al. Parkinson's disease sleep scale–validation of the revised version PDSS-2. Mov Disord 2011; **26**(4): 644–652.

34. Kurtis MM, et al. A review of scales to evaluate sleep disturbances in movement disorders. Front Neurol 2018; **9**: 369.

35. Hogl B, et al. Scales to assess sleep impairment in Parkinson's disease: critique and recommendations. Mov Disord 2010; **25**(16): 2704–2716.

36. Fernandez-Pajarin G, et al. Evaluating the efficacy of nocturnal continuous subcutaneous apomorphine infusion in sleep disorders in advanced Parkinson's disease: the APO-NIGHT study. J Parkinsons Dis 2016; **6**(4): 787–792.

37. Patel N, et al. Nighttime sleep and daytime sleepiness improved with pimavanserin during treatment of Parkinson's disease psychosis. Clin Neuropharmacol 2018; **41**(6): 210–215.

38. Fei L, Zhou D, Ding ZT. The efficacy and safety of rotigotine transdermal patch for the treatment of sleep disorders in Parkinson's disease: a meta-analysis. Sleep Med 2019; **61**: 19–25.

39. Stefansdottir S, et al. Subjective sleep problems in patients with early Parkinson's disease. Eur J Neurol 2012; **19**(12): 1575–1581.

40. Bušková J, et al. Sleep disturbances in untreated Parkinson's disease. J Neurol 2011; **258**(12): 2254–2259.

41. Happe S, et al. Association of daytime sleepiness with nigrostriatal dopaminergic degeneration in early Parkinson's disease. J Neurol 2007; **254**(8): 1037–1043.

42. Dhawan V, et al. The range and nature of sleep dysfunction in untreated Parkinson's disease (PD). A comparative controlled clinical study using the Parkinson's disease sleep scale and selective polysomnography. J Neurol Sci 2006; **248**(1–2): 158–162.

43. Suzuki K, et al. Evaluation of cutoff scores for the Parkinson's disease sleep scale-2. Acta Neurol Scand 2015; **131**(6): 426–430.

44. Muntean ML, et al. Clinically relevant cut-off values for the Parkinson's Disease Sleep Scale-2 (PDSS-2): a validation study. Sleep Med 2016; **24**: 87–92.

45. Trenkwalder C, et al. Rotigotine effects on early morning motor function and sleep in Parkinson's disease: a double-blind, randomized, placebo-controlled study (RECOVER). Mov Disord 2011; **26**(1): 90–99.

46. Martinez-Martin P, et al. The Parkinson's Disease Sleep Scale-2 (PDSS-2): validation of the Spanish version and its relationship with a roommate-based version. Mov Disord Clin Pract 2019; **6**(4): 294–301.

47. Liu H, et al. Rapid eye movement behavior disorder in drug-naïve patients with Parkinson's disease. J Clin Neurosci 2019; **59**: 254–258.

48. Evatt ML, et al. Dysautonomia rating scales in Parkinson's disease: sialorrhea, dysphagia, and constipation–critique and recommendations by Movement Disorders Task Force on rating scales for Parkinson's disease. Mov Disord 2009; **24**(5): 635–646.

49. Pavy-Le Traon A, et al. The Movement Disorders Task Force review of dysautonomia rating scales in Parkinson's disease with regard to symptoms of orthostatic hypotension. Mov Disord 2011; **26**(11): 1985–1992.

50. Visser M, et al. Assessment of autonomic dysfunction in Parkinson's disease: the SCOPA-AUT. Mov Disord 2004; **19**(11): 1306–1312.

51. Ashraf-Ganjouei A, et al. Autonomic dysfunction and white matter microstructural changes in drug-naïve patients with Parkinson's disease. PeerJ 2018; **6**: e5539.

52. Stanković I, et al. Longitudinal assessment of autonomic dysfunction in early Parkinson's disease. Parkinsonism Relat Disord 2019; 66: 74–79.

53. Jones JD, et al. Gastrointestinal symptoms are predictive of trajectories of cognitive functioning in de novo Parkinson's disease. Parkinsonism Relat Disord 2020; 72: 7–12.

54. Friedman JH, et al. Fatigue rating scales critique and recommendations by the Movement Disorders Society task force on rating scales for Parkinson's disease. Mov Disord 2010; 25(7): 805–822.

55. Brown RG, et al. The Parkinson fatigue scale. Parkinsonism Relat Disord 2005; 11(1): 49–55.

56. Nilsson MH, Bladh S, Hagell P. Fatigue in Parkinson's disease: measurement properties of a generic and a condition-specific rating scale. J Pain Symptom Manage 2013; 46(5): 737–746.

57. Stocchi F. Benefits of treatment with rasagiline for fatigue symptoms in patients with early Parkinson's disease. Eur J Neurol 2014; 21(2): 357–360.

58. Fernandez HH, et al. Scales to assess psychosis in Parkinson's disease: critique and recommendations. Mov Disord 2008; 23(4): 484–500.

59. Schrag A, et al. Depression rating scales in Parkinson's disease: critique and recommendations. Mov Disord 2007; 22(8): 1077–1092.

60. Leentjens AF, et al. Anxiety rating scales in Parkinson's disease: critique and recommendations. Mov Disord 2008; 23(14): 2015–2025.

61. Evans AH, et al. Scales to assess impulsive and compulsive behaviors in Parkinson's disease: critique and recommendations. Mov Disord 2019; 34(6): 791–798.

62. Leentjens AF, et al. The Parkinson Anxiety Scale (PAS): development and validation of a new anxiety scale. Mov Disord 2014; 29(8): 1035–1043.

63. Santangelo G, et al. Anxiety in early Parkinson's disease: validation of the Italian observer-rated version of the Parkinson Anxiety Scale (OR-PAS). J Neurol Sci 2016; 367: 158–161.

64. Leentjens AF, et al. Apathy and anhedonia rating scales in Parkinson's disease: critique and recommendations. Mov Disord 2008; 23(14): 2004–2014.

65. Starkstein SE, et al. Reliability, validity, and clinical correlates of apathy in Parkinson's disease. J Neuropsychiatry Clin Neurosci 1992; 4(2): 134–139.

66. Pedersen KF, et al. Psychometric properties of the Starkstein Apathy Scale in patients with early untreated Parkinson disease. Am J Geriatr Psychiatry 2012; 20(2): 142–148.

67. Terashi H, et al. Characteristics of apathy in treatment-naïve patients with Parkinson's disease. Int J Neurosci 2019; 129(1): 16–21.

68. Siciliano M, et al. Motor, behavioural, and cognitive correlates of fatigue in early, de novo Parkinson disease patients. Parkinsonism Relat Disord 2017; 45: 63–68.

69. Sawada H, Oeda T. Protocol for a randomised controlled trial: efficacy of donepezil against psychosis in Parkinson's disease (EDAP). BMJ Open 2013; 3(9): e003533.

70. Rieu I, et al. International validation of a behavioral scale in Parkinson's disease without dementia. Mov Disord 2015; 30(5): 705–713.

71. Visser M, et al. Assessment of psychiatric complications in Parkinson's disease: the SCOPA-PC. Mov Disord 2007; 22(15): 2221–2228.

72. Martinez-Martin P, et al. A short scale for evaluation of neuropsychiatric disorders in Parkinson's disease: first psychometric approach. J Neurol 2012; 259(11): 2299–2308.

73. Chaudhuri KR, et al. The nondeclaration of nonmotor symptoms of Parkinson's disease to health care professionals: an international study using the nonmotor symptoms questionnaire. Mov Disord 2010; 25(6): 704–709.

74. https://www.movementdisorders.org/MDS/MDS-Rating-Scales/MDS-Unified-Parkinsons-Disease-Rating-Scale-MDS-UPDRS.htm. Assessed on 25.08.2021.

Chapter 3

Non-Motor Symptoms in Late-Stage Parkinson's Disease

Umar Shuaib, Adam Margolius, Hubert H. Fernandez

Introduction

Late-stage Parkinson's disease (PD) poses a significant challenge to clinicians. In addition to this, there is a lack of clarity in even its terminology and definition. It has been termed as advanced, late-stage, end-stage, and even palliative PD [1–3]. As the term *late-stage* PD has become the most widespread, it will be used henceforth. The criteria for diagnosing late-stage PD too has varied, with initial literature using varying cut-offs of the Hoehn and Yahr (H&Y) staging to determine the degree of advancement [1–3]. There has been significant criticism to this approach; it was asserted that while H & Y is heavily weighted toward postural instability and lower limb problems, it may overlook other motor symptoms that contribute to the advancing state, and it excludes non-motor symptoms (NMS). It was also written with the assumption that severity of PD is most related to motor symptoms [4]. However, this ignores consistent findings that NMS and axial symptoms together are strongly associated with disease progression [5]. Later approaches have thus asserted that other features that measure functional independence should be integrated in the definition, such as medication-related complaints, NMS [6], and dependence on caregivers (e.g. scores less than 50% on the Schwab and England Activities of Daily Living Scale) [7].

There has been extensive energy and funding aimed at treating PD motor symptoms, but management of NMS has traditionally been lacking. This is largely due to an initial underestimation of the importance of these non-cardinal features; however, there is ample evidence to suggest the impact NMS have on late-stage PD patients. For example, a study found that non-levodopa responsive symptoms and NMS dominate at 15 years of disease [8], and another study showed only 4 of 15 late-stage symptoms of PD patients perceived as having a severe impact on their health status were actually motor. In a survey of 173 late-stage PD patients, four NMS and only one motor complication were listed as being important issues for them, showing significant shifts in perceived severity of symptoms in advanced disease progression (Table 3.1) [9]. Further emphasizing this notion is that NMS are more strongly associated with patient distress, caregiver burnout, and nursing home placement, with psychosis playing a particularly significant role in nursing home placement [2]. Furthermore, evidence has also shown that certain NMS milestones herald the timing of death, with visual hallucinations, falls, and dementia occurring 5.1, 4.1, and 3.3 years on average prior to demise, respectively [10]. Persistent orthostatic hypotension in dementia with Lewy bodies (DLB) and PD dementia patients has been shown to be an independent predictor of poor prognosis [11]. Levodopa has the propensity to further worsen orthostatic hypotension, in addition to its other side effects, in a third of patients [12]. Despite this significant impact, treatment of NMS is lagging behind that of motor symptoms in both quantity and quality of clinical trials, and particularly in fruition of efficacious treatments. Few symptoms respond to levodopa [12], further outlining the necessity of increased focus on this area.

Epidemiology

As awareness of the impact of NMS in PD has increased, there have been increasing efforts to assess its prevalence in PD (Table 3.2). Tools have been developed, such as the Non-motor Symptoms Questionnaire (NMSQuest), to screen for and assess the total burden of NMS. Earlier studies that attempted to assess the prevalence of NMS in a comprehensive manner were carried out in cohorts of PD as a whole, and focused analysis of patients with late-stage PD is limited. More recently there have been efforts to assess

Table 3.1 Rank of most bothersome PD-related complaints in 173 patients with disease duration of more than six years

Rank	Complaint	First choice (%)	Second choice (%)	Third choice (%)	Total score	Total score in early disease
1	Fluctuating medication response	15	8.1	5.1	115	8
2	Mood	7.5	12.1	8.7	96	28
3	Drooling	10.4	6.9	4	85	7
4	Sleep	9.8	5.2	8.1	83	15
5	Tremor	8.1	5.2	4	67	101
6	Pain	6.4	5.8	4	60	50
7	Bowel problems	4	4	6.4	46	17
8	Urinary problems	2.9	5.2	4	40	9
9	Falls	4	4	2.3	39	4
10	Appetite/weight	2.3	4.6	4.6	36	13
11	Slowness	3.5	3.5	2.3	34	112
12	Fatigue	2.3	2.9	5.2	21	3
13	Sexual dysfunction	4.6	1.2	0.6	29	10
14	Hallucinations/delusions	2.3	2.9	2.3	26	6
15	Restless legs	1.7	2.9	4	26	11
16	Speech	1.2	3.5	4.6	26	4
17	Compulsive behavior	3.5	1.2	1.7	25	5
18	Handwriting	2.3	1.7	2.9	25	18
19	Loss of smell/taste	1.7	1.7	4.6	23	30
20	Sweating	1.2	2.9	4	23	7
21	Stiffness	1.2	3.5	2.3	22	76
22	Swallowing	0	4.6	3.5	22	3
23	Freezing	2.3	1.7	1.7	21	4
24	Memory	1.2	1.7	5.2	21	6

Note: Adapted from Politis M, Wu K, Molloy S, et al. Parkinson's disease symptoms: the patient's perspective. Mov Disord 2010; 25 (11): 1646–1651. doi:10.1002/mds.23135

NMS prevalence in cohorts of late-stage PD, usually defined by H&Y 4–5 or by the presence of motor fluctuations.

Developed in 2006, the NMSQuest was the first single questionnaire designed to comprehensively assess NMS in PD. NMSQuest is a 30-item questionnaire, which can be completed by either patient or caregiver. Each individual item relates to a distinct NMS, and simply inquires about its presence or absence. The individual symptoms are divided into nine domains: digestive, urinary, apathy/attention/memory, hallucinations/delusions, depression/anxiety, sexual function, cardiovascular, sleep disorder, and miscellany. The items were selected by an expert panel, with the aid of the UK Parkinson's Disease Society survey of patients and caregivers, as well as a review of the literature available at the time. In 2006, a pilot study was published using the NMSQuest in 123 PD patients as well as 96 controls [13]. There was a significant relationship between NMS burden and H&Y stage. Patients with "severe" PD (defined as H&Y 4–5) had an average of 12.7 (out of 30) NMS, whereas "moderate" patients (H&Y 2.5–3) had an average of 10.4, and "mild"

Table 3.2 Prevalence of non-motor symptoms in select late-stage PD cohort studies

	Witjas et al. 2002 [24]	Hely et al. 2008 [22]	Coelho et al. 2010 [2]
N=	50	36	50
Age, mean ±SD (years)	66.2±8.5	74±7.9	74.1±7.0
Disease duration ±SD (years)	12.7±5.4	20 (range 19.8–22)	17.9±6.3
Hoehn and Yahr stage, mean	3.8 ("Off" state)	4.6 ("Off" state)	4.4 ("On" state)
Depression, n (%)	34 (68%)[a]	NR[b]	31 (62%)
Dementia, n (%)	NR[c]	25 (83%)[d]	25 (50%)
Visual hallucination, n (%)	23 (46%)[e]	23 (74%)	22 (44%)
Sympomatic orthostatic hypotension	NR	15 (48%)	13 (26%)

[a] "Sadness," reported in the "Off" state.

[b] Fifty percent were on antidepressant medications.

[c] Average MMSE in cohort was 27.1±2.5 (≤24 were excluded).

[d] Out of 30 living patients.

[e] In the "On" state.

patients (H&Y 1–2) had an average of 8.0. Further analysis of advanced PD patients was not done in this pilot study.

Subsequently a larger, international study of PD patients using the NMSQuest was published, with results gathered from 545 patients across six countries (US, UK, Italy, Germany, Japan, and Israel). The prevalence of NMS by domain increased significantly with disease progression (as defined by H&Y stage) for every domain with the exception of sexual function. In this study 8.8% of the population were considered to have "severe" disease (H&Y 4–5). These patients had an average of 13 NMS (±5.5) while "moderate" patients (H&Y 3) had an average of 12.0 (±5.2) and "mild" patients (H&Y 1–2.5) had an average of 8.8 (±4.9) [14].

In the following years, the NMSQuest has been utilized in many different countries and PD populations around the world. Although similar to the initial studies, analysis dedicated to late-stage PD remained limited [15–18].

Barone et al. assessed the prevalence of NMS in 1072 Italian PD patients using structured interviews in the PRIAMO (Parkinson and non-motor symptoms) study [19, 20]. NMS were divided into 12 domains (GI symptoms, pain, urinary symptoms, postural hypotension, sleep disorders, fatigue, apathy, attention/memory, skin disorders, psychic symptoms, respiratory symptoms, and "miscellaneous" (olfaction/taste,

sexual symptoms, weight changes), each of which contained up to ten individual items. The investigators found that the most frequently reported NMS in the PD population as a whole were fatigue (58.1%), anxiety (55.8%), leg pain (37.9%), insomnia (36.9%), urgency and nocturia (35%), drooling (31%), and difficulty with concentration (31%). All domains of symptoms correlated with disease severity (as defined by H&Y stage) except orthostatic symptoms (P=0.0774). For example, fatigue was reported in 37.7% of patients with mild disease (H&Y 1) and 81.6% of patients with advanced disease (H&Y 4–5). Similarly, urinary symptoms, apathy, attention/memory symptoms, and respiratory symptoms were reported in 43.1%, 24.6%, 37.7%, and 9.6% of patients with mild disease, and 89.8%, 49.0%, 65.3%, and 30.6% of patients with advanced disease, respectively [19]. However, it should be noted that of the 1072 patients enrolled in the study, only 49 (4.6%) were H&Y 4–5.

Riedel et al. assessed the prevalence of neuropsychiatric symptoms in a sample of 1449 PD patients, recruited across 315 sites in Germany [21]. Of the patients in this study, 17.1% were H&Y stage 4 or 5. The authors found that the risk of dementia, depression, and psychotic syndromes (hallucinations, delusions, paranoid ideation) each correlated with both age and disease severity. Depression was present in 44% of H&Y 4–5 patients, compared to 28.6% H&Y 3, and 14.7% H&Y 1–2. Dementia rates in these three groups were 50.6%, 32.2%, and 17.5%, and psychotic syndrome rates were 35.6%, 12.0%, and 4.4%, respectively [21].

The previously mentioned studies have been large, cross-sectional studies that look at the PD population as a whole. It is difficult to compare the studies to each other directly, given their different patient populations and methodologies. The NMSQuest studies utilized a brief questionnaire specific for NMS in PD, whereas the PRIAMO study was based on semi-structured interviews, and Riedel's study a battery of scales and study instruments. The PRIAMO study was conducted at only Italian centers, so therefore the results may not be as generalizable as the international patient population of the NMSQuest studies. Similarly, Riedel's study was conducted with patients seen in Germany. These studies were not designed to assess NMS burden in advanced PD patients specifically. Nonetheless, they provide valuable insight into NMS prevalence in the advanced PD population. Although the exact prevalence of various NMS in PD differs according to methodologies and patient population, it is clear that the total burden of NMS increases as the motor symptoms of the disease progress.

More recently, there have been numerous investigations of epidemiology of NMS in the advanced PD population, though they tend to be smaller in scale.

Hely et al. followed a cohort of 149 de novo Australian PD patients, with 20-year follow-up analysis published in 2008 [22]. Thirteen patients had atypical parkinsonian syndromes and were excluded from analysis. By year 20, 100 of 136 patients (74%) had died. Six patients were lost to follow-up. Of those living, the mean H&Y stage was 4.2 in the "On" state, and 4.6 in the "Off" state. NMS were frequent. Autonomic symptoms assessed included symptomatic postural hypotension present in 15 patients (48%), urinary incontinence in 22 (71%), fecal incontinence in 5 (17%), and constipation requiring daily laxatives in 12 (40%). Visual hallucinations occurred in 23 patients (74%). Other NMS reported included excessive daytime sleepiness in 21 patients (70%). Twenty-five of 30 (83%) surviving patients had dementia. Depression was

not formally assessed due to the high prevalence of cognitive impairment, but 15 (50%) were on antidepressant medication [22]. This study is one of the longest prospective studies of PD patients yet published.

Coelho and colleagues conducted a cross-sectional study of 50 PD patients with H&Y stage 4 or 5 in the "On" state [2]. The authors reported demographics, motor, and non-motor symptomatology. All patients had at least one neuropsychiatric symptom. Thirty-one patients (63%) reported depression. Visual hallucinations were present in 22 patients (44%) and an additional 22 patients previously had visual hallucinations which had resolved. Likewise, 16 patients (32%) reported delusions, and another 9 had a history of delusions. Symptoms of dysautonomia were present in nearly all (96%) patients, with constipation (82%) and urinary dysfunction (64%) being the most common. Depression was present in 31 patients (62%) and anxiety in 25 (50%). Other NMS of note include insomnia in 30 patients (60%) and drooling in 35 patients (70%).

Over time, it has become clear that NMS often co-existed during motor fluctuations due to chronic levodopa exposure [23]. Several studies assessed rates of NMS in the "Off" and "On" state, thereby observing the rates of fluctuation in various NMS. Witjas and colleagues administered a structured questionnaire to 50 PD patients with motor fluctuations [24]. The questionnaire assessed 54 separate NMS, divided into three subgroups: 26 dysautonomic, 21 cognitive/psychiatric, and 7 pain/sensory. The average age of the patients was 66.2 years (±8.5 years) and average H&Y stage was 3.8 in the "Off" state. Of note, patients with MMSE≤24 were excluded from this study. All patients in the study had at least one NMS, and all patients experienced some form of non-motor fluctuations (NMF). The most frequently occurring NMF were anxiety (66%), drenching sweats (64%), slowness of thinking (58%), and fatigue (56%). In the "Off" state, anxiety was present in 88% of patients, drenching sweats in 59%, slowness of thinking in 83%, and fatigue in 75%. Other NMS of note include visual hallucinations (present in 46% of patients in the "On" state), feelings of "sadness" (68%, in the "Off" state), and "diffuse pain" (89%, in the "Off" state). Of note, NMF have been shown to improve with subthalamic nucleus (STN) deep brain stimulation (DBS), with one series of 40 patients showing a reduction of total number of NMF from 15.6 preoperatively, to 6.6 one year after surgery [25].

Storch et al. administered questionnaires to 100 PD patients with motor fluctuations, done in both the "Off" and "On" states [26]. Mean H&Y stage in the "Off" state was 3.4±0.9, with 49% of the patients H&Y 4–5 in the "Off" state. Data were reported using a visual analog scale, ranging from 0% (no symptoms) to 100% (most severe symptom possible). The most frequent NMS present in this cohort included fatigue (88%) and problems with concentration/attention (67%).

There are difficulties in ascertaining the prevalence of NMS in PD, especially in the disease's advanced stages. Larger studies look at the PD population as a whole, and often detailed analysis by disease severity is not available. Defining "late-stage" PD can be difficult, as discussed previously in this chapter. While the prevalence of various NMS varies depending on the study population, it is clear that these symptoms are highly prevalent, and that NMS burden increases with advancing disease.

Quality of Life in Late-Stage Parkinson's Disease

While levodopa-responsive motor symptoms predominantly dictate the course of treatment in early PD, distress and disability later in the course of disease is primarily attributed to NMS and levodopa-resistant motor symptoms [5]. The latter mentioned features are the most reliable predictors for mortality and nursing home placement. More specifically, dementia, hallucinations, postural instability, and falls are the strongest independent predictors of institutionalization and death [5, 8]. Health-related quality of life (HRQoL), an individual's or group's perceived physical and mental health over time, is a scale commonly used to assess QoL. Pain, particularly that caused by muscle cramping or dystonia, and treatment refractory depression are intimately related features of late disease that create a vicious circle, feeding off one another to the extent of being found to be the most significant contributor to poor HRQoL in one study [27]. Another study found that nocturia, fatigue, and sialorrhea had the most impact on HRQoL [28]. Yet another study found fatigue, pain,

depression, and sleep have the strongest independent associations with distress [29]. Cognitive impairment, contrast sensitivity, and visual processing speed alongside motor symptoms are significantly impaired in patients who lose their ability to drive, which is a milestone of loss of independence that they find extremely distressing. While the individual symptoms mentioned above seem to vary, they share the commonality of being NMS, and neurologists and patients are often frustrated by the lack of efficacious treatment options.

Another measure closely related with patient QoL is caregiver burden. The burden of PD is largely borne by informal caregivers, who provide a large contribution to the healthcare system by delaying nursing home placement and improving patient outcomes [30]. This unfortunately takes a significant toll on caregivers; in one study, 44% of caregivers were found to be depressed, based on the Hospital Anxiety and Depression Scale [31]. They also report deterioration of physical and mental health as well as their social life [30], resulting in increased episodes of chronic illnesses and more frequent use of tranquillizers [32]. Depression, anxiety, agitation, sialorrhea, functional and cognitive impairment, hallucinations, as well as motor dysfunction in PD are strong predictors of caregiver distress [33]. Caregiver frustration, depression, and decreased QoL ultimately result in their burnout, and subsequently places an increased burden on the healthcare system.

As PD patients gradually deteriorate from independent living to ultimate nursing home placement, their healthcare costs begin to rise at a staggering rate. Old age, dementia, functional impairment, and hallucinations are strong independent predictors for nursing home admission, and high caregiver burden further increases this risk [34, 35]. Presence of hallucinations was found to be the strongest predictor of nursing home placement [35]. A study in the UK found that the strongest influence on direct cost of care is institutionalized care for late-stage patients, showing an increased expenditure of 500% [36]. There is also evidence to suggest that nursing home placement of late-stage PD patients is not only an irreversible process, but also associated with significantly increased mortality [37].

In addition to requiring increasing levels of care as their disease progresses, late-stage PD patients are also hospitalized more frequently, which provides another avenue of burden on the healthcare system. In a study that evaluated PD admissions, only 15% of patients were admitted primarily for management of motor symptoms, whereas 39% had complaints such as pneumonia and delirium that were indirectly attributed to late-stage illness [38]. Another study found that when ordered by frequency, the most common reasons for admission of late-stage PD patients were falls, pneumonia, urinary tract infections, reduced mobility, psychiatric complaints, heart failure, fracture, orthostatic hypotension, surgical reasons, upper gastrointestinal bleed, cerebrovascular attacks, and myocardial infarctions [39]. This preponderance of NMS-related complaints demonstrates further the important role NMS play in the hospitalization and healthcare expenditure of these patients. Moreover, not only do NMS directly increase the propensity for patients to require hospitalization, but dysphagia can further complicate inpatient PD medication dosing and contributes to the development of parkinsonism-hyperpyrexia syndrome and the ensuing morbidity and mortality that often accompanies it [40]. Ultimately, pneumonia resulting from aspiration has been the most common cause of death in these patients [41].

In conclusion, though motor symptoms predominate in the early course of Parkinson's disease, NMS often dictate the progression and burden of disease in late-stage disease. As the population continues to age and prevalence of PD increases, this will become increasingly important. Unfortunately, despite recent advances in our understanding of PD, and the recognition of the wide spectrum of its symptomatology and impact on each patient, the crude H&Y staging remains the predominant means through which progression is classified and analyzed. Moreover, research has thus far been inconsistent at best in developing efficacious treatments for the most burdensome NMS, particularly in the way of pharmacologic breakthroughs. The resulting burden placed on the overall well-being of late-stage PD patients, and in turn their families and the overall healthcare system, has become crippling. In fact, a strong argument can be made that developing new and more meaningful treatments for NMS has the greatest potential to improve clinical outcomes and alleviate burdens in multiple aspects of PD care.

References

1. Papapetropoulos S, Mash DC. Motor fluctuations and dyskinesias in advanced/end stage Parkinson's disease: a study from a population of brain donors. J Neural Transm 2007; **114** (3): 341–345. doi:10.1007/s00702-006-0603-6

2. Coelho M, Marti MJ, Tolosa E, et al. Late-stage Parkinson's disease: the Barcelona and Lisbon cohort. J Neurol 2010; **257** (9): 1524–1532. doi:10.1007/s00415-010-5566-8

3. Giles S, Miyasaki J. Palliative stage Parkinson's disease: patient and family experiences of healthcare services. Palliat Med 2009; **23** (2): 120–125. doi:10.1177/0269216308100773

4. Hoehn MM, Yahr MD. Parkinsonism: onset, progression, and mortality. Neurology 1967; 17(5).

5. Coelho M, Ferreira JJ. Late-stage Parkinson disease. Nat Rev Neurol. 2012; **8**(8): 435–442. doi:10.1038/nrneurol.2012.126

6. Jankovic J, Tolosa E. *Parkinson's Disease & Movement Disorders*. 6th ed. Wolters Kluwer; 2015.

7. Schwab RS, England AC. Projection technique for evaluating surgery in Parkinson's disease. In: Billingham FH and Donaldson MC (eds.). *Third Symposium on Parkinson's Disease*. Churchill Livingstone; 1969, 152–157.

8. Hely MA, Morris JGL, Reid WGJ, Trafficante R. Sydney multicenter study of Parkinson's disease: non-L-dopa-responsive problems dominate at 15 years. Mov Disord 2005; **20** (2): 190–199. doi:10.1002/mds.20324

9. Politis M, Wu K, Molloy S, Bain PG, Chaudhuri KR, Piccini P. Parkinson's disease symptoms: the patient's perspective. Mov Disord 2010; **25** (11): 1646–1651. doi:10.1002/mds.23135

10. Kempster PA, O'Sullivan SS, Holton JL, Revesz T, Lees AJ. Relationships between age and late progression of Parkinson's disease: a clinico-pathological study. Brain 2010; **133** (6): 1755–1762. doi:10.1093/brain/awq059

11. Stubendorff K, Aarsland D, Minthon L, Londos E. The impact of autonomic dysfunction on survival in patients with dementia with Lewy bodies and Parkinson's disease with dementia. PLoS One 2012; **7** (10): 3–8. doi:10.1371/journal.pone.0045451

12. Fabbri M, Coelho M, Guedes LC, et al. Response of non-motor symptoms to levodopa in late-stage Parkinson's disease: results of a levodopa challenge test. Parkinsonism Relat Disord 2017; **39**: 37–43. doi:10.1016/j.parkreldis.2017.02.007

13. Chaudhuri KR, Martinez-Martin P, Schapira AHV, et al. International multicenter

pilot study of the first comprehensive self-completed nonmotor symptoms questionnaire for Parkinson's disease: the NMSQuest study. Mov Disord 2006; 21 (7): 916–923. doi:10.1002/mds.20844

14. Martinez-Martin P, Schapira AHV, Stocchi F, et al. Prevalence of nonmotor symptoms in Parkinson's disease in an international setting; study using nonmotor symptoms questionnaire in 545 patients. Mov Disord 2007; 22 (11): 1623–1629. doi:10.1002/mds.21586

15. Azmin S, Khairul Anuar AM, Tan HJ, et al. Nonmotor symptoms in a Malaysian Parkinson's disease population. Parkinsons Dis 2014; 2014. doi:10.1155/2014/472157

16. Rodríguez-Violante M, Cervantes-Arriaga A, Villar-Velarde A, Corona T. Prevalence of non-motor dysfunction among Parkinson's disease patients from a tertiary referral center in Mexico City. Clin Neurol Neurosurg 2010; 2010. doi:10.1016/j.clineuro.2010.07.021

17. Crosiers D, Pickut B, Theuns J, et al. Non-motor symptoms in a Flanders-Belgian population of 215 Parkinson's disease patients as assessed by the non-motor symptoms questionnaire. Am J Neurodegener Dis 2012; 1 (2): 160–167.

18. Cosentino C, Nuñez Y, Torres L. Frequency of non-motor symptoms in Peruvian patients with Parkinson's disease. Arq Neuropsiquiatr 2013; 2013. doi:10.1590/0004-282x20130005

19. Barone P, Antonini A, Colosimo C, et al. The PRIAMO study: a multicenter assessment of nonmotor symptoms and their impact on quality of life in Parkinson's disease. Mov Disord 2009; 24 (11): 1641–1649. doi:10.1002/mds.22643

20. Antonini A, Colosimo C, Marconi R, Morgante L, Barone P. The PRIAMO study: background, methods and recruitment. Neurol Sci 2008; 29 (2): 61–65. doi:10.1007/s10072-008-0863-z

21. Riedel O, Klotsche J, Spottke A, et al. Frequency of dementia, depression, and other neuropsychiatric symptoms in 1,449 outpatients with Parkinson's disease. J Neurol 2010; 257 (7): 1073–1082. doi:10.1007/s00415-010-5465-z

22. Hely MA, Reid WGJ, Adena MA, Halliday GM, Morris JGL. The Sydney multicenter study of Parkinson's disease: the inevitability of dementia at 20 years. Mov Disord 2008; 2008. doi:10.1002/mds.21956

23. Martínez-Fernández R, Schmitt E, Martinez-Martin P, Krack P. The hidden sister of motor fluctuations in Parkinson's disease: a review on nonmotor fluctuations. Mov Disord 2016; 31 (8): 1080–1094. doi:10.1002/mds.26731

24. Witjas T, Kaphan E, Azulay JP, et al. Nonmotor fluctuations in Parkinson's disease: frequent and disabling. Neurology 2002; 2002. doi:10.1212/WNL.59.3.408

25. Witjas T, Kaphan E, Régis J, et al. Effects of chronic subthalamic stimulation on nonmotor fluctuations in Parkinson's disease. Mov Disord 2007; 22 (12): 1729–1734. doi:10.1002/mds.21602

26. Storch A, Schneider CB, Wolz M, et al. Nonmotor fluctuations in Parkinson disease: severity and correlation with motor complications. Neurology 2013; 80 (9): 800–809. doi:10.1212/WNL.0b013e318285c0ed

27. Roh JH, Kim BJ, Jang JH, et al. The relationship of pain and health-related quality of life in Korean patients with Parkinson's disease. Acta Neurol Scand 2009; 119 (6): 397–403. doi:10.1111/j.1600-0404.2008.01114.x

28. Martinez-Martin P, Rodriguez-Blazquez C, Kurtis MM, Chaudhuri KR. The impact of non-motor symptoms on health-related quality of life of patients with Parkinson's disease. Mov Disord 2011; 26 (3): 399–406. doi:10.1002/mds.23462

29. Sjödahl Hammarlund C, Hagell P, Nilsson MH. Motor and non-motor predictors of illness-related distress in Parkinson's disease. Parkinsonism Relat Disord 2012; 18 (3): 299–302. doi:10.1016/j.parkreldis.2011.10.015

30. Schrag A, Hovris A, Morley D, Quinn N, Jahanshahi M. Caregiver-burden in Parkinson's disease is closely associated with psychiatric symptoms, falls, and disability. Parkinsonism Relat Disord 2006; 12 (1): 35–41. doi:10.1016/j.parkreldis.2005.06.011

31. Ozdilek B, Gunal DI. Motor and non-motor symptoms in Turkish patients with Parkinson's disease affecting family caregiver burden and quality of life. J Neuropsychiatry Clin Neurosci 2012; 24 (4): 478–483. doi:10.1176/appi.neuropsych.11100315

32. O'Reilly F, Finnan F, Allwright S, Smith GD, Ben-Shlomo Y. The effects of caring for a spouse with Parkinson's disease on social, psychological and physical well-being. Br J Gen Pract 1996; 46 (410): 507–512.

33. Santos-García D, de la Fuente-Fernández R. Factors contributing to caregivers' stress and burden in Parkinson's disease. Acta Neurol Scand 2015; 131 (4): 203–210. doi:10.1111/ane.12305

34. Yaffe K, Fox P, Newcomer R, et al. Patient and caregiver characteristics and nursing home placement in patients with dementia. J Am Med Assoc 2002. doi:10.1001/jama.287.16.2090

35. Aarsland D, Larsen JP, Tandberg E, Laake K. Predictors of nursing home placement in

Parkinson's disease: a population-based, prospective study. J Am Geriatr Soc 2000; **48** (8): 938–942. doi:10.1111/j.1532-5415.2000.tb06891.x

36. Findley L, Aujla M, Bain PG, et al. Direct economic impact of Parkinson's disease: a research survey in the United Kingdom. Mov Disord 2003; **18** (10): 1139–1145. doi:10.1002/mds.10507

37. Goetz CG, Stebbins GT. Mortality and hallucinations in nursing home patients with advanced Parkinson's disease. Neurology 1995; **45** (4): 669–671. doi:10.1212/WNL.45.4.669

38. Temlett JA, Thompson PD. Reasons for admission to hospital for Parkinson's disease. Intern Med J 2006; **36** (8): 524–526. doi:10.1111/j.1445-5994.2006.01123.x

39. Woodford H, Walker R. Emergency hospital admissions in idiopathic's Parkinson's disease. Mov Disord 2005; **20** (9): 1104–1108. doi:10.1002/mds.20485

40. Jones SL, Hindle JV. Parkinson's disease in the acute hospital. Clin Med J 2011; **11** (1): 84–88. doi:10.7861/clinmedicine.11-1-84

41. Hely MA, Morris JGL, Traficante R, et al. The Sydney Multicentre Study of Parkinson's disease: progression and mortality at 10 years. J Neurol Neurosurg Psychiatry 1999; **67** (3): 300–307. doi:10.1136/jnnp.67.3.300

Neuropathology of Non-Motor Parkinson's Disease Symptoms

Helmut Heinsen and Lea Tenenholz Grinberg

Motor and Non-Motor Symptoms in the Course of Parkinson's Disease

Lewy body disease, an α-synucleinopathy, is the neuropathological counterpart of idiopathic Parkinson's disease and one of the most frequent neurodegenerative diseases in humans [1]. Parkinson's disease features compelling motor symptoms. Parkinson summarized these symptoms under the mixed Greek-Latin term *paralysis agitans* (shaking palsy) [2], and for decades, these motor symptoms described by Parkinson remained the most studied features of Lewy body disease.

However, autonomic dysfunctions and non-motor symptoms associated with Lewy body disease are frequent and often pre-date the onset of motor diseases [3]. Autonomic dysfunctions comprise constipation, bowel dysfunction, seborrheic face, dysphagia, dysarthria, impotence, urinary frequency, bladder dysfunction, orthostatic hypotension, and increased sweating. Other non-motor symptoms include sleep disorders (REM behavior disorder, vivid dreams, daytime drowsiness, sleep fragmentation cognitive impairment, bradyphrenia, tip-of-the-tongue (word-finding) phenomenon, depression, apathy, anhedonia, fatigue, behavioral and psychiatric problems, sensory symptoms including anosmia, ageusia, pain (shoulder, back), and paresthesias [4]. Progressive worsening of non-motor symptoms considerably contributes to the relentless decrease in quality of life in patients with Lewy body disease [5, 6, 7].

Similarly to the case of motor symptoms, patients with Lewy body disease manifest variable severity and distribution of non-motor symptoms, which prompted investigators to propose variants of idiopathic Parkinson's disease based on the presence/absence, characteristics, time course, and underlying neuropathology of non-motor symptoms [8, 9]. Finally, except for REM behavior disorder, which is an excellent predictor of underlying synucleinopathies, all of the motor and non-motor symptoms can also be caused by distinct neuropathological changes. Therefore, the final diagnosis of idiopathic Parkinson's disease and parkinsonian diseases is based on clinical features and neuropathological diagnoses [10]. Jellinger subdivides the latter into a total of 33 parkinsonian diseases caused by common neurodegenerative, uncommon neurodegenerative, and secondary factors [4]. Dickson et al. [11] focus on molecular pathological features of common and rare diseases and distinguish α-synucleinopathies from tauopathies, TDP-43-proteinopathies, and non-specific degeneration in the substantia nigra pars compacta.

Neuropathological Criteria

Before the introduction of immunohistochemical methods, macroscopically visible pallor of the substantia nigra and absence of vascular lesions in the basal ganglia in individuals older than 55 years manifesting progressive rigidity, tremor, and akinesia were considered as a strong indicator of idiopathic Parkinson's disease. The neuropathological diagnosis was confirmed by the presence of highly characteristic intraneuronal Lewy bodies in histological sections through the same region [12].

Abnormal α-Synuclein, Lewy Neurites, and Lewy Bodies

Lewy was the first to demonstrate the hyaline neuronal cytoplasmic inclusions in histological sections that were coined after him. Lewy bodies consist of a heterogeneous mixture of more than 90 proteins [13] (see Figure 4.1). α-synuclein, a ubiquitous protein that consists of 140 amino acids, is a major component of Lewy bodies. Missense mutation in *NCAM*, the gene that encodes α-synuclein, causes familial Parkinson's

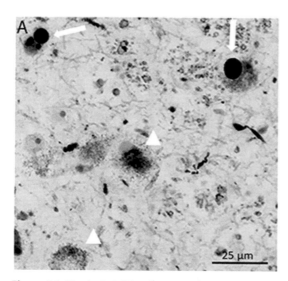 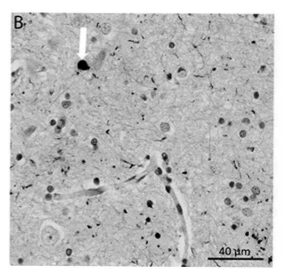

Figure 4.1 Histological slides of a case with Lewy body dementia immunostained for α-synuclein. (A) shows the substantia nigra; (B) the amygdala. Note the large number of Lewy neurites (in brown; see color plate). Arrows point to Lewy bodies and arrowheads to neuromelanin-containing neurons.

disease [14]. α-synuclein shows in presynaptic terminals and associates with presynaptic vesicles [15]. It likely plays a key role in dopaminergic synapses and the survival of dopaminergic neurons. Although widely distributed in the brain, the concentration of α-synuclein is heterogeneous. Noteworthy, regions enriched for α-synuclein (anterior cingulate cortex, medial temporal lobe) produce more Lewy body pathology than regions expressing low levels of physiological α-synuclein (cerebellum, primary visual cortex) [16].

For elusive reasons, physiological (cytosolic) α-synuclein is subject to conformational changes. The misfolded α-synuclein molecules form oligomers, which in turn form protofibrils that finally condense into insoluble fibrils. Fibrils constitute a major part of Lewy bodies.

In-vitro experiments have shown that α-synuclein assemblies can spread in anterograde and retrograde direction depending on their composition and structure [17, 18, 19, 20, 21]. Long-term in vivo imaging in transgenic mice supported the in-vitro observations by demonstrating a pathway in which early disordered inclusions mature into dense inclusions that lead to neuronal death [22]. In-vitro experiments with cell cultures and in-vivo experiments with transgenic animals suggest that pre-formed fibrils have seeding properties, meaning they can generate new fibrils, and contribute to

a prion-like spreading of the disease [23, 24]. Evidence shows that Lewy body pathology in humans may spread in a similar way. However, one must always keep in mind that knowledge about the deleterious role of Lewy body pathology is still imperfect. Autopsy studies showcase incidental Lewy body pathology in cognitively normal individuals lacking any sign of a movement disorder, neuropsychiatric features, or other CNS findings that would be attributed to Lewy body disease in other cases [25]. Also, the rate of substantia nigra neuronal loss seems to surpass the fraction of Lewy body positive neurons in substantia nigra pars compacta [26]. Thus, neuronal loss in Lewy body disease does not fit into a simple hypothesis of detrimental, beneficial, or neutral effects of Lewy body-affected neurons. Neuronal death results from a combination of several extrinsic and intrinsic factors that interplay over an extended time interval [27].

Improvements in methods for biochemical analyses and antibody purification contributed to extending our knowledge about the genesis, role, and fate of Lewy bodies in humans [28, 29]. Immunohistochemistry of phosphorylated α-synuclein unveiled inclusions of different morphology, including perikaryal Lewy bodies with halo (classical Lewy bodies) and without halo (cortical Lewy bodies), and perikaryal diffuse, granular, and polymorphic neuronal inclusions. Moreover, immunohistochemistry unveiled aggregation of α-synuclein in presynaptic terminals or as pale neurites in axon collaterals of hyperbranched axons, called Lewy neurites [30, 31, 32]. Chartier and Duyckaerts [33] summarize observations and conclusions of previous authors.

Staging of α-Synucleinopathies with Molecular Pathological Features

Analysis of Time Course, Spread, and Selective Vulnerability by Means of Standardized Antibodies

All neurodegenerative diseases spread in a non-random fashion following specific neuronal networks [34]. Braak, et al. [35] analyzed 100 μm-thick histological sections of brainstem and cerebrum immunostained against α-synuclein from brains of patients who were clinically diagnosed with Parkinson's disease, brains from cases with Lewy neurites or Lewy bodies, and age- and gender-matched control cases to examine the progression of Lewy body disease in the human brain. They confirmed a predictive spread of pathological α-synuclein that became the basis for a staging system (Figure 4.2). The authors distinguished six stages that parallel the brainstem-predominant type, the limbic or transitional type, and the diffuse cortical types proposed previously by Kosaka, et al. [36]. In subsequent publications, Braak et al. refined their staging system and discussed the systemic spread from the gut to the brain via dorsal motor nucleus of the vagus, the selective vulnerability of projection neurons with long-thin unmyelinated axons [37], spinal cord inclusions, and a dual-hit hypothesis [38]. According to this hypothesis, gut and nose provide entry access to the brain for microbial and/or other environmental factors, and the hitherto unknown agents trigger a progressing spreading of pathological α-synuclein. The comprehensive and seminal observations of Braak and co-workers were summarized in a monography [39].

The original Braak et al. staging system of idiopathic Parkinson's disease focused on supraspinal projection nuclei and coordination centers of the central nervous system. Previous reports described Lewy bodies [40] and coil-like glial inclusions in

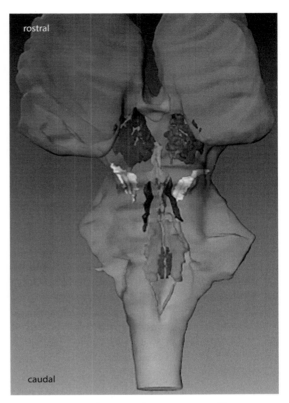

Figure 4.2 Three-dimensional reconstruction of key brainstem nuclei involved in early Lewy body disease. Braak stage 1: dorsal motor nucleus of the vagus (lower green); Braak stage 2: gigantocellular nucleus of the reticular formation (red), raphe magnus (purple) and locus coeruleus (lower black); Braak stage 3: dorsal raphe (upper green), pedunculopontine tegmental nucleus (yellow), and substantia nigra (upper black) (For the color version, please refer to the plate section.)

the spinal cord of cases with dementia with Lewy body and Parkinson's disease [41]. Other investigators extended these observations to the central and peripheral nervous system [42, 43, 44, 45, 46, 47]. Lewy pathology progresses in a caudo-rostral direction, including para- and prevertebral sympathetic ganglia, together with parasympathetic prevertebral and intramural ganglia. Neurons and neurites of the gastric Auerbach plexus show an increasing number of Lewy body profiles parallel to increases in the CNS stage [39].

The publication of Braak and co-workers had a considerable impact on the scientific community. It helped to broaden the view about Lewy body disease, transforming it from a disease affecting the substantia nigra leading to impaired dopaminergic basal ganglia innervation to multi-organ disease affecting the central nervous, the peripheral autonomic system, especially the cardiac, gastrointestinal, and urogenital systems [48].

Peripheral Nervous System

The involvement of the peripheral nervous system is believed to pre-date the involvement of the central nervous system. However, it is still unclear what is affected first: the sympathetic or the parasympathetic system? For an extensive review, see Orimo, et al. [49].

Dating the involvement of peripheral nervous system components by Lewy body pathology is challenging. First, most of the autopsied cases come from patients at the end-disease stage. Observations on cases with early stages of Lewy body disease are limited, contradictory, and subject to inconsistent methodology. Reduced neuron density in spinal intermediolateral nuclei was observed in patients with Parkinson's disease [50], but it is unclear if this is an early event as preganglionic spinal cord Lewy disease pathology in the same region could only be seen in stages 4 to 6 [46]. On the other hand, Bloch, et al. [42] and Oinas, et al. [45] reported rare cases with α-synucleinopathy restricted to the spinal cord or spinal cord and olfactory bulb. Routine immunohistochemical diagnosis is made with paraffin sections ranging in thickness between 5 and 8 μm, as opposed to the studies conducted by Braak and colleagues, which used 100-μm sections. Thus, the majority of studies focusing on Lewy body pathology in the peripheral nervous system are prone to underestimate pathological inclusion densities, particularly during initial stages with an overall low-density of inclusions.

The involvement of the peripheral nervous system could explain some of the non-motor symptoms seen in Parkinson's disease. However, the role of both pathophysiological and pathological α-synuclein in the peripheral nervous system is a matter of debate. Recently, Krämer, et al. [51] subjected 35 early-to-intermediate Parkinson's disease patients to a combination of different sympathetic tests and immunohistochemical investigation of phosphorylated α-synuclein biopsies from the thigh. Despite finding evidence of phosphorylated α-synuclein in peripheral nerve fibers, the authors failed to find adrenoreceptor sensitivity changes or dysfunction in the study subjects. They attribute decreased muscle sympathetic nerve activity to a central sympathetic impairment. Finally, Surmeier, et al. [27] concluded that the correlation between Lewy pathology and neuronal death is weak. These observations should be kept in mind when neuropathological changes are correlated with non-motor clinical symptomatology in the course of idiopathic Parkinson's disease.

Parkinson's disease patients show sympathetic denervation and increasing stage-dependent pathological α-synuclein in the heart [49, 52, 53]. Interestingly, as opposed to multiple system atrophy, another type of α-synucleinopathy in which orthostatic hypotension is early and severe, the clinical manifestation of cardiac and peripheral sympathetic deficiency are rather observed in later stages of Lewy body disease [54]. On the other hand, 123I-MIBG scintigraphy and 11 C-donepezil PET display uptake reductions suggesting postganglionic cardiac autonomic denervation from the early stages of Parkinson's disease. Besides peripheral autonomic failure, increasing supraspinal dysregulation of preganglionic neurons located in the intermediate reticular zone of the medulla could play a role in cardiovascular system symptoms [55].

Non-Motor Symptoms Associated with Braak et al. Stage 1 [39]

The first pathological evidence of Lewy body disease in the central nervous system is inclusions in neurites and neurons of the medullary dorsal IX/X motor nucleus, medullary intermediate reticular zone, preganglionic sympathetic projection neurons, lamina I of the spinal cord, and anterior olfactory nucleus. The caudal two-thirds of the esophagus, the complete stomach, and the gut until the left colonic flexure are under extrinsic efferent control of the dorsal nucleus of the vagus [56]. The more caudal parts of the gut are under the control of the sacral parasympathetic system and related pelvic ganglia.

Consequently, autonomic disorders including gastrointestinal complications like constipation, dysphagia and drooling, orthostatic hypotension, dysregulated sweating, urologic problems, and sexual dysfunction are common occurrences in Parkinson disease and dementia with Lewy bodies [57, 58, 59, 60, 61], even before the onset of the more characteristic motor symptoms. Kaufmann, et al. [62] report a case with autonomic failure 20 years prior to the progressive extrapyramidal syndrome.

Early Lewy pathology in the dorsal nucleus of the vagus could explain why drooling is reported by 70% of individuals with Parkinson's disease. Drooling is believed to result from decreased swallowing frequency and efficiency rather than increased saliva production, although a high frequency of synucleinopathy was found in the submandibular gland [44]. The usefulness of submandibular biopsies as a diagnostic tool for Lewy body disease is under investigation [63]. Esophageal dysmotility, delayed gastric emptying and retention, and constipation are frequently encountered in the early stages of Parkinson's disease.

Although some studies using gastrointestinal biopsies reported early involvement of submucosal and myenteric plexus in the gastrointestinal system [49], most used different methodology, thus data about the rostrocaudal gradient of Lewy body disease in the gut are incomplete [64].

Hyposmia or anosmia is most likely associated with early olfactory system α-synucleinopathy.

Braak et al. Stage 2

Stage 2 encompasses more regions of the medulla oblongata and the pontine tegmentum, including the serotoninergic lower raphe nuclei, the magnocellular reticular nuclei, the noradrenergic coeruleus-subcoeruleus complex of the medulla oblongata, and the pontine tegmentum under the term gain setting system. These nuclei modulate ascending and descending communication between higher-order rostral tel-, di-, and mesencephalic regions and the more caudal medulla oblongata and spinal cord centers.

Nuclei affected at this stage modulate many important physiological phenomena, including pain and sleep control. However, as these nuclei feature multifarious afferent and widespread efferent connections and employ volume transmission rather than classical wiring transmission, a clear-cut mechanistic clinicopathological explanation of early non-motor symptoms in the course of Parkinson's disease is elusive [65].

A wide spectrum of pain manifestations is reported by about half of Parkinson's disease patients, even in the premotor stage. Dorsal root c-fibers, which end on cells in dorsal horn lamina-

II neurons of the spinal cord, conduct painful stimuli. Braak, et al. [66] focus on detailed Lewy pathology in dorsal horn multipolar layer II neurons. These polymodal neurons do not project to the thalamus, but other lamina II cells may feed the spinothalamic tract, and collaterals of these cells could contact neurons in the gigantocellullar and the caudal raphe group [67]. In their function as a gain setting system, the brainstem gigantocellular reticular formation nucleus, the caudal raphe group, with the coeruleus/subcoeruleus complex could modify pain perception, processing, and transmission at the level of the spinal cord.

Braak et al. Stage 3

At this point, Lewy body pathology spreads to the mesencephalic tegmentum and basal forebrain including the central subnucleus of the amygdala, the substantia nigra and adjoining nuclei, non-thalamic nuclei with diffuse projections (magnocellular nuclei of the basal forebrain, pedunculopontine tegmental nucleus, and dorsal raphe nuclei and the hypothalamic tuberomammillary nucleus). The nuclei categorized as non-thalamic nuclei with diffuse projections differ from each other by their neurotransmitters. However, their long thin sparsely myelinated axons supply subcortical nuclei and extended regions of the cerebral cortex and the cerebellum.

Sleep disturbances are frequently observed non-motor symptoms in the course of Parkinson's disease. It is still a matter of debate whether animal models can replicate human sleep. Furthermore, the assessment of the literature comparing humans and animal models is complicated by the inconsistent terminology of the nuclear structures involved [68]. REM sleep is induced by a complex interplay of medullary REM-on (ventrolateral part of the periaqueductal gray matter, lateral pontine tegmentum) and REM-off structures (Ncl.subcoeruleus-stage II). These brainstem centers are either excited or inhibited by noradrenergic (locus coeruleus-stage II), serotoninergic (dorsal raphe nucleus-stage III), orexin (lateral hypothalamic area of the hypothalamus – staging uncertain, but likely early [69], acetylcholine (pedunculopontine nucleus, lateral dorsal tegmentum) afferents, and other transmitters including glutamate and GABA [68]. The pathophysiology of excessive daytime sleepiness (EDS) could be inferred from impaired activity of the ascending arousal system, including locus ceruleus, tubero-mammillary nuclei, and lateral hypothalamic area which are involved by Lewy body pathology from stage II onward.

REM-sleep behavior disorder (RBD) is defined by rapid eye movements, desynchronized electro-encephalographic activity, dreams, and muscle paralysis that preclude the individual from acting out the action of dreams [68]. A confirmed RBD diagnosis is practically pathognomonic of an α-synucleinopathy [70]. Much debate has occurred about the neuropathological basis of lack of atonia during REM sleep occurring in these patients. Degeneration of the gigantocellular reticular nucleus, the human homolog of the rodent's ventral gigantocellular nucleus has been implicated as a possible genesis for lack of atonia, although a recent neuropathological work showing severe degeneration of these neurons in Alzheimer's disease, a condition in very rare reports of RBD, challenges this assumption [71]. More recently, degeneration of the subcoeruleus neurons became an alternative to explain these symptoms [72, 73]. Pathologic motor behavior in RBD could be explained by decreased inhibitions of the brainstem and spinal cord motor neurons and an increased sensorimotor cortex excitation of the latter [68].

The prevalence of depression in Parkinson`s disease ranges from 7% to 70%, and a small percentage of Parkinson's disease patients shows depressive signs prior to the onset of motor symptoms [74]. The reasons for depression are unclear in humans, but they are deemed to have an important biological basis, including malfunction of the serotoninergic raphe nuclei, the noradrenergic locus coeruleus, and the dopaminergic ventral tegmental area, nuclei affected in the early stages. Depressed patients with Parkinson's disease have lower [11 C]RTI-32 (a marker of dopamine and noradrenaline) binding than non-depressed Parkinson's disease patients in the locus coeruleus and in several limbic regions [75]. CSF levels of dopamine and 5-hydroxytryptamine are also lower in patients with depression [76].

The decline of cholinergic magnocellular basal forebrain neurons and of histaminergic tubero-mammillary nuclei could be associated with deficits of neurotransmitters/modulators in the cerebral cortex and subsequent impairment of higher cognitive functions. In fact, cholinesterase inhibitors are beneficial for managing cognitive

and behavioral symptoms of dementia with Lewy body, another clinical manifestation of Lewy body disease [77, 78].

Braak et al. Stage 4

At this stage, more limbic structures are involved, including the amygdala and intralaminar thalamic nuclei, the anteromedial temporal limbic cortex (transentorhinal and entorhinal region), hippocampal formation, and the second sector of the Ammon's horn.

This stage also features full-fledged, typical motor symptoms of Parkinson's disease, including tremor, rigidity, and hypokinesia which can be observed at this stage.

Harding, et al. [79] showed a significant correlation between higher density of Lewy bodies in the basolateral nucleus of the amygdala and visual hallucinations.

Braak et al. Stages 5 and 6

In these terminal stages, the disease spreads to isocortical regions including the medial temporal lobe and higher-order sensory association areas, and also insula, claustrum, and basal ganglia. At stage 5, patients usually manifest severe motor disability, cognitive fluctuations, and may be wheel-chair-bound, or bedridden. In stage 6, the primary sensory and motor areas are additionally affected.

Pathoanatomical and Clinical Features Beyond the Current Staging Systems

Many neurodegenerative conditions develop cortical pathology, but with a distinct laminar distribution. Lewy body disease, Alzheimer's disease, chorea Huntington, and chorea-acanthocytosis show compelling differences on isocortical laminar pathology. In the first, pathological changes are enriched in the infragranular layers, whereas in the second, the supragranular layer III and the infragranular layer V show the highest amount of pathology. Both choreas show selective loss of layer IIIc pyramidal cells polymodal association cortices, layer V pyramidal cells, and lamina VI [80].

Few authors attempted to reproduce the staging system proposed by Braak et al. Jellinger [48] subdivides the authors into those pro and con. He concludes that "Braak's staging system is valid for PD patients with young onset, long duration with motor symptoms, but not for others, e.g., late-onset and rapid course PD" and calls for further studies. In a recent study on 280 cases from the Arizona Study of Aging and Neurodegenerative Disorders, Adler, et al. [81] categorized all cases into 1 through 5 Unified Staging System for Lewy Body Disorder (USSLB) stages. Criteria in stages IIa and IIb roughly correspond to prodromal and mild symptoms both in cases presenting as Parkinson's disease and those presenting as dementia with Lewy bodies. This staging system is in line with a recent hypothesis of Cersosimo [82] suggesting a caudo-rostral route for both Parkinson's disease and dementia with Lewy bodies, where he postulates an olfactory descending route in dementia with Lewy bodies which does not discard a possible dual hit in the etiology and pathogenesis of both diseases. Experimental model work suggests that different strains of pathological α-synuclein could use either glia or neurons for intracerebral spread [21]. Which of these spread mechanisms, if any, happen in the human brain is still a matter of debate [83, 84].

Recently, Seidel, et al. [85] have extended Braak stages 4 through 6 by a comprehensive neuropathological investigation of the brainstems of 11 synucleinopathy cases (6 cases with the clinical diagnosis of Parkinson's disease, 5 cases with dementia with Lewy bodies) and 5 control cases. The authors analyzed serial 100-μm-thick horizontal sections stained with aldehyde fuchsin and Darrow red for the demonstration of Nissl substance and neuronal lipofuscin and immunohistochemistry against α-synuclein. They distinguished the distribution pattern and density of Lewy bodies and neurites as well as coiled bodies. They reported Lewy bodies and neurites in all cranial nerve nuclei, premotor oculomotor, precerebellar and vestibular brainstem nuclei. These α-synucleinopathy deposits in the brainstem could contribute to the pathophysiology of tremor, gait, and postural instability, impaired balance and postural reflexes, and repeated falls. Moreover, their results support that sporadic Lewy body disease (either manifesting as Parkinson's disease or dementia with Lewy bodies) and familial Parkinson's disease caused by the *A30P* mutation are strictly related clinically as well as neuropathologically.

Lewy body disease features in many cases an asymmetrical degeneration of dopaminergic neurodegeneration and subsequent lateralization of motor symptoms. For more on lateralization, see Riederer, et al. [86]. However, most quantitative neuropathological studies were restricted to unilateral assessment [87, 88]. Studies assessing both substantia nigra sides pinpoint to an asymmetric neuron loss [89]. Noteworthy, healthy controls may show an asymmetry in neuronal number in the substantia nigra. Di Lorenzo Alho, et al. [90] report asymmetry of up to 53% in which either the right or the left showed more neurons in a sample of 15 control subjects ranging in age from 50 to 91 years. It is unclear if these baseline asymmetries could explain unilateral resilience or cognitive reserve in later stages of Lewy body disease. To our knowledge, neuronal number asymmetries in other brainstem nuclei involved in Lewy body disease were only reported for the preganglionic autonomic innervation of the feline heart [91]. After injection of the retrograde cholera toxin horseradish peroxidase-conjugated tracer into the AV-ganglion, three times more labeled neurons were encountered in the left rostral ventrolateral ambiguus and two times more labeled neurons in the right dorsal motor nucleus of the vagus. Further work is necessary to establish if other nuclei show asymmetry in humans and what would be the clinical consequences of such asymmetry.

Future Directions for Clinicopathological Studies in Lewy Body Disease Focusing on Non-Motor Neurons

Enhancing the focus on the earliest disease stages is likely to bring innovations that will help to stop the progress of Lewy body disease before disabling symptoms emerge. Longitudinal comprehensive neuropsychiatric, clinical, imaging, and autopsy studies provide invaluable contributions to the understanding of the neurobiological basis of non-motor symptoms in Lewy body disease. However, since such symptoms usually precede motor symptoms, large clinicopathological studies in the relatively healthy elderly would provide the best window of opportunity to dissect the basis for these symptoms in a brain with a limited amount of pathology. However, the recruitment of subjects with asymptomatic, or pre-motoric Lewy disease pathology is impractical in the absence of biomarkers.

Better biofluid biomarkers could help to screen individuals at pre-motor Lewy body disease for comprehensive longitudinal studies focusing on the timeline of symptom development. Pet tracers for abnormal tau- and beta-amyloid emerged in the past few years and are enabling research on Alzheimer's disease in pre-symptomatic individuals. A similar approach for detecting α-synuclein could bring valuable data on origin, onset, and time course of the spread of pathological α-synuclein inside and outside the central nervous system.

Systematic neuropathological studies of the suprarenal, the submandibular gland, and gut may shed light on the burden of α-synuclein in these systems. However, due to the size of these organs and the scarcity of α-synuclein deposits – for instance, the density of gut innervation decreases in a rostrocaudal manner [44, 92] – it is challenging to conduct such studies using traditional pathological methods. A systematic survey of the sympathetic and parasympathetic innervation of the heart represents a particular challenge [93, 94]. However, such studies could benefit from ultra-thick histological sections and serial sectioning to enhance the geometrical probability to encounter Lewy bodies and neurites in the peripheral nervous system and to correlate their number with Lewy pathology in the intermediolateral nucleus of the spinal cord or the dorsal motor nucleus of the vagus in the brainstem.

References

1. Ascherio A, Schwarzschild MA. The epidemiology of Parkinson's disease: risk factors and prevention. Lancet Neurol 2016; **15** (12): 1255–1270.

2. Parkinson J. An essay on the shaking palsy. 1817. J Neuropsychiatry Clin Neurosci 2002; **14** (2): 223–236; discussion 222.

3. Obeso JA, Stamelou M, Goetz CG, et al. Past, present, and future of Parkinson's disease: a special essay on the 200th Anniversary of the Shaking Palsy. Mov Disord 2017; **32** (9): 1264–1310.

4. Jellinger KA. Parkinson's disease. In Dickson DW and Weller RO (eds.). *Neurodegeneration: The Molecular Pathology of Dementia and Movement Disorders*. Wiley Blackwell; 2011, 194–224.

5. Hely MA, Reid WG, Adena MA, et al. The Sydney multicenter study of Parkinson's disease: the inevitability of dementia at 20 years. Mov Disord 2008; **23** (6): 837–844.

6. Lim SY, Lang AE. The nonmotor symptoms of Parkinson's disease: an overview. Mov Disord 2010; **25** (3): S123–S130.

7. Martinez-Martin P, Rodriguez-Blazquez C, Kurtis MM, et al. The impact of non-motor symptoms on health-related quality of life of patients with Parkinson's disease. Mov Disord 2011; **26** (3): 399–406.

8. Rajput AH, Voll A, Rajput ML, et al. Course in Parkinson disease subtypes: a 39-year clinicopathologic study. Neurology 2009; **73** (3): 206–212.

9. Selikhova M, Williams DR, Kempster PA, et al. A clinico-pathological study of subtypes in Parkinson's disease. Brain 2009; **132** (Pt 11): 2947–2957.

10. Lang AE, Lozano AM. Parkinson's disease. First of two parts. N Engl J Med 1998; **339** (15): 1044–1053.

11. Dickson DW, Braak H, Duda JE, et al. Neuropathological assessment of Parkinson's disease: refining the diagnostic criteria. Lancet Neurol 2009; **8**(12): 1150–1157.

12. Lewy FH. Zur pathologischen Anatomie der Paralysis agitans. Deutsche Zeitschrift für Nervenheilkunde 1914; **50** (1–4 Siebente Jahresversammlung der Gesellschaft Deutscher Nervenärzte in: Breslau am 29. September bis 1. Oktober 1913): 50–55.

13. Wakabayashi K, Tanji K, Odagiri S, et al. The Lewy body in Parkinson's disease and related neurodegenerative disorders. Mol Neurobiol 2013; **47** (2): 495–508.

14. Flagmeier P, Meisl G, Vendruscolo M, et al. Mutations associated with familial Parkinson's disease alter the initiation and amplification steps of α-synuclein aggregation. Proc Natl Acad Sci USA 2016; **113** (37): 10328–10333.

15. Burre J. The synaptic function of alpha-synuclein. J Parkinson's Dis 2015; **5**(4): 699–713.

16. Erskine D, Patterson L, Alexandris A, et al. Regional levels of physiological α-synuclein are directly associated with Lewy body pathology. Acta Neuropathol 2018; **135** (1): 153–154.

17. Peelaerts W, Bousset L, Van der Perren A, et al. Alpha-Synuclein strains cause distinct synucleinopathies after local and systemic administration. Nature 2015; **522** (7556): 340–344.

18. Villar-Piqué A, Lopes da Fonseca T, Sant'Anna R, et al. Environmental and genetic factors support

the dissociation between α-synuclein aggregation and toxicity. Proc Natl Acad Sci USA 2016; **113** (42): E6506–E6515.

19. Bieri G, Gitler AD, Brahic M. Internalization, axonal transport and release of fibrillar forms of alpha-synuclein. Neurobiol Dis 2018; **109** (B): 219–225.

20. Melki R. How the shapes of seeds can influence pathology. Neurobiol Dis 2018; **109** (Pt B): 201–208.

21. Peelaerts W, Bousset L, Baekelandt V, Melki R. α-Synuclein strains and seeding in Parkinson's disease, incidental Lewy body disease, dementia with Lewy bodies and multiple system atrophy: similarities and differences. Cell Tissue Res 2018; **373** (1): 195–212.

22. Osterberg VR, Spinelli KJ, Weston LJ, et al. Progressive aggregation of alpha-synuclein and selective degeneration of Lewy inclusion-bearing neurons in a mouse model of parkinsonism. Cell Rep 2015; **10** (8): 1252–1260.

23. Borghammer P. How does parkinson's disease begin? Perspectives on neuroanatomical pathways, prions, and histology. Mov Disord 2018; **33** (1): 48–57.

24. Vargas JY, Grudina C, Zurzolo C. The prion-like spreading of α-synuclein: from in vitro to in vivo models of Parkinson's disease. Ageing Res Rev 2019; **50**: 89–101.

25. Markesbery WR, Jicha GA, Liu H, Schmitt FA. Lewy body pathology in normal elderly subjects. J Neuropathol Exp Neurol 2009; **68** (7): 816–822.

26. Greffard S, Verny M, Bonnet AM, et al. A stable proportion of Lewy body bearing neurons in the substantia nigra suggests a model in which the Lewy body causes neuronal death. Neurobiol Aging 2010; **31** (1): 99–103.

27. Surmeier DJ, Obeso JA, Halliday GM. Selective neuronal vulnerability in Parkinson disease. Nat Rev Neurosci 2017; **18** (2): 101–113.

28. McKeith IG, Dickson DW, Lowe J, et al. Diagnosis and management of dementia with Lewy bodies: third report of the DLB Consortium. Neurology 2005; **65** (12): 1863–1872.

29. Beach TG, White CL, Hamilton RL, et al. Evaluation of alpha-synuclein immunohistochemical methods used by invited experts. Acta Neuropathol 2008; **116** (3): 277–288.

30. Duda JE. Olfactory system pathology as a model of Lewy neurodegenerative disease. J Neurolog Sci 2010; **289** (1–2): 49–54.

31. Kanazawa T, Adachi E, Orimo S, et al. Pale neurites, premature alpha-synuclein aggregates with centripetal extension from axon collaterals. Brain Pathol 2012; **22** (1): 67–78.

32. Colom-Cadena M, Pegueroles J, Herrmann AG, et al. Synaptic phosphorylated α-synuclein in dementia with Lewy bodies. Brain 2017; **140** (12): 3204–3214.

33. Chartier S, Duyckaerts C. Is Lewy pathology in the human nervous system chiefly an indicator of neuronal protection or of toxicity? Cell Tissue Res 2018; **373** (1): 149–160.

34. Seeley WW, Crawford RK, Zhou J, Miller BL, Greicius MD. Neurodegenerative diseases target large-scale human brain networks. Neuron 2009; **62** (1): 42–52.

35. Braak H, Del Tredici K, Rüb U, et al. Staging of brain pathology related to sporadic Parkinson's disease. Neurobiol Aging 2003; **24** (2): 197–211.

36. Kosaka K, Tsuchiya K, Yoshimura M. Lewy body disease with and without dementia: a clinicopathological study of 35 cases. Clin Neuropathol 1988; **7** (6): 299–305.

37. Braak H, Rüb U, Gai WP, Del Tredici K. Idiopathic Parkinson's disease: possible routes by which vulnerable neuronal types may be subject to neuroinvasion by an unknown pathogen. J Neural Transm 2003; **110** (5): 517–536.

38. Hawkes CH, Del Tredici K, Braak H. Parkinson's disease: a dual-hit hypothesis. Neuropathol Applied Neurobiol 2007; **33** (6): 599–614.

39. Braak H, Del Tredici K. Neuroanatomy and pathology of sporadic Parkinson's disease. Adv Anatomy Embryol Cell Biol 2009; **201**: 1–119.

40. Oyanagi K, Wakabayashi K, Ohama E, et al. Lewy bodies in the lower sacral parasympathetic neurons of a patient with Parkinson's disease. Acta Neuropathol 1990; **80** (5): 558–559.

41. Hishikawa N, Hashizumeb Y, Yoshida M, Sobue G. Clinical and neuropathological correlates of Lewy body disease. Acta Neuropathol 2003; **105** (4): 341–350.

42. Bloch A, Probst A, Bissig H et al. Alpha-synuclein pathology of the spinal and peripheral autonomic nervous system in neurologically unimpaired elderly subjects. Neuropathol Applied Neurobiol 2006; **32** (3): 284–295.

43. Klos KJ, Ahlskog JE, Josephs KA, et al. Alpha-synuclein pathology in the spinal cords of neurologically asymptomatic aged individuals. Neurology 2006; **66** (7): 1100–1102.

44. Beach TG, Adler CH, Sue LI, et al. Multi-organ distribution of phosphorylated alpha-synuclein histopathology in subjects with Lewy body disorders. Acta Neuropathol 2010; **119** (6): 689–702.

45. Oinas M, Paetau A, Myllykangas L, et al. Alpha-synuclein pathology in the spinal cord autonomic

nuclei associates with alpha-synuclein pathology in the brain: a population-based Vantaa 85+study. Acta Neuropathol 2010; **119** (6): 715–722.

46. Del Tredici K, Braak H. Spinal cord lesions in sporadic Parkinson's disease. Acta Neuropathol 2012; **124** (5): 643–664.

47. Tamura T, Yoshida M, Hashizume Y, Sobue G. Lewy body-related α-synucleinopathy in the spinal cord of cases with incidental Lewy body disease. Neuropathology 2012; **32** (1): 13–22.

48. Jellinger KA. Is Braak staging valid for all types of Parkinson's disease? J Neural Transm 2019; **126** (4): 423–431.

49. Orimo S, Ghebremedhin E, Gelpi E. Peripheral and central autonomic nervous system: does the sympathetic or parasympathetic nervous system bear the brunt of the pathology during the course of sporadic PD? Cell Tissue Res 2018; **373** (1): 267–286.

50. Wakabayashi K, Takahashi, H. The intermediolateral nucleus and Clarke's column in Parkinson's disease. Acta Neuropathol 1997; **94**: 287–289.

51. Krämer HH, Lautenschläger G, de Azevedo M, et al. Reduced central sympathetic activity in Parkinson's disease. Brain Behav 2019; **9** (12): e01463.

52. Orimo S, Oka T, Miura H, et al. Sympathetic cardiac denervation in Parkinson's disease and pure autonomic failure but not in multiple system atrophy. J Neurol Neurosurg Psychiatry 2002; **73** (6): 776–777.

53. Orimo S, Takahashi A, Uchihara T, et al. Degeneration of cardiac sympathetic nerve begins in the early disease process of Parkinson's disease. Brain Pathol 2007; **17** (1): 24–30.

54. Cersosimo MG, Benarroch EE. Autonomic involvement in Parkinson's disease: pathology, pathophysiology, clinical features and possible peripheral biomarkers. J Neurolog Sci 2012; **313** (1–2): 57–63.

55. Braune S, Reinhardt M, Schnitzer R, et al. Cardiac uptake of [123I]MIBG separates Parkinson's disease from multiple system atrophy. Neurology 1999; **53** (5): 1020–1025.

56. Travagli RA, Hermann GE, Browning KN, Rogers RC. Brainstem circuits regulating gastric function. Ann Rev Physiol 2006; **68**: 279–305.

57. Quigley EMM. Gastrointestinal dysfunction in Parkinson's disease. Semin Neurol 1996; **16** (03): 245–250.

58. Adler CH. Nonmotor complications in Parkinson's disease. Mov Disord 2005; **20** (Suppl 11): S23–S29.

59. Jost WH. Gastrointestinal dysfunction in Parkinson's disease. J Neurolog Sci 2010; **289** (1–2): 69–73.

60. Lebouvier T, Coron E, Chaumette T, et al. Routine colonic biopsies as a new tool to study the enteric nervous system in living patients. Neurogastroenterol Motility 2010; **22** (1): e11–e14.

61. Derkinderen P, Rouaud T, Lebouvier T, et al. Parkinson disease: the enteric nervous system spills its guts. Neurology 2011; **77** (19): 1761–1767.

62. Kaufmann H, Nahm K, Purohit D, Wolfe D. Autonomic failure as the initial presentation of Parkinson disease and dementia with Lewy bodies. Neurology 2004; **63** (6): 1093–1095.

63. Beach TG, Adler CH, Dugger BN, et al. Submandibular gland biopsy for the diagnosis of Parkinson disease. J Neuropathol Exp Neurol 2013; **72** (2): 130–136.

64. Ruffmann C, Parkkinen L. Gut feelings about -synuclein in gastrointestinal biopsies: biomarker in the making? Mov Disord 2016; **31** (2): 193–202.

65. Taber KH. Hurley RA. Volume transmission in the brain: beyond the synapse. J Neuropsychiatry Clin Neurosci 2014; **26** (1): iv–4.

66. Braak H, Sastre M, Bohl JRE, et al. Parkinson's disease: lesions in dorsal horn layer I, involvement of parasympathetic and sympathetic pre- and postganglionic neurons. Acta Neuropathol 2007; **113** (4): 421–429.

67. Nieuwenhuys R, Voogd J, van Huijzen C. *The Human Central Nervous System*. Springer; 2008.

68. Iranzo A. The REM sleep circuit and how its impairment leads to REM sleep behavior disorder. Cell Tissue Res 2018; **373** (1): 245–266.

69. Fronczek R, Overeem S, Lee SYY, et al. Hypocretin (orexin) loss in Parkinson's disease. Brain 2007; **130** (Pt 6): 1577–1585.

70. Ferman TJ, Boeve BF, Smith GE, et al. Inclusion of RBD improves the diagnostic classification of dementia with Lewy bodies. Neurology 2011; **77** (9): 875–882.

71. Eser RA, Ehrenberg AJ, Petersen C, et al. Selective vulnerability of brainstem nuclei in distinct tauopathies: a postmortem study. J Neuropathol Exp Neurol 2018; **77** (2): 149–161.

72. Boeve BF, St Louis EK, Kantarci K. Neuromelanin-sensitive imaging in patients with idiopathic rapid eye movement sleep behaviour disorder. Brain 2016; **139** (Pt 4): 1005–1007.

73. Dauvilliers Y, Schenck CH, Postuma RB, et al. REM sleep behaviour disorder. Nat Rev Dis Primers 2018; **4** (1): 19.

74. Grinberg LT, Rueb U, Alho AT, Heinsen H. Brainstem pathology and non-motor symptoms in PD. J Neurolog Sci 2010; **289** (1–2): 81–88.

75. Remy P, Doder M, Lees A, et al. Depression in Parkinson's disease: loss of dopamine and noradrenaline innervation in the limbic system. Brain 2005; **128** (Pt 6): 1314–1322.

76. Lian TH, Guo P, Zuo LJ, et al. An investigation on the clinical features and neurochemical changes in Parkinson's disease with depression. Front Psychiatry 2019; **9**: 723.

77. O'Brien JT, Holmes C, Jones M, et al. Clinical practice with anti-dementia drugs: a revised (third) consensus statement from the British Association for Psychopharmacology. J Psychopharmacol 2017; **31** (2): 147–168.

78. Hershey LA, Coleman-Jackson R. Pharmacological management of dementia with Lewy bodies. Drugs Aging 2019; **36** (4): 309–319.

79. Harding AJ, Stimson E, Henderson JM, Halliday GM. Clinical correlates of selective pathology in the amygdala of patients with Parkinson's disease. Brain 2002; **125**: 2431–2445.

80. Liu J, Heinsen H, Grinberg LT, et al. Pathoarchitectonics of the cerebral cortex in chorea-acanthocytosis and Huntington's disease. Neuropathol Applied Neurobiol 2019; **45** (3): 230–243.

81. Adler CH, Beach TG, Zhang N, et al. Unified staging system for Lewy body disorders: clinicopathologic correlations and comparison to Braak staging. J Neuropathol Exp Neurol 2019; **78** (10): 891–899.

82. Cersosimo MG. Propagation of alpha-synuclein pathology from the olfactory bulb: possible role in the pathogenesis of dementia with Lewy bodies. Cell Tissue Res 2018; **373** (1): 233–243.

83. Steiner JA, Quansah E, Brundin P. The concept of alpha-synuclein as a prion-like protein: ten years after. Cell Tissue Res 2018; **373** (1): 161–173.

84. Tamgüney G, Korczyn A. A critical review of the prion hypothesis of human synucleinopathies. Cell Tissue Res 2018; **373** (1): 213–220.

85. Seidel K, Mahlke J, Siswanto S, et al. The brainstem pathologies of Parkinson's disease and dementia with Lewy bodies. Brain Pathol 2015; **25** (2): 121–135.

86. Riederer P, Jellinger KA, Kolber P, et al. Lateralisation in Parkinson disease. Cell Tissue Res 2018; **373** (1): 297–312.

87. Pakkenberg B, Møller A, Gundersen HJG, et al. The absolute number of nerve cells in substantia nigra in normal subjects and in patients with Parkinson's disease estimated with an unbiased stereological method. J Neurol Neurosurg Psychiatry 1991; **54**: 30–33.

88. Rudow G, O'Brien R, Savonenko AV, et al. Morphometry of the human substantia nigra in ageing and Parkinson's disease. Acta Neuropathol 2008; **115** (4): 461–470.

89. Kempster PA, Gibb WR, Stern GM, Lees AJ. Asymmetry of substantia nigra neuronal loss in Parkinson's disease and its relevance to the mechanism of levodopa related motor fluctuations. J Neurol Neurosurg Psychiatry 1989; **52** (1): 72–76.

90. Di Lorenzo Alho AT, Suemoto CK, Polichiso L, et al. Three-dimensional and stereological characterization of the human substantia nigra during aging. Brain Struct Funct 2016; **221** (7): 3393–3403.

91. Massari VJ, Johnson TA, Gatti PJ. Cardiotopic organization of the nucleus ambiguus? An anatomical and physiological analysis of neurons regulating atrioventricular conduction. Brain Res 1995; **679**: 227–240.

92. Coon EA, Cutsforth-Gregory JK, Benarroch EE. Neuropathology of autonomic dysfunction in synucleinopathies. Mov Disord 2018; **33** (3): 349–358.

93. Pauza DH, Skripka V, Pauziene N, Stropus R. Morphology, distribution, and variability of the epicardiac neural ganglionated subplexuses in the human heart. Anat Rec 2000; **259** (4): 353–382.

94. Ghebremedhin E, Del Tredici K, Langston JW, Braak H. Diminished tyrosine hydroxylase immunoreactivity in the cardiac conduction system and myocardium in Parkinson's disease: an anatomical study. Acta Neuropathol 2009; **118** (6): 777–784.

Neuroimaging Studies in Non-Motor Parkinson's Disease Symptoms

David J. Brooks

Introduction

It is now accepted that Parkinson's disease (PD) is a multi-system disorder associated not only with progressive asymmetric limb bradykinesia, rigidity, rest tremor, and later postural impairment and gait difficulties, but also with dementia, depression, daytime somnolence, REM sleep behavior disorder, and autonomic dysfunction [1]. Pathologically PD is characterized by neuronal inclusions of abnormally aggregated α-synuclein in the form of Lewy bodies and neurites [2]. These target the nigro-striatal and meso-frontal dopaminergic projections impairing limb movement and executive functions, respectively. They also cause cholinergic neuronal loss from the nucleus basalis leading to attentional and memory deficits, serotonergic neuronal loss from the median raphe nuclei leading to affective and sleep disorders, and noradrenergic neuronal loss from the locus ceruleus resulting in REM sleep behavior disorder (RBD), depression, and anxiety.

In addition to the direct effects of α-synuclein pathology on brain function, PD patients are at higher risk of concomitant Alzheimer pathology [3]. This can now be detected with PET imaging ahead of onset of dementia.

Structural imaging with MRI can now detect the presence of substantia nigra compacta (SNC) and nucleus basalis cell loss in PD along with melanin loss from the locus ceruleus and the SNC [4, 5]. Volumetric MRI can also detect cortical thinning when present in early PD cases [6]. Functional MRI (fMRI) using BOLD sequence acquisition allows functional brain networks to be identified. The functionally connected regions show synchronized slow oscillations in their levels of oxygenation. These inter-regional correlations can be identified with independent component analysis (ICA). Reduced connectivity of the executive network and increased connectivity of

the default mode network has been reported in PD [7]. Alternatively, graph theory can be used to identify functional nodes and hubs across the brain and the strength of the pathways connecting them. Graph theory shows a clustering of nodes and hubs with raised connectivity of short and reduced connectivity of longer pathways – the so-called small world pattern [8].

Radiotracer-based functional imaging (PET and SPECT) now has a menu of ligands available for examining the terminal function of dopamine, serotonin, noradrenaline, and acetylcholine neurons and for detecting the presence of inflammation in the form of microglial activation and Alzheimer pathology (extracellular β-amyloid fibrillary plaques and intracellular paired helical tau fibrils forming neurofibrillary tangles). PET tracers are usually labeled with the short-lived ^{11}C ($t_{1/2}$ 20 minutes) or ^{18}F ($t_{1/2}$ 110 minutes) radioisotopes whereas SPECT tracers are labelled with longer-lived ^{123}I ($t_{1/2}$ 13.2 hours) or ^{99m}Tc ($t_{1/2}$ 6 hours) isotopes. ^{11}C-labelled compounds need to be produced on site with a cyclotron and hot cells whereas ^{18}F-tracers and SPECT ligands can be imported from external production sites. Some of the radiotracers in common use are detailed in Table 5.1.

Imaging Mechanisms of Cognitive Impairment in Parkinson's Disease

If patients with PD survive for over two decades with the disorder their prevalence of dementia can be as high as 80% though the overall prevalence averages at around 40%. The incidence of dementia is six times higher than that of age-matched healthy people and increases exponentially with age [9]. It has been suggested that the presence of aggregated α-synuclein inclusions may stimulate aggregation of β-amyloid leading to concomitant Alzheimer pathology [3]. Cognitive deficits associated with PD can take the form of a dysexecutive

Table 5.1 PET and SPECT markers of non-motor symptoms in PD

System	Target	Tracer	Non-motor symptoms
Glucose	Hexokinase	^{18}F-FDG	dementia, atypical PD
Dopamine	transporters	^{123}I-FP-CIT	depression, anxiety
		^{123}I-beta-CIT	fatigue, hyposmia,
		^{18}F-FP-CIT	apathy, dementia
		^{11}C-methylphenidate	
		^{11}C-RTI-32	
		^{11}C-CFT	
		^{11}C-PE2I	
	AADC	^{18}F-6-fluorodopa	
	VMAT2	^{11}C/^{18}F-DTBZ	
	D2 sites	^{11}C-raclopride	OCD, addiction
		^{11}C-PHNO	
Noradrenaline	transporters	^{11}C-MeNER	REM sleep behavior disorder
		^{11}C-RTI-32	depression, anxiety
Adrenaline	transporters	^{123}I-MIBG	cardiac sympathetic function
Serotonin	transporters	^{11}C-DASB	fatigue, somnolence,
		^{123}I-FP-CIT	depression, apathy
		^{123}I-beta-CIT	
	HT1A	^{11}C-WAY100635	depression, tremor
		^{18}F-MPPF	
	HT2A	^{18}F-setoperone	
		^{18}F-altanserin	
Cholinergic	AChE	^{11}C-NMP4A	attention and memory loss
		^{11}C-PMP	depression
		^{11}C-donepezil	dysautonomia
Opioid	μ, γ, δ	^{11}C-diprenorphine	pain
	μ	^{11}C-carfentenil	
Inflammation	TSPO	^{11}C-PK11195	cognitive deficits
		^{11}C-PBR28	
		^{18}F-DPA714	
Amyloid plaque	β-amyloid	^{11}C-PiB	cognitive deficits
		^{18}F-florbetaben	
		^{18}F-flutametamol	
		^{18}F-florbetapir	
Tau tangles	P-tau	^{18}F-flortaucipir	cognitive deficits
		^{18}F-MK6240	
		^{18}F-PI-2620	

syndrome or impairment of visuospatial capacities, attentional control, and short-term memory. However, language function is relatively preserved in contrast to Alzheimer's disease (AD). Degeneration of the medial substantia nigra and ventral tegmental area with loss of mesolimbic and mesocortical dopaminergic projections is associated with executive problems such as planning, sorting, and decision-making [10]. Direct involvement of the cortex by Lewy body pathology which targets the cingulate and cortical association areas along with cholinergic cell loss from the nucleus basalis of Meynert is associated with memory and attentional deficits and visual perception problems [11]. Neuroinflammation in the form of microglial activation and incidental Alzheimer and vascular pathology can also be present and contribute to cognitive deficits.

Structural Changes

The gray matter atrophy patterns in 67 PD patients with no cognitive impairment (PD-NC) and 23 patients with mild cognitive impairment (PD-MCI) have been examined with MRI [12]. Gray matter volume differences have been examined using voxel-based morphometry and the relationships between cognitive performance in specific domains and regional atrophy have been interrogated. The PD-MCI patients had reduced global cognition that correlated with cortical gray matter loss – see Figure 5.1. They also exhibited impaired executive function, attention, memory, and language abilities linked with gray matter loss in the left insular, left superior frontal and left middle temporal areas. There was a significant positive correlation between left insular atrophy and executive-attention dysfunction. The authors concluded that domain-specific cognitive impairment in mild PD could be linked with distinct areas of gray matter atrophy and this was demonstrable early in the disease course.

Diffusion tensor imaging has been used to interrogate microstructural correlates of impairments across cognitive domains in PD [13]. Fractional anisotropy (FA) – that is, the directionality of water flow – and mean water diffusivity (MD)

were assessed in 16 PD cases using region of interest (ROI) and voxel-based analyses. Executive function correlated positively with FA increases and inversely with MD decreases in frontal white matter tracts. Language and attentional performance correlated with the level of frontal FA and attention was linked with cingulate integrity. Memory impairment was associated with reductions in MD within the fornix. The authors concluded that in PD patients specific patterns of white matter diffusivity underlie their impairments in distinct cognitive domains.

Glucose Metabolic Changes

Resting ^{18}F-deoxyglucose (FDG) uptake reflects brain hexokinase activity and is a marker of regional synaptic activity in humans. A cohort of 79 newly diagnosed PD patients (mean clinical disease duration 8 months) had FDG-PET while taking their usual medication [14]. Statistical parametric mapping software (SPM12) localized reduced glucose metabolism in the occipital and inferior parietal lobes – see Figure 5.2. The PD patients had cognitive testing at baseline with the Cognitive Drug Research (CDR) and CANTAB computerized batteries, the Mini-Mental State Examination (MMSE), and the Montreal Cognitive Assessment (MoCA), and were retested after 18 months. Low ratings on memory-based tasks were associated with reduced FDG uptake in posterior parietal and temporal regions while attentional performance was associated with frontal deficits. Baseline parietal FDG uptake normalized to cerebellar uptake predicted MMSE and MoCA scores 18 months later after controlling for the baseline score level. These workers concluded

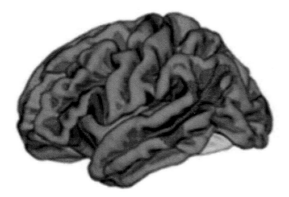
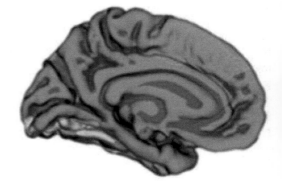

Figure 5.1 A cortical surface map showing where there is a significant correlation between gray matter thickness and MoCA cognitive ratings in Parkinson's disease [12]. (For the color version, please refer to the plate section.)

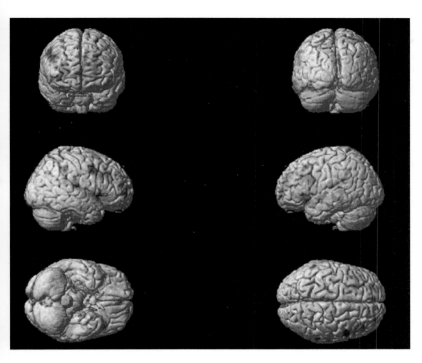

Figure 5.2 A cortical surface map showing areas of significantly reduced glucose metabolism in non-demented Parkinson's disease patients [14]. (For the color version, please refer to the plate section.)

that reduced baseline parietal metabolism is associated with high risk of future cognitive decline.

Series of more advanced PD patients who later developed dementia (PDD) have shown more extensively reduced baseline FDG uptake involving frontal as well as temporoparietal association areas [15, 16]. In a longitudinal PET study, 23 PD patients without dementia had an FDG scan at baseline and again after a four-year follow-up [17]. At their four-year follow-up, six patients (26%) had developed dementia. The PDD converters had significant baseline glucose hypometabolism in the visual primary and association cortex, the posterior cingulate, and caudate nucleus compared with healthy controls. Non-converters had only mild baseline hypometabolism targeting the primary occipital cortex. These findings suggest that early metabolic changes in visual association and posterior cingulate cortex may predict the PD cases which will progress to dementia.

Dementia with Lewy bodies (DLB) is characterized by dementia, parkinsonism, and fluctuating confusion accompanied by visual hallucinations and psychosis. The dementia is present at onset or within the first year of parkinsonism. Yong and colleagues have compared patterns of glucose metabolism in PD patients without dementia [18], PD cases with later dementia (PDD), and patients fulfilling consensus criteria for DLB. Compared with normal controls, both PDD and DLB patients showed significant metabolic decreases in the parietal lobe, occipital lobe, temporal lobe, frontal lobe, and anterior cingulate. When DLB patients and PDD patients were compared to PD patients without dementia, both the dementia groups showed relative reductions of glucose metabolism in inferior and medial frontal lobes bilaterally and the right parietal lobe. These metabolic deficits were greater in DLB patients. A direct comparison between DLB and PDD showed a relative metabolic decrease in anterior cingulate in patients with DLB. These findings support the concept that PDD and DLB have a similar underlying pattern of cortical dysfunction reminiscent of AD, although the anterior cingulate and occipital lobe are more involved in PDD and DLB.

Dopaminergic Dysfunction

The role of the mesolimbic and mesocortical dopaminergic projections in PD dementia has been investigated with ^{18}F-dopa PET. Regional

[18] F-dopa uptake, measured as an influx-constant Ki, reflects the presynaptic decarboxylation of the radiotracer by aromatic amino acid decarboxylase (AADC) and the density of the axonal terminal plexus. In an early series, Rinne and colleagues showed that performance on tests of working memory and attention correlated with head of caudate [18] F-dopa uptake [19]. [18] F-dopa PET has been used to investigate the influence of the dopaminergic system on levels of performance by PD-MCI subjects on executive tasks [20]. Sixteen non-demented PD subjects performed the Tower of London (TOL) spatial planning task and a verbal working memory task (VWMT). Statistical parametric mapping (SPM) localized a significant association between right caudate [18] F-dopa uptake (Ki) and TOL scores and between left anterior putamen Ki and VWMT performance. These findings support a role of striatal dopaminergic depletion in the early impairment of executive functions seen in PD. They suggest that spatial and verbal executive tasks require integrity of the right and left striatum, respectively, and imply that the pattern of cognitive changes manifest by a patient with PD may reflect differential dopamine loss in the two striatal complexes.

Using [18] F-dopa PET, Ito and colleagues assessed changes in dopaminergic function in PD and PDD patients matched for age, disease duration, and disease severity [21]. Compared to the PD patients without dementia, the PDD patients showed [18] F-dopa uptake reductions in the right caudate and bilaterally in the ventral striatum and the anterior cingulate.

Striatal and cortical dopaminergic changes in patients with PD-MCI compared with cognitively normal PD have also been examined by Christopher and colleagues [22]. [11] C-dihydrotetrabenazine (DTBZ) PET was used to measure striatal vesicular monoamine transporter (VMAT2) binding in dopamine nerve terminals while [11] C-FLB 457 PET was used to determine cortical D2 receptor availability – a marker of synaptic dopamine levels. The PD-MCI cases showed severe dopamine depletion in rostral striatum and reduced D2 receptor availability in both insulae compared to cognitively normal PD and healthy subjects. Levels of insular D2 binding predicted executive competence of PD patients. These workers concluded that there is a crucial and direct role for insular dopaminergic modulation in facilitating cognitive function.

^{123}I-FP-CIT SPECT, a marker of dopamine transporter (DAT) binding, has been used to assess the extent and pattern of dopamine transporter loss in patients with DLB compared with PDD [23]. Striatal transporter loss in patients with DLB was of a similar magnitude to that seen in non-demented PD while the PDD group of patients showed a greater reduction in striatal ^{123}I-FP-CIT binding. Compared with PD patients, where a selective and asymmetric targeting of putamen was observed, patients with DLB and PDD showed a more global striatal reduction in ^{123}I-FP-CIT binding with loss of the caudate-putamen gradient seen in PD. A significant correlation between the Mini-Mental State Examination scores and ^{123}I-FP-CIT binding was observed in PD patients with dementia, supporting the hypothesis that rostral striatal dopaminergic loss contributes to the cognitive impairment of these patients.

In summary, while putamen dopamine terminal dysfunction is a feature of PD, DLB, and PDD, imaging findings support the concept that executive deficits and dementia in PD is associated with impaired mesolimbic, mesocortical, and caudate dopaminergic function.

Cholinergic Changes

Cholinergic terminal function can be assessed by measuring synaptic acetylcholine esterase (AChE) activity or cholinergic terminal vesicle transporter density. The PET ligands [11] C-MP4A and [11] C-PMP are substrates for AChE [24, 25]. Global cortical [11] C-MP4A binding was found to be reduced by 11% in non-demented PD but by 30% in PDD [24]. Loss of [11] C-MP4A uptake targeted the posterior cortex in PD but spread to involve all cortex in PDD. The parietal ^{11}C-MP4A signal was significantly lower in PDD than PD and loss of frontal and temporo-parietal ^{11}C-MP4A binding correlated with reductions in striatal [18] F-dopa uptake.

Levels of cortical AChE activity measured with [11] C-PMP PET have shown a significant correlation with WAIS-III Digit Span scores, a test of working memory and attention, and ratings with tests of attention and executive function, such as the Trail Making B and the Stroop Colour Word test in a combined group of PD and PDD patients [25]. Cortical AChE deficiency did not correlate with motor disability in these subjects, however, loss of their thalamic ^{11}C-PMP signal, reflecting loss of cholinergic projections from the pedunculopontine nucleus, correlated with severity of their gait disorder.

The SPECT tracer ^{123}I-iodobenzovesamicol (^{123}I-BVM), an acetylcholine vesicle transporter marker, has been used to detect cholinergic terminal dysfunction in PD patients with and without dementia. PD patients without dementia showed selectively reduced binding of ^{123}I-BVM in parietal and occipital cortex, whereas PDD patients had globally reduced cortical binding [26].

In conclusion, cortical cholinergic terminal dysfunction is associated with significant cognitive decline in PD. These imaging findings rationalize the use of AChE inhibitors in PDD.

Post-synaptic muscarinic acetylcholine receptor availability has also been assessed in PD with ^{11}C-NMPB PET [27]. Frontal cortex ^{11}C-NMPB uptake was significantly raised in the PD patients – a PDD case showed the highest binding in frontal and temporal areas. It was concluded that loss of ascending cholinergic input to the cortex from the nucleus basalis led to the increased availability of the muscarinic receptors. However, in a separate study of PDD subjects, ^{123}I-iodo-quinuclidinyl-benzilate (QNB) SPECT showed reduced muscarinic binding in frontal and temporal lobes bilaterally, possibly reflecting cortical intrinsic neuron loss due to local Lewy body disease. Interestingly, the PDD patients showed a significant elevation of ^{123}I-QNB binding in the occipital lobe, possibly reflecting a loss of cholinergic input. This last finding could be a contributor to the visual disturbances that are frequent in PDD [28].

Imaging Coincident Alzheimer Pathology in Parkinson's Disease

The PET tracer ^{11}C-PIB is a neutral thioflavin T analogue that shows high nanomolar affinity for extracellular fibrillar β-amyloid (Aβ) plaques in Alzheimer brain slices but only low affinity for intracellular neurofibrillary tau tangles or Lewy bodies [29]. ^{11}C-PIB PET has been used to determine the prevalence of raised cortical β-amyloid in PD, PDD, and DLB. A majority of DLB patients show raised ^{11}C-PIB binding in their association cortical areas, particularly targeting frontal and cingulated cortices, the levels approaching those seen in Alzheimer patients [30]. Cortical Aβ is

also seen in around 50% of PDD patients while non-demented PD cases show a prevalence that is around 20–30% similar to that seen as an incidental finding in elderly healthy subjects [31, 32, 33]. The pattern and extent of increased cortical ^{11}C-PIB binding has been reported to be similar in PDD and Lewy body dementia [34].

Some neuropathological studies have proposed that Lewy body disease is the primary substrate driving cognitive impairment progression in PD whereas others have highlighted the significant levels of Alzheimer neurofibrillary and Aβ plaque pathology that demented PD patients exhibit [11, 35]. Gomperts and colleagues have reported that the presence of amyloid plaques in PD does not determine the nature of cognitive deficits that may be present but rather increases their risk of progression to dementia compared with patients who are amyloid free [36].

[18F]-florbetaben is a PET stilbene ligand for β-amyloid fibrils. In a small series it was reported that only 29% of seven DLB cases and none of the five non-demented PD patients investigated showed cortical [18F]-florbetaben retention [37]. These findings are against ß-amyloid deposition being the primary pathogenesis of dementia in Lewy body disorders.

[18]F-flortaucipir PET is a marker of paired helical tau fibril load though also shows off-target binding to neuromelanin and metalloproteins. In a series of 15 non-demented PD cases it was reported that no increased cortical ^{18}F-flortaucipir binding was evident though reduced nigral signal was seen due to the melanin loss present [38]. Lee et al. have used ^{18}F-flortaucipir PET to investigate patterns of tau accumulation across the spectrum of Lewy body diseases [39]. Their study included 12 PD patients with normal cognition, a combined group of 22 PD-MCI and PDD cases, and 18 DLB patients. Participants also had ^{18}F-florbetaben PET to determine amyloid load and cortical signals were compared between the LB cases, 25 healthy controls, and 25 Alzheimer patients. Overall, the DLB patients showed non-significantly increased ^{18}F-flortaucipir binding in sensorimotor, visual, and the parieto-temporal cortices. However, when only amyloid-positive DLB patients were considered there was a significantly increased tau load in these regions. Tau binding in temporal cortex was less prominent in DLB than in Alzheimer's disease while sensorimotor and visual cortex binding was greater. Amyloid-negative LB patients did not show

increased [18] F-flortaucipir binding whether cognitive impairment was present or absent. These workers concluded that the pattern of tau tangles in DLB and AD are distinct and that the presence of amyloid deposition plays an important role in the accumulation of neocortical tau in Lewy body diseases.

Winer and colleagues have compared tau tangle load in 15 patients with PD who were cognitively normal (PD-CN), 15 PD-MCI, and 49 healthy control (HC) participants and also evaluated the relationships between β-amyloid (Aβ), tau, and cognition [40]. Five PD-CN and one PD-MCI patients (21%) were Aβ-positive on [11] C-PiB PET compared with 24 of 49 HCs. Whole-brain [18] F-flortaucipir uptake was similar in the groups of PD-CN cases, PD-MCI cases, and Aβ-negative controls. However, cortical tau was significantly elevated in Aβ-positive PD patients relative to Aβ-negative patients. The authors concluded that patterns of cortical Aβ and tau deposition are related to Aβ status and age in PD-CN, PD-MCI, and age-matched healthy subjects. They concluded that cognitive deficits in PD without overt dementia are not due to concomitant Alzheimer disease.

Microglia Activation

Inflammation in the form of activated microglia is a non-specific response to brain injury. The activated cells can adopt a protective phenotype promoting neuronal survival by releasing growth factors, walling off necrotic tissue, and stripping and remodeling synapses [41]. They can also adopt a cidal phenotype causing further neurodegeneration through the release of a variety of cytokines and neurotoxic factors. The isoquinoline [11] C-*-PK11195 PET is an in vivo marker of the translocator protein (TSPO) expressed by the mitochondria of activated microglia [42, 43]. Studies have reported significant increases in [11] C-*-PK11195 binding in nigra, striatum, and association cortical areas in PD patients compared to healthy normal controls [44, 45]. Edison and colleagues have reported that PDD patients showed increased [11] C-*-PK11195 binding in anterior and posterior cingulate, striatum, frontal, temporal, parietal, and occipital cortical regions compared with normal controls and more extensive cortical microglial activation than non-demented PD patients [33]. In PDD the levels of cortical microglial activation were inversely

correlated with Mini-Mental State Examination scores suggesting that neuroinflammation may contribute to the cognitive impairment in these patients.

Imaging Mechanisms of Depression in Parkinson's Disease

Depressive symptoms are common in PD patients and depression has a reported prevalence that varies from 10% to 45% depending on the criteria used for diagnosis [46]. Depressive symptoms may precede the onset of motor symptoms in PD patients but the nature of depression differs from endogenous depression in that guilt is not generally a feature. The pathophysiological substrates of PD depression remain obscure and the syndrome responds variably to drug treatment. A reactive response to a frustrating and incurable disorder cannot be excluded and may certainly play a significant role. It also seems likely that depression in PD could result from degeneration of monoaminergic transmitter pathways innervating limbic structures.

Brain Structural Changes

A voxel-based morphometry (VBM) study of PD patients with and without depression has shown gray matter decreases in the bilateral orbitofrontal cortex, the right superior temporal pole, and the limbic system of depressed PD patients [47]. It has also been reported that white matter volume is reduced in the anterior cingulate bundle and inferior orbitofrontal region in depressed PD patients [48]. Severity of depressive features in these patients significantly correlated with white matter volume loss in the right inferior orbitofrontal lobe.

Diffusion tensor imaging (DTI) revealed bilateral abnormalities of water diffusivity in the anterior cingulate in depressed PD patients [49]. Compared to non-depressed PD patients, depressed patients were found to have reduced directionality (fractional anisotropy) of water diffusivity in bilateral mediodorsal thalamic regions, indicating a loss of nerve fibers, the severity of which negatively correlated with the scores of depressive features [50]. These structural changes all point to degeneration of limbic structures being associated with depression in PD.

Functional Imaging Changes

Mayberg and colleagues were the first group to study depressed PD cases with FDG-PET and reported reduced glucose metabolism in the caudate and the inferior frontal lobe of depressed compared with non-depressed PD patients and control subjects [51]. Subsequently, reduced glucose metabolic activity has been reported in the striatum, thalamus, amygdala, hippocampus, anterior cingulate, and orbitofrontal and insula cortex of depressed PD cases [52]. Levels of brain glucose metabolism were correlated with the severity of the depressive features.

Dopaminergic Function

A difficulty when comparing imaging findings in depressed with non-depressed PD patients is that depression can worsen apparent bradykinesia making it difficult to match groups for levels of locomotor disability. Depressed PD patients have shown relatively decreased dopamine transporter (DAT) binding of the whole striatum [53] and the left caudate nucleus [54]. Weintraub and colleagues reported an association between depressive symptom scores in PD and left anterior putamen DAT binding with ^{99m}Tc-TRODAT-1 SPECT [55]. ^{11}C-RTI-32 PET, a marker of DAT and noradrenergic transporter binding, detected reduced ventral striatal and limbic signal in depressed PD cases [56]. These findings all implicate a loss of monoaminergic function in the limbic system being related to the depressive features in PD. It is well recognized clinically that levodopa can improve depression as PD patients switch from an "off" to an "on" state.

Serotonergic Function

^{11}C-DASB PET measures brain serotonin transporter (SERT) availability and shows signal loss in non-depressed PD patients in orbitofrontal cortex (–22%), caudate (–30%), putamen (–26%), and midbrain (–29%) [57]. Politis and co-workers have used ^{11}C-DASB PET to interrogate SERT availability in antidepressant-naïve PD patients with depressive symptomatology [58]. They divided their 34 PD patients into two groups of ten with depression and 24 without depression and compared their SERT availability with depressivity ratings on the BDI-II and HAM-D scales. They reported that the depressed PD cases had elevated ^{11}C-DASB binding in their amygdala, hypothalamus, caudal raphe nuclei, and posterior cingulate cortex compared to PD patients without depression. Their raised SERT binding levels correlated with depressivity ratings and these workers suggested that reduced synaptic levels of serotonin in depressed cases resulted in their increased SERT availability. In other brain areas – striatum, rostral raphe, prefrontal cortex, and insula – the SERT availability was found to be reduced.

^{123}I-β-CIT is a tropane analogue which binds with nanomolar affinity to dopamine, noradrenaline, and serotonin transporters. Midbrain binding of ^{123}I-β-CIT one hour after intravenous injection primarily reflects SERT availability [59]. Using ^{123}I-β-CIT SPECT, Kim and colleagues reported reduced striatal DAT binding in a cohort of 45 PD patients with early disease [60]. However, these workers were unable to detect differences in midbrain uptake of this radioligand in depressed compared with non-depressed PD patients and there was no correlation between brainstem ^{123}I-β-CIT binding and Hamilton Depression Rating Scale scores.

^{11}C-WAY100635 PET is a marker of serotonin 5-HT$_{1A}$ receptor binding. These sites are located both presynaptically on 5-HT cell bodies in the midbrain raphe nuclei, where they inhibit serotonin release, and postsynaptically on cortical pyramidal neurons and glia. 5-HT$_{1A}$ sites are concentrated in the hippocampus and cingulate with only a low density in the striatum and they are absent in the cerebellum. A 25% reduction of ^{11}C-WAY 100635 binding in the midbrain raphe of PD patients compared with healthy controls has been reported [61]. However, the raphe uptake of ^{11}C-WAY 100635 was similar in PD patients with and without a history of depression. The results from both the ^{123}I-β-CIT SPECT and ^{11}C-WAY 100635 PET studies fail to support a major role for serotonergic loss in causing PD depression.

More recently, postsynaptic serotonergic system in PD patients with and without depression has been assessed with ^{18}F-MPPF PET, another marker of 5-HT$_{1A}$ receptor binding. Compared with non-depressed PD patients, depressed patients exhibited reduced tracer uptake in the left hippocampus, the right insula, the left superior temporal cortex, and the orbitofrontal cortex [62]. As HT$_{1A}$ sites are expressed by cortical pyramidal cells, these findings most likely reflect dysfunction of intrinsic limbic

53

neurons in PD with depression rather than reflecting loss of serotonergic projections.

To summarize, imaging findings are inconsistent but, overall, evidence is against serotonergic dysfunction playing a major role in the etiology of depressive symptoms in PD. However, it may be that a subgroup of depressed PD patients could benefit from SSRIs. Further investigations are required to establish whether serotonergic neurotransmission in the neocortex is decreased in SSRI responsive cases.

Noradrenergic and Cholinergic Dysfunction

The role of the noradrenergic system in PD depression has been investigated with ^{11}C-RTI 32 PET, a marker of both noradrenaline (NAT) and dopamine (DAT) transporter binding. PD patients show reduced binding of ^{11}C-RTI 32 in both striatal, brainstem, thalamus, and limbic areas. Remy and colleagues compared ^{11}C-RTI 32 PET findings in PD patients with and without depression matched for age, disability, disease duration, and doses of anti-parkinsonian medications [63]. Compared to those without depression, patients with depression showed a significant reduction of ^{11}C-RTI 32 binding in the noradrenergic locus ceruleus, the thalamus, and several regions of the limbic system, including the amygdala, ventral striatum, and anterior cingulate. Severity of anxiety in PD correlated inversely with ^{11}C-RTI 32 uptake in all these regions, whereas apathy was only inversely correlated with the radiotracer binding in the ventral striatum. These results suggest that depression and anxiety in Parkinson's disease are associated with both loss of noradrenaline innervation and selective loss of dopaminergic projections to the limbic system.

The relationship between ratings of depressive symptoms and cortical AChE activity in subjects with PD has been investigated [64]. Eighteen PD cases, including six with coexistent dementia, had ^{11}C-PMP PET and AChE levels were compared with Cornell Scale for Depression in Dementia (CSDD) ratings. The PD patients had raised scores on the CSDD and there was a significant inverse correlation between cortical ^{11}C-PMP uptake and CSDD scores – even after controlling for Mini-Mental State Examination scores as a confound. The authors concluded that depressive symptomatology in PD is associated with cortical cholinergic denervation, especially when dementia is also present.

Imaging Mechanisms of Fatigue in Parkinson's Disease

Recent PET studies have thrown light on the neurobiology of fatigue in PD. Untreated PD patients who complained of fatigue have shown similar striatal dopamine transporter availability to patients without fatigue, so dopamine loss does not appear per se to lead to fatigue in PD [65]. PD patients with and without fatigue have been assessed with both ^{18}F-dopa and ^{11}C-DASB PET to assess the integrity of their brain dopaminergic and serotonergic projections [66]. The PD patients with chronic fatigue showed significantly lower SERT binding than the patients without fatigue in ventral basal ganglia, anterior cingulate, and amygdala. These workers also saw significant decreases in caudate and insular ^{18}F-dopa Ki in the cohort of PD patients with fatigue compared to those without fatigue. These findings suggest that the presence of fatigue in PD is primarily associated with loss of serotoninergic input to the basal ganglia and limbic circuits and provide a rationale for its treatment with strategies to increase brain levels of serotonin.

Mechanisms of Sleep Disorders in Parkinson's Disease

A majority of PD patients develop sleep disorders as their condition progresses and these are associated with a significant deterioration in quality of life [67]. The sleep disorders can be categorized as nocturnal insomnia, excessive daytime somnolence (EDS), and parasomnias including REM sleep behavior disorder (RBD), vivid dreaming, and somnambulism. The pathogenesis of these disorders involves dysfunction of sleep centers in the brainstem, hypothalamus, and superchiasmatic nucleus and they are exacerbated by dopamine replacement therapies [68]. Brainstem centers mediating sleep hygiene include the noradrenergic locus ceruleus, serotoninergic dorsal raphe, and the dopaminergic ventral tegmental area.

Happe and colleagues have reported a significant inverse correlation between ratings of excessive daytime sleepiness with the Epworth Sleepiness Scale (ESS) and striatal ^{123}I-FP-CIT binding in early PD patients [69]. There was no correlation of ESS scores with age, disease duration, or UPDRS motor disability scores. These data suggest dopaminergic nigrostriatal degeneration is associated with daytime sleepiness even in early PD. An [18] F-dopa PET study measured striatal and midbrain dopamine storage capacity in PD patients with sleep disorders and reported a significant inverse correlation between mesopontine [18] F-dopa Ki and duration of REM sleep measured with polysomnography [70]. The authors suggested that monoaminergic activity in the rostral brainstem regulates the duration of nocturnal REM sleep in PD but, as [18] F-dopa is taken up by dopaminergic, noradrenergic, and serotonergic nerve terminals, it remained uncertain which of these transmitters was most relevant.

Parkinson's disease patients with and without EDS have been scanned with both [18] F-dopa and [11] C-DASB PET to assess the integrity of monoaminergic terminals function and serotonin transport availability in their sleep regulatory centers [71]. The EDS patients showed significant decreases in [11] C-DASB binding in thalamus, locus ceruleus, rostral raphe, and hypothalamus compared to healthy volunteers – see Figure 5.3. They also had significantly reduced [18] F-dopa uptake in locus ceruleus, rostral raphe, and the ventral tegmental area. The same structures, with the exception of the locus ceruleus, were preserved in the PD group without EDS. A direct comparison between patients with

and without EDS showed relative reductions in thalamic, rostral raphe, frontal and insular cortical [11] C-DASB binding in the EDS cases. These findings suggest that reductions in serotonergic and noradrenergic tone contribute to development of EDS in PD.

Kotagal et al. have recently reported that the presence of RBD in PD patients is associated with cholinergic system degeneration in neocortical, limbic cortical, and thalamic areas [72]. A majority of RBD cases progress to develop synucleinopathies – generally PD or DLB and less frequently multiple system atrophy within a time span of 5–12 years [73, 74, 75]. It is now considered that RBD represents a prodromal phenotype of PD/DLB and so provides a means of studying the earliest disease stage. Serial FP-CIT SPECT scans have shown progressive nigrostriatal dysfunction over 3 years before the onset of parkinsonism in RBD patients [76]. Around one-third of PD cases have evidence of RBD when examined with polysomnography.

Pathological involvement of the noradrenergic locus ceruleus occurs in PD and widespread reduction in noradrenaline is found at post-mortem. MRI can detect a loss of neuromelanin in the locus ceruleus in PD while [11] C-MeNER PET is a marker of noradrenaline transporter availability. Sommerauer and co-workers used these imaging modalities to study the association of RBD in PD

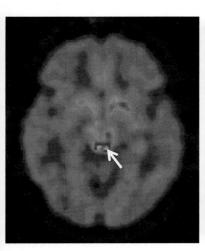 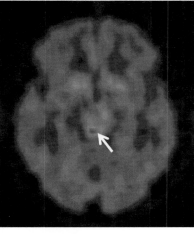

PD without excessive daytime somnolence ESS < 10

PD with excessive daytime somnolence ESS > 10

Figure 5.3 Reduced [11] C-DASB binding in the thalamus and median raphe of PD patients with excessive daytime somnolence. Picture courtesy of N. Pavese. (For the color version, please refer to the plate section.)

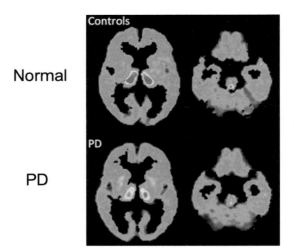

Figure 5.4 Reduced [11] C-MeNER binding in the thalamus and locus ceruleus of PD patients with REM sleep behavior disorder. Picture courtesy of M. Sommerauer. (For the color version, please refer to the plate section.)

with loss of their noradrenergic function [77]. Thirty non-demented PD patients (16 with RBD on polysomnography) had imaging of their locus ceruleus with a neuromelanin-sensitive MRI sequence and brain noradrenaline transporter availability measured with [11] C-MeNER PET. They found that the PD patients with RBD showed decreased locus ceruleus neuromelanin and reduced thalamic and locus ceruleus binding of [11] C-MeNER – see Figure 5.4 – which correlated with the duration of REM sleep without atonia. The presence of RBD in PD was associated with a higher prevalence of cognitive impairment, slowed EEG activity, and orthostatic hypotension. These workers concluded that the presence of RBD in PD was associated with reduced noradrenergic function and was linked to both cognitive deterioration and orthostatic hypotension.

Imaging Autonomic Denervation in Parkinson's Disease

Sympathetic Dysfunction

[123]I-metaiodobenzylguanidine (MIBG) scintigraphy and [18] F-fluorodopamine PET are both markers of sympathetic nerve terminal function. Decreased myocardial uptake of these tracers has been reported in PD patients even in early stages when cardiovascular reflexes are still intact [78].

However, MIBG scintigraphy is not a sensitive marker of early PD as 50% of Hoehn and Yahr stage I cases still show normal tracer binding. An [11] C-metahydroxyephedrine PET study has suggested that there is a segmental pattern of cardiac sympathetic denervation in PD, proximal lateral left ventricular wall function being most severely affected and the anterior and proximal septal wall function remaining relatively preserved [79].

Oka and colleagues have examined the association between myocardial ^{123}I-MIBG uptake and orthostatic hypotension, pulse and blood pressure changes during the Valsalva maneuver, and erect and supine plasma norepinephrine concentrations in PD patients [80]. Mean myocardial ^{123}I-MIBG uptake was significantly lower in PD patients with orthostatic hypotension and an abnormal Valsalva response. However, no correlation was found between the fall in systolic blood pressure on head-up tilt and baroreflex sensitivity or plasma norepinephrine concentrations. These results indicate that: 1) cardiac sympathetic dysfunction is only present in half of Hoehn and Yahr stage 1 PD cases, and 2) when present in PD, cardiac sympathetic dysfunction is not necessarily associated with altered cardiovascular reflexes.

Parasympathetic Dysfunction

Parkinson's disease is also associated with parasympathetic dysfunction resulting in constipation and gastroparesis which can occur ahead of motor problems. It has been suggested that pathological α-synuclein aggregations may first originate in the bowel due to pathogenic changes in the microbiome and then, in a prion-like fashion, trigger formation of further aggregates in the brainstem, the pathology ascending via the vagus nerve [81]. Histologically cholinergic neurons have been visualized by immunostaining for acetylcholinesterase. Donepezil is a high-affinity antagonist of acetylcholinesterase in clinical use to boost acetylcholine levels in dementias. 5-[C-11]-methoxy-donepezil provides a PET marker of acetylcholinesterase activity in both brain and peripheral organs and has been used to study PD [82]. Twelve patients with established disease had clinical severity of their motor disability, constipation, and gastroparesis documented. Heart rate variability on ECG and gastric emptying time was measured in all subjects. The PD cases showed significantly decreased [11] C-donepezil binding in the small intestine and

● Healthy control

■ PD patient

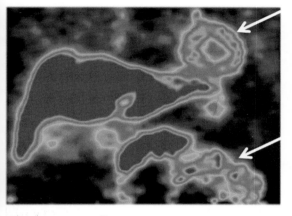
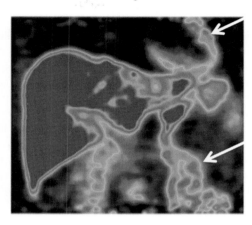

Figure 5.5 Reduced ^{11}C-donepezil uptake in the intestine and myocardium of a PD patient relative to a healthy control. Picture courtesy of P. Borghammer. (For the color version, please refer to the plate section.)

pancreas with a smaller decrease in the myocardium – see Figure 5.5. No correlations were found between ^{11}C-donepezil uptake and severity of constipation, gastric emptying time, or heart rate variability. This dissociation may reflect the fact that intrinsic cholinergic neurons of the enteric nervous system largely remain intact in PD. A follow-up ^{11}C-donepezil PET study imaged 19 early PD cases and again found significantly reduced uptake in the small intestine but now the colon and kidneys were also involved [83]. These workers concluded that widespread parasympathetic denervation is evident even in early cases of PD.

Imaging Changes and Hyposmia in Parkinson's Disease

Olfactory dysfunction (hyposmia) affects up to 60% of PD patients and often precedes their motor symptoms by several years, providing a potential marker of subclinical disease. Diffusion-weighted MRI has shown abnormal water diffusivity in olfactory tracts in PD [84]. Olfaction is preserved in atypical causes of PD and so olfactory function tests may be a useful tool for the differential diagnosis of parkinsonian syndromes.

PET and SPECT have been used to correlate the presence of olfactory and dopaminergic dysfunction in subjects either with PD or at risk for the disorder. Putamen DAT binding, measured with [99mTc]TRODAT-1 SPECT, correlated with ratings on the University of Pennsylvania Smell Identification Test (UPSIT) [85].

[11]C-beta-CFT PET has been used to correlate DAT availability with UPSIT scores in PD [86]. The total UPSIT scores were significantly reduced in the PD patients and there was a significant correlation between dorsal striatal ^{11}C-beta-CFT uptake and total UPSIT ratings. In a subsequent study. the same authors observed that hippocampal DAT binding correlated with UPSIT scores [87]. They suggested that the mesolimbic dopamine innervation of the hippocampus could play a role in the development of selective hyposmia in PD.

The relationship between individual UPSIT scores and measures of motor disability (disease duration, stage, and severity), non-motor function (cognitive function, depression, anxiety, and sleep) and severity of nigrostriatal dysfunction has also been investigated in PD patients. UPSIT scores correlated positively with striatal DAT binding and negatively with years of disease duration and UPDRS motor score. These findings suggest that the olfactory impairment in PD may not be stationary in the early motor stages but continues to progress over time.

Patients with idiopathic hyposmia have been followed over 4 years [88]. Olfactory testing was combined with transcranial sonography of the substantia nigra and ^{123}I-FP-CIT SPECT at baseline. By 4 years, 7% of the individuals with idiopathic hyposmia had developed clinical PD and another 6% had soft motor symptoms and signs. Reduction of striatal ^{123}I-beta-CIT binding was present in seven out of 40 (17.5%) hyposmic relatives of PD patients who had no parkinsonian symptoms. Four out of these seven (57%) subjects with reduced striatal ^{123}I-beta-CIT binding converted to clinical PD over a two-year follow-up. In summary, combining the findings from these studies suggests that a combination of olfactory testing and neuroimaging techniques may provide a prediction tool for the risk of developing PD, although the sensitivity of these modalities is relatively low and will only become of real value when neuroprotective agents are available for PD.

Conclusions

Neuroimaging has been instrumental in demonstrating in vivo the multisystem dysfunction that is present in PD even in the earliest cases. It also allows different aspects of disease progression to be monitored and emphasizes that the dopaminergic system is only one component of the mechanism involved in causing dementias, affective disorders, sleep disturbance, and autonomic dysfunction in PD. The demonstration of cholinergic loss in the dementia of PD has rationalized the early use of acetylcholinesterase inhibitors such as rivastigmine. While noradrenergic and serotonergic dysfunction have been shown to be present in REM sleep behavior disorder and daytime somnolence and fatigue, the development of effective replacement therapies is still awaited.

Other neurotransmitter systems may also be relevant to PD such as dysfunction of opioid and cannabinoid transmission. PET radioligands to image activity of both these systems in the brain are now available. Opioid imaging may be relevant to the pain syndromes experienced by PD cases while dysfunction of cannabinoid transmission has been associated with depression and psychosis. Development of new tracers will hopefully lead to a better understanding and rational treatment of PD non-motor complications.

References

1. Chaudhuri KR, Healy DG, Schapira AH. Non-motor symptoms of Parkinson's disease: diagnosis and management. Lancet Neurol 2006; 5: 235–245.

2. Braak H, Tredici KD, Rub U, et al. Staging of brain pathology related to sporadic Parkinson's disease. Neurobiol Aging 2003; 24: 197–211.

3. Irwin DJ, Lee VM, Trojanowski JQ. Parkinson's disease dementia: convergence of alpha-synuclein, tau and amyloid-beta pathologies. Nat Rev Neurosci 2013; 14: 626–636.

4. Ofori E, Pasternak O, Planetta PJ, et al. Increased free water in the substantia nigra of Parkinson's disease: a single-site and multi-site study. Neurobiol Aging 2015; 36: 1097–1104.

5. Sommerauer M, Fedorova TD, Hansen AK, et al. Evaluation of the noradrenergic system in Parkinson's disease: an 11 C-MeNER PET and neuromelanin MRI study. Brain 2018; 141: 496–504.

6. Wilson H, Niccolini F, Pellicano C, Politis M. Cortical thinning across Parkinson's disease stages and clinical correlates. J Neurol Sci 2019; 398: 31–38.

7. Baggio HC, Segura B, Sala-Llonch R, et al. Cognitive impairment and resting-state network connectivity in Parkinson's disease. Hum Brain Mapp 2015; 36: 199–212.

8. Baggio HC, Sala-Llonch R, Segura B, et al. Functional brain networks and cognitive deficits in Parkinson's disease. Hum Brain Mapp 2014; 35: 4620–4634.

9. Emre M. Dementia associated with Parkinson's disease. Lancet Neurol 2003; 2: 229–237.

10. Rinne JO, Rummukainen J, Lic M, et al. Dementia in Parkinson's disease is related to neuronal loss in the medial substantia nigra. Ann Neurol 1989; 26: 47–50.

11. Aarsland D, Perry R, Brown A, et al. Neuropathology of dementia in Parkinson's disease: a prospective, community-based study. Ann Neurol 2005; 58: 773–776.

12. Mak E, Zhou J, Tan LC, et al. Cognitive deficits in mild Parkinson's disease are associated with distinct areas of grey matter atrophy. J Neurol Neurosurg Psychiatry 2014; 85: 576–580.

13. Zheng Z, Shemmassian S, Wijekoon C, et al. DTI correlates of distinct cognitive impairments in Parkinson's disease. Hum Brain Mapp 2014; 35: 1325–1333.

14. Firbank MJ, Yarnall AJ, Lawson RA, et al. Cerebral glucose metabolism and cognition in newly diagnosed Parkinson's disease: ICICLE-PD study. J Neurol Neurosurg Psychiatry 2017; 88: 310–316.

15. Peppard RF, Martin WRW, Carr GD, et al. Cerebral glucose metabolism in Parkinson's disease with and without dementia. Arch Neurol 1992; 49: 1262–1268.

16. Vander-Borght T, Minoshima S, Giordani B, et al. Cerebral metabolic differences in Parkinson's and Alzheimer's disease matched for dementia severity. J Nucl Med 1997; **38**: 797–802.

17. Bohnen NI, Koeppe RA, Minoshima S, et al. Cerebral glucose metabolic features of Parkinson disease and incident dementia: longitudinal study. J Nucl Med 2011; **52**(6): 848–855.

18. Yong SW, Yoon JK, An YS, Lee PH. A comparison of cerebral glucose metabolism in Parkinson's disease, Parkinson's disease dementia and dementia with Lewy bodies. Eur J Neurol 2007; **14**: 1357–1362.

19. Rinne JO, Portin R, Ruottinen H, et al. Cognitive impairment and the brain dopaminergic system in Parkinson disease: [18 F]fluorodopa positron emission tomographic study. Arch Neurol 2000; **57**: 470–475.

20. Cheesman AL, Barker RA, Lewis SJ, et al. Lateralisation of striatal function: evidence from 18 F-dopa PET in Parkinson's disease. J Neurol Neurosurg Psychiatry 2005; **76**: 1204–1210.

21. Ito K, Nagano-Saito A, Kato T, et al. Striatal and extrastriatal dysfunction in Parkinson's disease with dementia: a 6-[18 F]fluoro-L-dopa PET study. Brain 2002; **125**: 1358–1365.

22. Christopher L, Marras C, Duff-Canning S, et al. Combined insular and striatal dopamine dysfunction are associated with executive deficits in Parkinson's disease with mild cognitive impairment. Brain 2014; **137**: 565–575.

23. O'Brien JT, Colloby S, Fenwick J, et al. Dopamine transporter loss visualized with FP-CIT SPECT in the differential diagnosis of dementia with Lewy bodies. Arch Neurol 2004; **61**: 919–925.

24. Hilker R, Thomas AV, Klein JC, et al. Dementia in Parkinson disease: functional imaging of cholinergic and dopaminergic pathways. Neurology 2005; **65**: 1716–1722.

25. Bohnen NI, Kaufer DI, Hendrickson R, et al. Cognitive correlates of cortical cholinergic denervation in Parkinson's disease and parkinsonian dementia. J Neurol 2006; **253**: 242–247.

26. Kuhl DE, Minoshima S, Fessler JA, et al. In vivo mapping of cholinergic terminals in normal aging, Alzheimer's disease, and Parkinson's disease. Ann Neurol 1996; **40**: 399–410.

27. Asahina M, Suhara T, Shinotoh H, et al. Brain muscarinic receptors in progressive supranuclear palsy and Parkinson's disease: a positron emission tomographic study. J Neurol Neurosurg Psychiat 1998; **65**: 155–163.

28. Colloby SJ, Pakrasi S, Firbank MJ, et al. In vivo SPECT imaging of muscarinic acetylcholine receptors using (R,R) 123I-QNB in dementia with Lewy bodies and Parkinson's disease dementia. Neuro Image 2006; **33**: 423–429.

29. Bacskai BJ, Frosch MP, Freeman SH, et al. Molecular imaging with Pittsburgh Compound B confirmed at autopsy: a case report. Arch Neurol 2007; **64**: 431–434.

30. Rowe CC, Ng S, Ackermann U, et al. Imaging beta-amyloid burden in aging and dementia. Neurology 2007; **68**: 1718–1725.

31. Edison P, Rowe CC, Rinne JO, et al. Amyloid load in Parkinson's disease dementia and Lewy body dementia measured with [11 C]PIB positron emission tomography. J Neurol Neurosurg Psychiatry 2008; **79**: 1331–1338.

32. Jokinen P, Scheinin N, Aalto S, et al. [(11)C]PIB-, [(18)F]FDG-PET and MRI imaging in patients with Parkinson's disease with and without dementia. Parkinsonism Relat Disord 2010; **16**: 666–670.

33. Edison P, Ahmed I, Fan Z, et al. Microglia, amyloid, and glucose metabolism in Parkinson's disease with and without dementia. Neuropsychopharmacol 2013; **38**: 938–949.

34. Foster ER, Campbell MC, Burack MA, et al. Amyloid imaging of Lewy body-associated disorders. Mov Disord 2010; **25**: 2516–2523.

35. Kempster PA, O'Sullivan SS, Holton JL, et al. Relationships between age and late progression of Parkinson's disease: a clinico-pathological study. Brain 2010; **133**: 1755–1762.

36. Gomperts SN, Locascio JJ, Rentz D, et al. Amyloid is linked to cognitive decline in patients with Parkinson disease without dementia. Neurology 2013; **80**: 85–91.

37. Villemagne VL, Ong K, Mulligan RS, et al. Amyloid imaging with (18)F-florbetaben in Alzheimer disease and other dementias. J Nucl Med 2011; **52**: 1210–1217.

38. Hansen AK, Knudsen K, Lillethorup TP, et al. In vivo imaging of neuromelanin in Parkinson's disease using 18 F-AV-1451 PET. Brain 2016; **139**: 2039–2049.

39. Lee SH, Cho H, Choi JY, et al. Distinct patterns of amyloid-dependent tau accumulation in Lewy body diseases. Mov Disord 2018; **33**: 262–272.

40. Winer JR, Maass A, Pressman P, et al. Associations between Tau, beta-amyloid, and cognition in Parkinson disease. JAMA Neurol 2018; **75**: 227–235.

41. Kim SU, de Vellis J. Microglia in health and disease. J Neurosci Res 2005; **81**: 302–313.

42. Banati RB, Newcombe J, Gunn RN, et al. The peripheral benzodiazepine binding site in the brain in multiple sclerosis: quantitative in vivo imaging of microglia as a measure of disease activity. Brain 2000; **123**: 2321–2337.

43. Wilms H, Claasen J, Rohl C, et al. Involvement of benzodiazepine receptors in neuroinflammatory and neurodegenerative diseases: evidence from activated microglial cells in vitro. Neurobiol Dis 2003; **14**: 417–424.

44. Ouchi Y, Yoshikawa E, Sekine Y, et al. Microglial activation and dopamine terminal loss in early Parkinson's disease. Ann Neurol 2005; **57**: 168–175.

45. Gerhard A, Pavese N, Hotton G, et al. In vivo imaging of microglial activation with [(11)C](R)-PK11195 PET in idiopathic Parkinson's disease. Neurobiol Dis 2006; **21**: 404–412.

46. Burn DJ. Beyond the iron mask: towards better recognition and treatment of depression associated with Parkinson's disease. Mov Disord 2002; **17**: 445–454.

47. Feldmann A, Illes Z, Kosztolanyi P, et al. Morphometric changes of gray matter in Parkinson's disease with depression: a voxel-based morphometry study. Mov Disord 2008; **23**: 42–46.

48. Kostic VS, Agosta F, Petrovic I, et al. Regional patterns of brain tissue loss associated with depression in Parkinson disease. Neurology 2010; **75**: 857–863.

49. Matsui H, Nishinaka K, Oda M, et al. Depression in Parkinson's disease. Diffusion tensor imaging study. J Neurol 2007; **254**: 1170–1173.

50. Li W, Liu J, Skidmore F, et al. White matter microstructure changes in the thalamus in Parkinson disease with depression: a diffusion tensor MR imaging study. Am J Neuroradiol 2010; **31**: 1861–1866.

51. Mayberg H, Starkstein S, Preziosi S, et al. Frontal lobe hypometabolism is associated with depression in Parkinson's disease. Neurology 1989; **39** Suppl 274.

52. Mentis M, Edwards C, Krch D, et al. Metabolic abnormalities associated with cognitive dysfunction in Parkinson's disease. Neurology 1999; **52** Supp 2: A221.

53. Meyer JH, Krüger S, Wilson AA, et al. Lower dopamine transporter binding potential in striatum during depression. Neuroreport 2001; **12**: 4121–4125.

54. Martinot M, Bragulat V, Artiges E, et al. Decreased presynaptic dopamine function in the left caudate of depressed patients with affective flattening and psychomotor retardation. Am J Psychiatry 2001; **158**: 314–316.

55. Weintraub D, Newberg AB, Cary MS, et al. Striatal dopamine transporter imaging correlates with anxiety and depression symptoms in Parkinson's disease. J Nucl Med 2005; **46**: 227–232.

56. Remy P, Doder M, Lees AJ, et al. Depression in Parkinson's disease: loss of dopamine and noradrenaline innervation in the limbic system. Brain 2005; **128**: 1314–1322.

57. Guttman M, Boileau I, Warsh J, et al. Brain serotonin transporter binding in non-depressed patients with Parkinson's disease. Eur J Neurol 2007; **14**: 523–528.

58. Politis M, Wu K, Loane C, et al. Depressive symptoms in PD correlate with higher 5-HTT binding in raphe and limbic structures. Neurology 2010; **75**: 1920–1927.

59. Laruelle M, Baldwin RM, Malison RT, et al. SPECT imaging of dopamine and serotonin transporters with [123I]beta-CIT: pharmacological characterization of brain uptake in nonhuman primates. Synapse 1993; **13**: 295–309.

60. Kim SE, Choi JY, Choe YS, et al. Serotonin transporters in the midbrain of Parkinson's disease patients: a study with 123I-beta-CIT SPECT. J Nucl Med 2003; **44**: 870–876.

61. Doder M, Rabiner EA, Turjanski N, et al. Brain serotonin HT1A receptors in Parkinson's disease with and without depression measured by positron emission tomography and 11 C-WAY100635. Mov Disord 2000; **15** Supp 3: 213.

62. Ballanger B, Klinger H, Eche J, et al. Role of serotonergic 1A receptor dysfunction in depression associated with Parkinson's disease. Mov Disord 2012; **27**: 84–89.

63. Remy P, Doder M, Lees AJ, et al. Depression in Parkinson's disease is associated with impaired catecholamine terminal function in the midbrain, thalamus, and anterior cingulate cortex. Neurology 2002; **58** Supp 3: A488.

64. Bohnen NI, Kaufer DI, Hendrickson R, et al. Cortical cholinergic denervation is associated with depressive symptoms in Parkinson's disease and parkinsonian dementia. J Neurol Neurosurg Psychiatry 2007; **78**: 641–643.

65. Schifitto G, Friedman JH, Oakes D, et al. Fatigue in levodopa-naive subjects with Parkinson disease. Neurology 2008; **71**: 481–485.

66. Pavese N, Metta V, Bose SK, et al. Fatigue in Parkinson's disease is linked to striatal and limbic serotonergic dysfunction. Brain 2010; **133**: 3434–3443.

67. Chaudhuri KR. Nocturnal symptom complex in PD and its management. Neurology 2003; **61**: S17–23.

68. Rye DB. Modulation of normal and pathologic motoneuron activity during sleep: insights from the neurology clinic, Parkinson's disease, and comments on parkinsonian-related sleepiness. Sleep Med 2002; **3** Suppl: S43–49.

69. Happe S, Baier PC, Helmschmied K, et al. Association of daytime sleepiness with nigrostriatal dopaminergic degeneration in early Parkinson's disease. J Neurol 2007; **254**: 1037–1043.

70. Hilker R, Razai N, Ghaemi M, et al. [18 F] fluorodopa uptake in the upper brainstem measured with positron emission tomography correlates with decreased REM sleep duration in early Parkinson's disease. Clin Neurol Neurosurg 2003; **105**: 262–269.

71. Pavese N. Imaging the aetiology of sleep disorders in dementia and Parkinson's disease. Curr Neurol Neurosci Rep 2014; **14**: 501.

72. Kotagal V, Albin RL, Muller ML, et al. Symptoms of rapid eye movement sleep behavior disorder are associated with cholinergic denervation in Parkinson disease. Ann Neurol 2012; **71**: 560–568.

73. Iranzo A, Molinuevo JL, Santamaria J, et al. Rapid-eye-movement sleep behaviour disorder as an early marker for a neurodegenerative disorder: a descriptive study. Lancet Neurol 2006; **5**: 572–577.

74. Postuma RB, Gagnon JF, Vendette M, Montplaisir JY. Idiopathic REM sleep behavior disorder in the transition to degenerative disease. Mov Disord 2009; **24**: 2225–2232.

75. Postuma RB, Gagnon JF, Rompré S, Montplaisir JY. Severity of REM atonia loss in idiopathic REM sleep behavior disorder predicts Parkinson disease. Neurology 2010; **74**: 239–244.

76. Iranzo A, Valldeoriola F, Lomena F, et al. Serial dopamine transporter imaging of nigrostriatal function in patients with idiopathic rapid-eye-movement sleep behaviour disorder: a prospective study. Lancet Neurol 2011; **10**: 797–805.

77. Sommerauer M, Fedorova TD, Hansen AK, et al. Evaluation of the noradrenergic system in Parkinson's disease: an 11 C-MeNER PET and neuromelanin MRI study. Brain 2018; **141**: 496–504.

78. Takatsu H, Nishida H, Matsuo H, et al. Cardiac sympathetic denervation from the early stage of Parkinson's disease: clinical and experimental studies with radiolabeled MIBG. J Nucl Med 2000; **41**: 71–77.

79. Wong KK, Raffel DM, Koeppe RA, et al. Pattern of cardiac sympathetic denervation in idiopathic Parkinson disease studied with 11 C hydroxyephedrine PET. Radiology 2012; **265**: 240–247.

80. Oka H, Yoshioka M, Onouchi K, et al. Characteristics of orthostatic hypotension in Parkinson's disease. Brain 2007; **130**: 2425–2432.

81. Hawkes CH, Del Tredici K, Braak H. Parkinson's disease: a dual-hit hypothesis. Neuropathol Appl Neurobiol 2007; **33**: 599–614.

82. Gjerloff T, Fedorova T, Knudsen K, et al. Imaging acetylcholinesterase density in peripheral organs in Parkinson's disease with C-11-donepezil PET. Brain 2015; **138**: 653–663.

83. Fedorova TD, Seidelin LB, Knudsen K, et al. Decreased intestinal acetylcholinesterase in early Parkinson disease: an 11 C-donepezil PET study. Neurology 2017; **88**: 775–781.

84. Scherfler C, Schocke MF, Seppi K, et al. Voxel-wise analysis of diffusion weighted imaging reveals disruption of the olfactory tract in Parkinson's disease. Brain 2006; **129**: 538–542.

85. Siderowf A, Newberg A, Chou KL, et al. [99mTc] TRODAT-1 SPECT imaging correlates with odor identification in early Parkinson disease. Neurology 2005; **64**: 1716–1720.

86. Bohnen NI, Gedela S, Kuwabara H, et al. Selective hyposmia and nigrostriatal dopaminergic denervation in Parkinson's disease. J Neurol 2007; **254**: 84–90.

87. Bohnen NI, Gedela S, Herath P, et al. Selective hyposmia in Parkinson disease: association with hippocampal dopamine activity. Neurosci Lett 2008; **447**: 12–16.

88. Ponsen MM, Stoffers D, Booij J, et al. Idiopathic hyposmia as a preclinical sign of Parkinson's disease. Ann Neurol 2004; **56**: 173–181.

Mild Cognitive Impairment

Amos D. Korczyn

Introduction

For many years Parkinson's disease (PD) was regarded primarily as a motor disorder and attempts to discover treatments focused on therapies for rigidity, bradykinesia, and tremor. The brain pathology studies concentrated on the nigrostriatal pathways and dopamine. It was the success of the dopamine replacement therapies which opened the way to discuss the non-motor manifestations of the disease, particularly mental health manifestations and dementia.

Cognitive impairment is very frequent in PD and actually may eventually affect all patients if they live long enough [1], causing additional suffering to patients and caregivers. It is not clear what the anatomical basis of cognitive impairment is, but it is thought to reflect α-synuclein deposition in the cortex and particularly in the limbic system, although most PD patients also bear β-amyloid and TDP-43 deposits once they become demented. These changes, however, do not correlate with the degree of cognitive decline and studies measuring neuronal loss and synapse degeneration are required, as indeed is the case also in Alzheimer's disease (AD) [2].

Parkinson's disease is a heterogeneous disease and actually the Parkinsonian syndrome contains many disorders, each of which is etiologically different (e.g. genetic and sporadic), with different clinical manifestations, including cognitive profile [3].

As in other neurodegenerative diseases, the cognitive decline in PD is rather insidious and thus it is useless to talk about its time of onset except in very general terms. However, the processes underlying the movement disorders and the mental changes are independent of each other and the deficits do not appear in a given order. In most cases, Parkinsonism is first to appear whereas in others cognitive decline comes first. This latter condition is frequently referred to as dementia with Lewy bodies (DLB) although whether PD and DLB are the same disease or different entities is a matter of debate [4].

The first clinical mental manifestations in either PD or DLB may be mnemonic, similar to those seen in AD. In AD, the existence of mild memory decline is termed amnestic mild cognitive impairment (aMCI) [5]. The term has been borrowed for PD and approved by the Movement Disorders Society (MDS) [6].

The original MCI criteria, as applied to AD, have not been perfect. Their accuracy in predicting conversion to dementia was low, around 50%. Some of the factors responsible for the low predictive power are obvious. They did not formally exclude patients with depression. It may be that even subsyndromal depression may lead to memory deficits or at least complaints of such. The duration of the stated cognitive decline is not mentioned in the criteria but is an important variable. Obviously, the same memory impairment has completely different implications if it developed recently or several years ago without deteriorating, etc. Another aspect is that there is usually no information on the baseline performance of these individuals, which would help to decide whether a certain degree of cognitive impairment is actually due to a decline. A more basic difficulty lies in the definition which requires that in order to be diagnosed as having MCI, the performance should be below that of the "normal" decline due to age. This definition is illogical because it accepts a "normal" cognitive decline with age. Thus, by this definition, the majority of so-called normal subjects are expected to lose cognitive abilities progressively until they become demented, without passing through a stage of MCI.

A practical, but rather significant, problem is the lack of agreement concerning the tool employed to objectively measure the cognitive function, and the cut-off point used to determine whether a person is below the expected. Commonly used is a threshold value of 1.5 SD below the mean "normal," yet this is inappropriate since in many cases the normative data are unavailable (e.g. for people with specific scholastic achievements, particularly those with higher education or those involved in academic professions, or subjects who have been diagnosed as having attention deficit hyperactivity disorder (ADHD) when younger), and in any case SD can only be applied if a normal distribution of values in the population exists, which may not apply in the case of cognitive function. Moreover, the assumption of a "normal distribution" implies that a certain proportion of the population exists below any given threshold value, without being affected by disease.

In PD, the difficulties in diagnosing MCI are even more significant. First, depression is very common in this population, even at the premotor stage complicating the diagnosis; another important factor in diagnosing MCI in the context of AD is independence in daily activities. Obviously, PD patients may need assistance because of their motor disabilities and it is impossible to determine what the relative contribution of motor impairment and of cognitive decline is. In the formal PD MCI definition suggested by the MDS there is no reference to any of these issues [6]. As in the case of AD, there is no consensus about a formal neuropsychological test. The arbitrarily proposed tests, MMSE and MoCA, have never been properly validated in MCI-PD. The difficulty is that these tests have been developed to measure the cognitive state of patients with AD-type dementia, and they lack sensitivity in the near normal range. In PD, the typical cognitive decline does not start with episodic memory but rather with executive functions like attention, verbal fluency, and processing speed [7]. In all these respects, the Addenbrooke's Cognitive Examination [8] may be somewhat advantageous. The poor sensitivity and specificity of the diagnosis of MCI-PD is reflected by the findings that up to 28% of diagnosed patients revert to normal cognition on re-examination [9] and only 50% progressed to dementia over 5 years [10].

It should be noted, as mentioned above, that MCI-PD is not a strict neurological entity. Even at autopsy, most patients will have additional pathologies, including beta amyloid, neurofibrillary tangles, TDP-43, vascular changes etc., in addition to synuclein deposition [11]. This heterogeneity is reflected by the clinical phenotype, rate of progression, etc. [12, 13].

Biomarkers

Several attempts have been made to identify biomarkers for MCI-PD [14]. To a large extent, these will show the same biomarkers associated with the α-synucleinopathy, which is expected and not very useful. Other biomarkers which can be found may be related to comorbid conditions, such as AD. What would be important is to identify biomarkers which are associated with cognitive decline. For this purpose, a comparison needs to be made between PD patients with MCI and those with completely normal cognition; however, these are more difficult to find. Thus, an important factor would be to identify factors associated with rate of decline. Such are not yet available.

Therapy

The cognitive decline reflects the neurodegenerative process which is likely to be associated with α-synuclein deposition. Thus, attempts to slow the degenerative process may attempt to target the synucleinopathy, and steps in this direction may benefit all the different manifestations of the disease, including cognition. However, the mere fact that cognitive impairment in PD is independent of the motor decline implies that treatment can be developed that will spare just the dopaminergic neurons and thus improve motor function. Similarly, since the cholinergic system is tightly associated with cognition, it may be that drugs protecting the nucleus basalis of Meynert might help to save cognition. Indeed, cholinesterase inhibitors, particularly Rivastigmine, have a beneficial effect in dementia with Lewy bodies (DLB), although the effect shown is merely symptomatic [15].

Of course, the identification of cognitive decline is scientifically important because it may help to discover the underlying processes which have caused or contributed to the cognitive decline. This is particularly relevant for the attempts to find therapies which may slow the cognitive decline or stop it altogether.

Investigations

While there are still no biological changes which are specific to the cognitive changes of PD, some measures should be taken to identify factors which may exacerbate the condition. PD patients are not immune to additional pathologies, such as metabolic changes or vascular lesions. Neuroimaging may identify subclinical strokes, white matter changes, or cerebral atrophy, including normal pressure hydrocephalus. Blood studies may detect inflammation, vitamin deficiencies, etc.

Management

Parkinson's disease patients with dementia need to be treated, and this applies also to those whose cognition is mildly impaired. With these limitations, what is the benefit of making a diagnosis of MCI in PD patients? The patients themselves are aware of their cognitive problems, by definition. Lacking available specific therapy, giving them the stamp of MCI will only increase their stress, which is definitely not helpful. Rather, attempts should be made to identify in each person individual factors which may contribute to the cognitive decline. These include biological ones, such as cardiovascular and metabolic disorders, as well as psychological ones, particularly loneliness and stress.

Parkinson's disease patients are particularly susceptible to loneliness, an established risk factor for dementia. Associated with it is depression which can be ameliorated (although drugs have not so far been studied specifically for depression in PD). While no drug is available to treat MCI in general (and in PD, in particular), some can, in fact, impair cognition further, particularly those with anti-muscarinic activities such as tricyclic antidepressants, particularly amitriptyline.

Hearing impairment has been reported to be a risk factor for dementia. Exercise is important in PD and should be encouraged even more in people with cognitive decline. Maintenance of normal blood pressure is important and in particular, hypotension should be ruled out. Lack of sufficient nocturnal sleep and sleep apnea could cause suboptimal cognitive function.

Parkinson's disease patients in general, but particularly those with incipient cognitive decline, should be encouraged to plan for the future. For those whose cognition is deteriorating, this may be their last chance to express their wishes, and in particular, to dictate advanced directives.

One of the main targets in treating older people in general, and those with PD in particular, is improving their quality of life. This is important even more so when dealing with people whose cognition is deteriorating. Encouragement to participate in social and intellectual activities, if enjoyed and satisfying, can be helpful and should be encouraged.

References

1. Hely MA, Reid WG, Adena MA, Halliday GM, Morris JG. The Sydney multicenter study of Parkinson's disease: the inevitability of dementia at 20 years. Mov Disord 2008; 23(6): 837–844. doi: 10.1002/mds.21956.PMID: 18307261

2. Andrade-Moraes CH, Oliveira-Pinto AV, Castro-Fonseca E, et al. Cell number changes in Alzheimer's disease relate to dementia, not to plaques and tangles. Brain 2013; 136(Pt12): 3738–3752. doi: 10.1093/brain/awt273. Epub 2013 Oct 17.PMID: 24136825

3. Korczyn AD. Parkinson's disease: one disease entity or many? J Neural Transm Suppl 1999; 56: 107–111. doi: 10.1007/978-3-7091-6360-3_5.PMID: 10370905

4. Jellinger KA, Korczyn AD. Are dementia with Lewy bodies and Parkinson's disease dementia the same disease? BMC Med 2018 6; 16(1): 34. doi: 10.1186/s12916-018-1016-8.PMID: 29510692

5. Petersen RC, Smith GE, Waring SC, et al. Mild cognitive impairment: clinical characterization and outcome. Arch Neurol 1999; 56(3): 303–308. doi: 10.1001/archneur.56.3.303.PMID: 10190820

6. Litvan I, Aarsland D, Adler CH, et al. MDS Task Force on mild cognitive impairment in Parkinson's disease: critical review of PD-MCI. Mov Disord 2011; 26(10): 1814–1824. doi: 10.1002/mds.23823. Epub 2011 Jun 9.PMID: 21661055

7. Weintraub D, Simuni T, Caspell-Garcia C, et al. Cognitive performance and neuropsychiatric symptoms in early, untreated Parkinson's disease. Parkinson's Progression Markers Initiative. Mov Disord 2015; 30(7): 919–927. doi: 10.1002/mds.26170. Epub 2015 Mar 4.PMID: 25737166

8. McColgan P, Evans JR, Breen DP, et al. Addenbrooke's Cognitive Examination-Revised for mild cognitive impairment in Parkinson's disease. Mov Disord 2012; 27(9): 1173–1177. doi: 10.1002/mds.25084. Epub 2012 Jun 25.PMID: 2273339

9. Pedersen KF, Larsen JP, Tysnes OB, Alves G. Natural course of mild cognitive impairment in Parkinson disease: a 5-year population-based study. Neurology 2017; 88(8): 767–774. doi: 10.1212/WNL.0000000000003634. Epub 2017 Jan 20.PMID: 28108638

10. Domellöf ME, Ekman U, Forsgren L, Elgh E. Cognitive function in the early phase of Parkinson's disease: a five-year follow-up. Acta Neurol Scand 2015; **132**(2): 79–88. doi: 10.1111/ane.12375.Epub 2015 Feb 3.PMID: 25644230

11. Adler CH, Caviness JN, Sabbagh MN, et al. Heterogeneous neuropathological findings in Parkinson's disease with mild cognitive impairment. Acta Neuropathol 2010; **120**(6): 827–828. doi: 10.1007/s00401-010-0744-4. Epub 2010 Sep 14.PMID: 20838798

12. Korczyn AD, Gurevich T. Parkinson's disease: before the motor symptoms and beyond. J Neurol Sci 2010; **289** (1–2): 2–6. doi: 10.1016/j.jns.2009.08.032. Epub 2009 Oct 3.PMID: 19801155

13. Korczyn AD. Is there a need to redefine Parkinson's disease? J Neurol Sci 2011; **310** (1–2): 2–3. doi: 10.1016/j.jns.2011.07.011. Epub 2011 Aug 16.PMID: 2184917610

14. Delgado-Alvarado M, Gago B, Navalpotro-Gomez I, Jiménez-Urbieta H, Rodriguez-Oroz MC. Biomarkers for dementia and mild cognitive impairment in Parkinson's disease. Mov Disord 2016; **31**(6): 861–881. doi: 10.1002/mds.26662. Epub 2016 May 19. PMID: 27193487

15. Emre M, Aarsland D, Albanese A, et al. Rivastigmine for dementia associated with Parkinson's disease. Engl J Med 2004; **351** (24): 2509–2518. doi: 10.1056/NEJMoa041470.PMID: 15590953

Cognitive Dysfunction in Parkinson's Disease

Damon Salzman and Shakeel Tabish

In 1817, the English surgeon Dr. James Parkinson penned his now classic work, "An Essay on the Shaking Palsy." He describes the condition as, "an involuntary tremulous motion, with lessened muscular power, in parts not in action, and even when supported; with a propensity to bend the trunk forwards, and to pass from a walking to a running pace; the senses and intellects being uninjured" [1].

The description of this paralysis agitans (later renamed as Parkinson's disease by Jean Marie Charcot) has largely remained unchanged today over 200 years later. However, we now realize that the latter part, that the senses and intellect being uninjured, is incorrect. This chapter will summarize the prevalence, incidence, pathophysiology, and the scope of the cognitive changes that are seen in this disease.

Prevalence

The World Health Assembly published the "Global action plan on the public response to dementia 2017–2025," and defined dementia as a syndrome – usually of a chronic or progressive nature – in which there is deterioration in cognitive function (i.e. the ability to process thought) beyond what might be expected from normal aging. It affects memory, thinking, orientation, comprehension, calculation, learning capacity, language, and judgement. Consciousness is not affected. The impairment in cognitive function is commonly accompanied, and occasionally preceded, by deterioration in emotional control, social behavior, or motivation [2].

It affects roughly 50 million people worldwide from all causes. While the most frequent cause is Alzheimer's disease (AD), other common pathologies include vascular dementia, dementia with Lewy bodies, and frontotemporal degeneration. While AD is relatively common, comprising approximately 70%, dementia due to Parkinson's

disease (PDD) is relatively rare as a primary cause at 3.6%.

Regardless of cause, the care of people with dementia has a significant social and financial impact on society. The direct social and medical costs, as well as the costs of informal care and loss of work productivity by caregivers, has an estimated annual cost of US $818 billion dollars. This cost is borne not only by a significant burden on societal and government institutions, but also by the families of the affected individuals. Indeed, the physical, emotional, and financial pressures can cause great stress to families and carers.

Incidence

While PDD is an uncommon cause of dementia, cognitive involvement in Parkinson's disease is becoming more widely recognized. Cognitive status in Parkinson's disease runs the gamut from normal mentation for age to mild cognitive impairment (MCI) to dementia. MCI is considered an intermediate condition between "normal aging" and dementia. While relatively uncommon at the time of diagnosis, the cumulative incidence of dementia increases with age and the duration of PD and can be as high as 80–90% by age 90 years [9].

A number of authors have looked more specifically at the prevalence over the years. Jeffrey Cummings' group published a paper in 1988 which reviewed 27 studies which included 4336 PD patients, where the prevalence of overt dementia was found to be 39.9% [5].

In 2004, Thomas Foltynie's group looked at the prevalence of MCI in a UK-based cohort [12]. The prevalence of mild cognitive impairment is estimated to be around 36% in PD patients based on the study done in this group. In this study, researchers selected a cohort of newly diagnosed patients with parkinsonism and Parkinson's disease in the UK over a two-year period. The patients participated in a detailed clinical assessment either at home or in an outpatient clinic; 36% had evidence of cognitive impairment based on their performance in the Mini-Mental State Examination, a pattern recognition task, and the Tower of London task.

In 2005, Dr. Aarsland et al. of Kings College London performed a meta-analysis of studies published in Pubmed related to PD prevalence. Twelve studies of the prevalence of PD or PDD (1,767 patients included) and 24 prevalence studies of dementia subtypes (4,711 patients included) were incorporated. The study showed that prevalence of dementia in PD ranged between 24% and 31% [4, 8].

In 2012, a task force of the Movement Disorder Society proposed a standardized set of criteria to diagnose MCI in Parkinson's disease. Two levels of criteria were described in the paper – the first level is an abbreviated assessment, while the second level was a comprehensive battery that allowed the division of MCI patients into multiple subtypes depending on the affected domains. Studies which have utilized these criteria have reported frequencies of MCI in PD patients between 14.8% and 42.5% in newly diagnosed patients.

Clinical Risk Factors

Given the significant impact of cognitive impairment in PD and the societal cost, it has been necessary for researchers to look at risk factors of this formerly under-recognized malady. Several groups have examined this question and found a number of associations. We list a number of the more commonly found associations here [7, 8, 10, 14, 16, 17, 18].

a) Age of the patient
b) Later age of onset of PD
c) Longer duration of PD symptoms
d) Presence of hallucinations
e) Akinetic dominant PD/bradykinesia
f) Severity of extrapyramidal symptoms
g) Cardiovascular autonomic dysfunction, including orthostatic hypotension
h) REM behavior disorder (RBD)

While it is beyond the scope of this chapter to delve into the underlying relationship of these factors and how they may contribute to the cognitive decline, a few of these will be touched on now and a few others will be described later on in this chapter.

Akinetic Dominant/Bradykinesia

In 2012, Poletti et al. published a paper looking at the relationship between cognitive impairment and motor symptoms of Parkinson's disease. In the study, 132 drug-naïve PD patients were compared with 100 healthy controls and followed for at least 3 years. Unsurprisingly, cognitive testing demonstrated MCI prevalence was higher in the PD patients than healthy controls. It was also noted that MCI PD patients had more severe bradykinesia scores than non-MCI PD patients and patients who had tremor as their main symptom had better performance on cognitive tasks [10].

Autonomic Dysfunction

Autonomic dysfunction (Autd) may occur in as many as 40% of people with PD [16]. It is defined as having at least two of the following symptoms or signs for at least 6 months.

1) Urinary urgency, increased daytime frequency, and nocturia without hesitancy
2) Constipation
3) Symptoms of upper gastrointestinal tract dysfunction, including nausea, bloating, and early satiety
4) Orthostatic hypotension
5) Sweating abnormalities
6) Erectile dysfunction in males

Studies have failed to demonstrate specific neuropathology to the central systems that would account for the AutD in patients with PD. Rather, it appears that this stems from damage to peripheral processes in the nervous system.

Interesting to note, AutD, like cognitive impairment, appears more common in patients with akinetic dominant PD. The implications of this are not clear. Two possibilities are that the mechanisms that lead to both AutD and cognitive impairment are identical and speak to a more widespread disease process. Another possibility is that the AutD is an independent risk factor for cognitive impairment, possibly due to fluctuations in cerebral perfusion or other processes.

REM Sleep Behavior Disorder

REM sleep behavior disorder (RBD) is a REM-related parasomnia during which people will not only act out their dreams, but the nature of those dreams may become violent. It occurs because of the failure to inhibit spinal motor neurons during REM sleep. It has been linked to the neurodegenerative disorders associated with α-synuclein positive intracellular inclusions, for example, parkinsonism, Lewy body dementia, and multiple system atrophy (MSA).

Several brainstem pontine regions have been implicated in RBD pathophysiology including the peri-locus ceruleus region, pedunculo-pontine nucleus, and laterodorsal tegmental nucleus. Supra-spinal mechanism handles REM atonia. During REM sleep, nuclei from the pons excite neurons in the medulla, which then transmit descending inhibitory projections to spinal alpha motor neurons resulting in hyperpolarization and muscle atonia. It is the disinhibition of these neurons that leads to muscle activity during the REM stage of sleep. The presence of RBD may pre-date the clinical presentation of Parkinson's by several years. In a case series, about half of the patients with RBD converted to a neurologic disorder within 12 years [17].

Duration and Severity of Symptoms

A number of studies have linked the duration and severity of the extrapyramidal symptoms to the presence and severity of cognitive impairment. In this author's opinion, this may be that as the amount of the dysfunctional α-synuclein protein deposition leads to the motor symptoms, a proportional amount also affects the various cognitive pathways. However, as we shall see when we look at the pathophysiology of this, it may be more complex than the simplistic explanation that we have proposed.

Genetic Risk Factors

Parkinson's-associated cognitive issues also have links to genetic aberrations. These mutations serve as independent risk factors in the development of these issues. Here we will briefly discuss those genes.

a) *GBA* gene (glucocerebrosidase gene). Studies show that patients with *GBA* mutations have an earlier age at onset of PD and are more likely to have cognitive dysfunction. Monocyte-associated inflammatory mediators might be elevated in these patients and these play a role in the development of cognitive issues [19, 21].

b) *SCNA* gene (α-synuclein gene). Patients with *SCNA* gene duplications and triplications have been found to develop PD and cognitive impairment along with autonomic dysfunction in early stages of the disease [22].

c) *MAPT* gene (microtubule-associated tau protein gene). *MAPT* H1/H2 genotypes have been found to be an independent predictor of dementia risk in PD [24].

d) Catechol-O-methyltransferase gene (*COMT* Val(158)Met). This gene has been implicated in cognitive dysfunction in patients with PD. Patients with this mutation were found to have significant difficulty with Tower of London performance, a fronto-striatal-based executive task, which was dynamic, such that the ability to solve this task changed with disease progression [24].

Pathogenesis

Historically it was thought that the dementia of PD was due to concomitant Alzheimer's disease or vascular dementia. However, research over recent years has shown that this is not the case. The exact mechanism by which cognitive decline and dementia happens in PD is not clearly understood. However, workers in this field have proposed several mechanisms that may play a role either alone or in conjunction to develop cognitive dysfunction, and ultimately PDD.

Lewy Body Pathology and Disease

As discussed in the genetic risk factors, α-synuclein and tau protein gene mutations have been implicated in the development of cognitive issues in PD. Indeed, Lewy bodies (LB) are largely collections of α-synuclein protein fibrils. It comes as no surprise that LB pathology seems to be the main mechanism that leads to the development of PDD.

In 2007, a study was published in the *Annals of Neurology* [23] that observed that cognitive decline and the development of PDD were strongly associated with the inversion polymorphism containing *MAPT*. A novel synergistic interaction was described between the *MAPT* inversion polymorphism and the single nucleotide polymorphism rs356219 from the 3′ region of *SNCA*. This data supports the hypothesis that tau and α-synuclein are involved in shared or converging pathways in the pathogenesis of PD. It further suggests that the tau inversion influences the development of cognitive impairment and dementia in patients with idiopathic PD.

In another study MAPT H1/H2 genotypes were found to be an independent predictor of dementia [24].

A study published by Dr. Aarsland's group in 2005 [4] detailed 21 patients with PD who were followed prospectively until their death. Even though 18 had dementia, none of the subjects fulfilled the Braak and Braak or NIA-Reagan Institute criteria for AD. However, all had limbic or neocortical LB disease. The LB score was the only pathological measure significantly associated with the annual decline on the MMSE in the univariate analyses, even after controlling for age, sex, and years of education. This prospective, community-based study clearly demonstrated that the main substrate of dementia in PD is LB disease, with only modest levels of concurrent AD pathology identified.

In a study in 2002, 13 patients with PD who developed PDD 4 years after PD onset were selected and post-mortem examination was performed showing diffuse or transitional LB disease as primary pathology substrate for dementia [26]. Twenty-six other studies have shown that LB densities in the entorhinal cortex and in the anterior cingulate cortex were significantly associated with CDR (clinical dementia rating scale). This suggests LB formation in limbic areas may be crucial for development of PDD [27].

Cholinergic Pathway

Studies have shown that there is loss of cortical AChE activity greater in PDD than in AD. Analysis of cognitive data in these PDD patients showed decreased performance on tests of attention and executive functioning [42]. This accords with the findings of another study where brain tissue from PD patients was compared with age-matched healthy controls. Cognitive decline in these PD patients was associated with reduced CHAT activity in the prefrontal cortex [44].

In another paper, a decrease in neocortical (particularly temporal) choline acetyltransferase correlated with the number of neurons in the nucleus basalis of Meynert. This suggests that primary cholinergic neuron degeneration relates, either directly or indirectly, to declining cognitive function in Parkinson's disease [45]. This is further supported by anticholinergic drug use in PD patients with associated cognitive decline [46].

Structural Changes in Parkinson's Disease Dementia

Studies have shown that dementia in Parkinson's disease is associated with structural neocortical changes in the brain when compared with normal controls, especially in both temporal and frontal lobes as well as the left parietal lobe. Gray matter reductions were found in frontal, parietal, limbic, and temporal lobes in patients with PDD compared with those with PD without dementia [37].

Clinical Presentation

Dementia with Lewy bodies and PDD share many similarities as both have underlying LB pathology [62, 63]. The time course and presentation of symptoms mainly differentiate the two disorders. However, in clinical practice it is generally recommended to diagnose PDD when dementia has developed in an already established PD patient, whereas DLB is generally diagnosed when dementia precedes or develops within a year of motor symptoms. This view is further endorsed by a report of the DLB consortium:

> DLB should be diagnosed when dementia occurs before or concurrently with parkinsonism, and PD-D should be used to describe dementia that occurs in the context of well-established PD. The appropriate term will depend upon the clinical situation and generic terms such as Lewy Body disease are often helpful. In research studies in which distinction is made between DLB and PD-D, the 1-year rule between the onset of dementia and parkinsonism for DLB should be used [64].

General tools used to evaluate MCI and PDD in PD patients include cognitive assessment tools such as MMSE, MoCA, and DRS Beck Depression Inventory among others. Tools to assess quality of life include PDQ and the HRQoL.

Before we discuss the symptoms of PDD, we will review the diagnostic criteria of PDD as defined by the Movement Disorder Society Task Force [64].

Parkinson's Disease Dementia Clinical Features

I Core Features

A diagnosis of Parkinson's disease, according to the UK Parkinson's Disease Society Brain Bank Clinical Diagnostic Criteria, is as follows:

Diagnosis of Parkinsonian Syndrome

Bradykinesia (slowness of initiation of voluntary movement with progressive reduction in speed and amplitude of repetitive actions).

And at least one of the following:

a) Muscular rigidity
b) 4–6 Hz rest tremor
c) Postural instability not caused by primary visual, vestibular, cerebellar, or proprioceptive dysfunction.

Exclusion Criteria for Parkinson's Disease

History of repeated strokes with stepwise progression of Parkinsonian features

History of repeated head injury

History of definite encephalitis

Oculogyric crises

Neuroleptic treatment at onset of symptoms

More than one affected relative

Sustained remission

Strictly unilateral features after three years

Supranuclear gaze palsy

Cerebellar signs

Early severe autonomic involvement

Early severe dementia with disturbances of memory, language, and praxis

Babinski sign

Presence of a cerebral tumor or communicating hydrocephalus on CT scan

Negative response to large doses of levodopa (if malabsorption excluded)

MPTP exposure

Supportive Prospective Positive Criteria for Parkinson's Disease: Three or More Required for Diagnosis of Definite Parkinson's Disease

Unilateral onset

Rest tremor present

Progressive disorder

Persistent asymmetry affecting the side of onset most

Excellent response (70–100%) to levodopa

Severe levodopa-induced chorea

Levodopa response for five years or more

Clinical course of ten years or more

MPTP, 1-methyl-4-phenyl-1,2,3,6-tetrahydropyridine

A Dementia Syndrome with Insidious Onset and Slow Progression, Developing within the Context of Established Parkinson's Disease and Diagnosed by History, Clinical, and Mental Examination, Is Defined as:

- Impairment in more than one cognitive domain
- Representing a decline from premorbid level
- Deficits severe enough to impair daily life (social, occupational, or personal care), independent of the impairment ascribable to motor or autonomic symptoms.

II Associated Clinical Features

Cognitive Features

- Attention: Impaired. Impairment in spontaneous and focused attention, poor performance in attentional tasks; performance may fluctuate during the day and from day to day
- Executive functions: Impaired. Impairment in tasks requiring initiation, planning, concept formation, rule finding, set shifting or set maintenance; impaired mental speed (bradyphrenia)
- Visuospatial functions: Impaired. Impairment in tasks requiring visual-spatial orientation, perception, or construction
- Memory: Impaired. Impairment in free recall of recent events or in tasks requiring learning new material, memory usually improves with cueing, recognition is usually better than free recall
- Language: Core functions largely preserved. Word finding difficulties and impaired comprehension of complex sentences may be present.

Behavioral Features

- Apathy: decreased spontaneity; loss of motivation, interest, and effortful behavior
- Changes in personality and mood including depressive features and anxiety
- Hallucinations: mostly visual, usually complex, formed visions of people, animals, or objects

- Delusions: usually paranoid, such as infidelity, or phantom boarder (unwelcome guests living in the home) delusions
- Excessive daytime sleepiness.

III Features Which Do Not Exclude Parkinson's Disease Dementia, but Make the Diagnosis Uncertain

- Co-existence of any other abnormality which may by itself cause cognitive impairment, but judged not to be the cause of dementia, e.g. presence of relevant vascular disease in imaging
- Time interval between the development of motor and cognitive symptoms not known.

IV Features Suggesting Other Conditions or Diseases as Cause of Mental Impairment, Which, When Present Make It Impossible to Reliably Diagnose Parkinson's Disease Dementia

Cognitive and behavioral symptoms appearing solely in the context of other conditions such as:

Acute Confusion due to

a) Systemic diseases or abnormalities
b) Drug intoxication
c) Major depressive disorder according to DSM V

Features compatible with "probable vascular dementia" criteria according to NINDS-AIREN (dementia in the context of cerebrovascular disease as indicated by focal signs in neurological exam such as hemiparesis, sensory deficits, and evidence of relevant cerebrovascular disease by brain imaging AND a relationship between the two as indicated by the presence of one or more of the following: onset of dementia within 3 months after a recognized stroke, abrupt deterioration in cognitive functions, and fluctuating, stepwise progression of cognitive deficits).

Probable Parkinson's Disease Dementia

a) Core features: both must be present
b) Associated clinical features:

- Typical profile of cognitive deficits including impairment in at least two of the four core cognitive domains (impaired attention which may fluctuate, impaired executive functions, impairment in visuospatial functions, and impaired free recall memory which usually improves with cueing)
- The presence of at least one behavioral symptom (apathy, depressed or anxious mood, hallucinations, delusions, excessive daytime sleepiness) supports the diagnosis of Probable PDD, lack of behavioral symptoms, however, does not exclude the diagnosis

c) None of the group III features present
d) None of the group IV features present

Possible Parkinson's Disease Dementia

a) Core features: both must be present
b) Associated clinical features:

- Atypical profile of cognitive impairment in one or more domains, such as prominent or receptive-type (fluent) aphasia, or pure storage-failure type amnesia (memory does not improve with cueing or in recognition tasks) with preserved attention
- Behavioral symptoms may or may not be present
- OR

c) One or more of the group III features present
d) None of the group IV features present

Cognitive Symptoms

There are many domains of cognition that are impaired in PDD but it mainly affects attention, visuospatial, executive functions, and construction/praxis. We will briefly discuss their pattern of involvement below.

Attention

This is defined as the ability to focus selectively on a selected stimulus, sustaining that focus, and shifting it at will; the ability to concentrate. Attention is generally impaired in PDD and is of fluctuating nature as compared to AD. This has been shown in studies involving letter cancellation tests and studies assessing variability in performance over time in a series of reaction time tasks [64, 65, 66].

Memory

Memory is defined as the ability to recover or to process information about past events or knowledge. Memory complaints are generally less common presenting problems in PDD as compared to DLB and AD. However, in more severe forms of dementia there is generally no difference between them. Patients generally have deficits in impaired cued recall. They also have deficits in both verbal and non-verbal recognition memory including visual recognition. However, the degree of impairment is less severe in PDD as compared to AD. Generally, recognition is less affected in PDD as compared to recall memory [64, 67].

Executive Functions

These are the mental processes that enable us to focus attention, plan, remember instructions, and juggle multiple tasks successfully. Executive functions are impaired in PDD more than AD. Verbal fluency, both phonemic and semantic, is generally impaired in PDD when evaluated by the initiation and the preservation part of the Dementia Rating Scale (DRS). Concept formulation is also noted to be impaired in PDD. Visual reasoning is another domain that is more affected in PDD as compared to AD [62, 68].

Construction and Praxis

Praxis is the process by which a skill is enacted. Construction and drawing tasks involve both cognitive functions and motor functions. Hence a deficit of either can contribute to problems in completing these tasks. Clock drawing tests are usually impaired in PDD and patients usually make more planning errors during the test. However, it provides limited information in discriminating PDD from AD and DLB as it is impaired in all three [62, 69].

Visuospatial Functions

Visual perception was measured in a study by performing tests of visual discrimination, space motion and object form perception on PD, PDD, DLB, and AD patients. Visual perception was impaired in both PDD and DLB patients. Therefore, substantial visuospatial impairments help to differentiate PDD and DLB from patients with AD [62, 70].

Language

Aphasia is defined as the loss or impairment of ability to understand or express language. Clinically evident aphasia is generally rare in PDD. As mentioned above in the section on executive function, verbal fluency is impaired in PDD. Indeed, the preservation of core language function helps to differentiate PDD from AD [62].

Behavioral and Neuropsychiatric Symptoms

Hallucinations and Delusions

Hallucinations are common in both PD and PDD. They are a major predictor of PDD [7]. They are seen in both PDD and DLB, but are more common in PDD. Hence it can be concluded that the presence of hallucinations is a marker of LB pathology. Patients with PDD usually have visual and auditory hallucinations. Visual hallucinations are complex and usually are anonymous people but can also be family members, body parts, or animals. They are usually colorful, static, and centrally located [62, 71]. Less frequently described, but increasingly recognized, are tactile hallucinations. These are frequently unpleasant and are more commonly described as the feeling of an animal (such as a snake wrapped around the leg) or insects (often crawling) on the skin [62].

Delusions are less common than hallucinations, however, both can co-exist as well. Delusions are usually of a paranoid nature and phantom boarder (a type of delusional misidentification syndrome in which the patient believes that someone uninvited is residing in his or her home despite evidence to the contrary).

Mood Disturbances

The rate of major depression has been reported to be 13% in PDD patients as compared to 9% in AD patients [72]. Anxiety occurs at the same rate in PDD as in non-demented patients and often both disorders coexist [62]. Irritable mood, anger, and aggression are commonly seen in AD [62, 73]. However, these are not commonly seen in PDD. Apathy is also seen in PDD, up to 50%, more than nondemented patients [74].

Interestingly, Dr. Thaler and colleagues at Tel Aviv University published an article in *Parkinsonism and Related Disorders* in 2012 entitled "Appreciation of humor is decreased among patients with Parkinson's Disease" [3]. It is speculated that this may be due to disruption of the mesolimbic dopaminergic pathways. Further it was found that the perception of humor was most impaired with visual presentation, and least impaired when listening to jokes.

Sleep Disorders

Fatigue and sleepiness are common symptoms of Parkinson's disease. RBD is seen in both PD and PDD [17, 18]. It is also shown that presence of RBD leads to more cognitive impairment and PDD development in PD. Obstructive sleep apnea and sleep disordered breathing has been found to not only increase the risk of developing PD but is also a consequence of the disease. Even, in the absence of overt sleep disorders, excessive daytime sleepiness is also associated with PDD [62, 75].

Management

Management of PDD may be conveniently divided into two categories: nonpharmacologic and pharmacologic strategies.

Nonpharmacologic Strategies

While it is beyond the scope of this chapter to discuss these in depth, a few of these will be touched on here. In this author's experience, education of the patient and the caregiver cannot be emphasized enough. Giving people an understanding of the scope and nature of the disease is of great importance. Explaining this earlier on leads to significant ongoing reduction in anxiety and more realistic expectations as the disease progresses. Referring people to appropriate support groups or community resources may also provide assistance. Assuring proper sleep and nutritional needs are met also positively impacts a patient's mental and physical therapy. Looking for and treating comorbid conditions, as well as looking for medications that may affect mentation are all clear and straightforward guidelines to dealing with PDD patients.

Pharmacologic Strategies

Cholinesterase Inhibitors

Cholinesterase inhibitors are prescribed for cognitive impairment in PDD. They also help with hallucinations. The main problem with their use is side effects such as worsening tremor, nausea, and vomiting. They are generally given a trial period of 2–3 months and if there is no improvement, they may be gradually reduced as they can lead to sudden behavioral and cognitive worsening.

Rivastigmine

A placebo-controlled study involving 541 patients was carried out; 410 completed the study. These were patients with mild-moderate dementia that developed at least 2 years after clinical diagnosis of PD. They were assigned to either group randomly. The study showed that rivastigmine was responsible for moderate improvement in dementia. However, it was also associated with higher rates of nausea, vomiting, and tremor [76].

Donepezil

A randomized placebo-controlled double-blind study was done that looked at the effects of donepezil in 550 patients with PDD. After 24 weeks, donepezil was associated with improvement in measures of executive function and attention but failed to meet primary endpoints [77].

Memantine

Approved by the FDA in 2003, memantine is an N-methyl-D-aspartate receptor antagonist primarily used in the management of AD. It is different from cholinesterase inhibitors as it works by a separate mechanism. It blocks the effects of glutamate, a neurotransmitter in the brain that leads to neuronal excitability and excessive stimulation in AD.

There was a double-blind placebo-controlled study done involving patients in outpatient clinics with PDD or DLB in Norway, Sweden, and the UK over 24 weeks. The primary endpoint was met in that there was improvement in the Clinical Global Impression of Change (CGIC). This study showed that memantine carries promise in treatment of dementia in PD. However, memantine can lead to worsening of neuropsychiatric symptoms such as hallucinations [78].

Antipsychotics

Visual hallucinations and delusions are common symptoms in PDD. These are caused by the disease process itself but also exacerbated by anticholinergic and antiparkinsonism medications. The first step in management of psychosis should be stopping anticholinergic medications. Although antiparkinsonism medications cannot be stopped, their dose should be reduced to help with psychotic symptoms. If these measures do not work, then low-dose antipsychotics can be used for symptomatic management. Quetiapine and clozapine are preferred over others.

A novel strategy in the treatment of hallucinations and delusions is the use of pimavanserin. It is a first-in-class, atypical antipsychotic that does not affect the dopaminergic system. It acts as an inverse agonist and antagonist at the serotonergic 5-HT-2a and 2 c, with no appreciable activity at 5-HT-2b, dopamine (including D2), calcium channel, histamine, or muscarinic cholinergic receptors. It was approved in 2016 by the FDA for the treatment of PD-related psychosis.

Sleep-Related Agents

The treatment of RBD and fatigue will be treated elsewhere in this volume, though for the sake of completeness we will touch on it briefly here.

REM sleep behavior disorder is a troubling condition and can be a significant source of distress to both the patient and bed partner. Melatonin in doses of 3–12 mg at bedtime have been utilized successfully to prevent the night-time symptoms of RBD and is frequently the first-line treatment. While effective in roughly only half of all cases, it has the advantage of not promoting daytime fatigue; it is relatively inexpensive and very safe. In addition, there is no addictive potential. Benzodiazepines such as clonazepam or lorazepam are the therapeutic mainstay. While more effective than melatonin, there is a more significant chance of daytime fatigue and possibly a greater chance of falling with the medication. The relative risks and benefits must be weighed. Medications which may worsen or potentiate the RBD should be removed or reduced as possible, in particular SSRI antidepressants, and replaced with other agents such as bupropion.

Daytime fatigue may be addressed by the judicious use of stimulant medication such as modafinil, armodafinil, or low doses of methylphenidate or amphetamines. Additionally, some of the medications used to treat PD such as levodopa/carbidopa, or some of the dopamine agonists may produce daytime sleepiness and dosage modifications as tolerated.

Mood Agents

There are many treatment options for depression that work well in people with PD. There are several types of antidepressants, including selective serotonin reuptake inhibitors (SSRIs), tricyclic antidepressants, and selective norepinephrine reuptake inhibitors (SNRIs). In this author's experience, bupropion appears particularly beneficial, and some studies have suggested that it has a positive effect on some of the motor symptoms of PD as well.

Many people also experience relief from their depression through psychological counseling, such as cognitive behavioral therapy. In addition, regular exercise has been shown to ease symptoms of depression.

Conclusion

While not part of the original description by James Parkinson, the cognitive and psychological changes of PD have become more widely recognized. While much work has been done to better define and delineate their cause, more research is needed. Further, with greater understanding, our hope is that better treatments will arise to treat this disorder and lead to improved quality of life for both patients and families.

References

1. Parkinson J. *An Essay on the Shaking Palsy*. Sherwood, Neely and Jones; 1817.

2. World Health Organization. *Global Action Plan on the Global Response to Dementia* 2017–2025. Geneva; 2017.

3. Thaler A, Posen J, Giladi N, et al. Appreciation of humor is decreased among patients with Parkinson's disease. Parkinsonism Relat Disord 2012; **18**(2): 144–148.

4. Aarsland D, Zaccai J, Brayne C. A systematic review of prevalence studies of dementia in Parkinson's disease. Mov Disord 2005; **20**: 1255–1263.

5. Cummings JL. Intellectual impairment in Parkinson's disease: clinical, pathologic, and biochemical correlates. Top Geriatr 1988; **1**(1): 24–36.

6. Aarsland D, Andersen K, Larsen JP, et al. Risk of dementia in Parkinson's disease. Neurology Mar 2001; **56**(6): 730–736.

7. Hobson P, Meara J. Risk and incidence of dementia in a cohort of older subjects with Parkinson's disease in the United Kingdom. Mov Disord 2004; **19**: 1043–1049.

8. Aarsland D, Andersen K, Larsen JP, Lolk A. Prevalence and characteristics of dementia in Parkinson disease: an 8-year prospective study. Arch Neurol 2003; **60**(3): 387–392.

9. Butler TC, van den Hout A, Matthews FE, et al. Dementia and survival in Parkinson disease: a 12-year population study. Neurology Mar 2008; **70**(13): 1017–1022.

10. Poletti M, Frosini D, Pagni C, et al. Mild cognitive impairment and cognitive-motor relationships in newly diagnosed drug-naive patients with Parkinson's disease. J Neurol Neurosurg Psychiatry 2012; **83**: 601–606.

11. Muslimović D, Post B, Speelman JD, Schmand B. Cognitive profile of patients with newly diagnosed Parkinson disease. Neurology 2005; **65**(8): 1239–1245.

12. Foltynie T, Brayne CEG, Robbins TW, Barker RA. The cognitive ability of an incident cohort of Parkinson's patients in the UK. The CamPaIGN Study. Brain 2004; **127**(3): 550–560.

13. Mayeux R, Denaro J, Hemenegildo N, et al. A population-based investigation of Parkinson's disease with and without dementia: relationship to age and gender. Arch Neurol 1992; **49**(5): 492–497.

14. Levy G, Schupf N, Tang MX, et al. Combined effect of age and severity on the risk of dementia in Parkinson's disease. Ann Neurol 2002; **51**: 722–729.

15. Anang JBM, Gagnon JF, Bertrand JA, et al. Predictors of dementia in Parkinson disease: a prospective cohort study. Neurology 2014; **83**(14): 1253–1260.

16. Anang JBM, Gagnon JF, Bertrand JA, et al. Predictors of dementia in Parkinson disease: a prospective cohort study. Neurology 2014; **83**(14): 1253–1260.

17. Jozwiak N, Postuma RB, Montplaisir J, et al. REM sleep behavior disorder and cognitive impairment in Parkinson's disease. Sleep 2017; **40**(8): zsx101.

18. Anang JBM, Gagnon JF, Bertrand JA, et al. Predictors of dementia in Parkinson disease: a prospective cohort study. Neurology 2014; **83**(14): 1253–1260.

19. Alcalay RN, Caccappolo E, Mejia-Santana H, et al. Cognitive performance of GBA mutation carriers with early-onset PD. Neurology 2012; **78**(18): 1434–1440.

20. Chahine LM, Qiang J, Ashbridge E, et al. Clinical and biochemical differences in patients having Parkinson disease with vs without GBA mutations. JAMA Neurol 2013; **70**(7): 852–858.

21. Liu G, Boot B, Locascio JJ, et al. Specifically neuropathic Gaucher's mutations accelerate cognitive decline in Parkinson's. Ann Neurol 2016; **80**: 674–685.

22. Obi T, Nishioka K, Ross OA, et al. Clinicopathologic study of a SNCA gene duplication patient with Parkinson disease and dementia. Neurology 2008; **70**(3): 238–241.

23. Goris A, Williams-Gray CH, Clark GR, et al. Tau and α-synuclein in susceptibility to, and dementia in, Parkinson's disease. Ann Neurol 2007; **62**: 145–153.

24. Williams-Gray CH, Evans JR, Goris AN, et al. The distinct cognitive syndromes of Parkinson's disease: 5 year follow-up of the CamPaIGN cohort. Brain 2009; **132**(11): 2958–2969.

25. Aarsland D, Perry R, Brown A, et al. Neuropathology of dementia in Parkinson's disease: a prospective, community-based study. Ann Neurol 2005; **58**: 773–776.

26. Apaydin H, Ahlskog JE, Parisi JE, et al. Parkinson disease neuropathology: later-developing dementia and loss of the levodopa response. Arch Neurol 2002; **59**(1): 102–112.

27. Kövari E, Gold G, Herrmann FR, et al. Lewy body densities in the entorhinal and anterior cingulate cortex predict cognitive deficits in Parkinson's disease. Acta Neuropathol 2003; **106**: 83–88.

28. Edison P, Rowe CC, Rinne JO, et al. Amyloid load in Parkinson's disease dementia and Lewy body dementia measured with [11 C] PIB positron emission tomography. J Neurol Neurosurg Psychiatry 2008; **79**: 1331–1338.

29. Petrou M, Bohnen NI, Müller MLTM, et al. Aβ-amyloid deposition in patients with Parkinson disease at risk for development of dementia. Neurology 2012; **79**(11): 1161–1167.

30. Kotzbauer PT, Cairns NJ, Campbell MC, et al. Pathologic accumulation of α-synuclein and Aβ in Parkinson disease patients with dementia. Arch Neurol 2012; **69**(10): 1326–1331.

31. Irwin DJ, White MT, Toledo JB, et al. Neuropathologic substrates of Parkinson disease dementia. Ann Neurol 2012; **72**: 587–598.

32. Hall H, Reyes S, Landeck N, et al. Hippocampal Lewy pathology and cholinergic dysfunction are associated with dementia in Parkinson's disease. Brain 2014; **137**(9): 2493–2508.

33. Siderowf A, Xie SX, Hurtig H, et al. CSF amyloid β 1–42 predicts cognitive decline in Parkinson disease. Neurology 2010; **75**(12): 1055–1061.

34. Alves G, Lange J, Blennow K, et al. CSF Aβ42 predicts early-onset dementia in Parkinson disease. Neurology 2014; **82**(20): 1784–1790.

35. Burton EJ, McKeith IG, Burn DJ, O'Brien JT. Brain atrophy rates in Parkinson's disease with and without dementia using serial magnetic

resonance imaging. Mov Disord 2005; **20**: 1571–1576.

36. Nagano-Saito A, Washimi Y, Arahata Y, et al. Cerebral atrophy and its relation to cognitive impairment in Parkinson disease. Neurology 2005; **64**(2): 224–229.

37. Beyer MK, Janvin CC, Larsen JP, et al. A magnetic resonance imaging study of patients with Parkinson's disease with mild cognitive impairment and dementia using voxel-based morphometry. J Neurol Neurosurg Psychiatry 2007; **78**: 254–259.

38. Melzer TR, Watts R, MacAskill MR, et al. Grey matter atrophy in cognitively impaired Parkinson's disease. J Neurol Neurosurg Psychiatry 2012; **83**: 188–194.

39. Mori H. Pathological substrate of dementia in Parkinson's disease – its relation to DLB and DLBD. Parkinsonism Relat Disord 2005; **11**: S41–S45.

40. Ballard C, Ziabreva I, Perry R, et al. Differences in neuropathologic characteristics across the Lewy body dementia spectrum. Neurology 2006; **67**(11): 1931–1934.

41. Shimada H, Hirano S, Shinotoh H, et al. Mapping of brain acetylcholinesterase alterations in Lewy body disease by PET. Neurology 2009; **73**(4): 273–278.

42. Bohnen NI, Kaufer DI, Hendrickson R, et al. Cognitive correlates of cortical cholinergic denervation in Parkinson's disease and parkinsonian dementia. J Neurol 2006; **253**: 242–247.

43. Bohnen NI, Kaufer DI, Ivanco LS, et al. Cortical cholinergic function is more severely affected in Parkinsonian dementia than in Alzheimer disease: an in vivo positron emission tomographic study. Arch Neurol 2003; **60**(12): 1745–1748.

44. Mattila PM, Röyttä M, Lönnberg P, et al. Choline acetyltransferase activity and striatal dopamine receptors in Parkinson's disease in relation to cognitive impairment. Acta Neuropathol 2001; **102**: 160–166.

45. Perry EK, Curtis M, Dick DJ, et al. Cholinergic correlates of cognitive impairment in Parkinson's disease: comparisons with Alzheimer's disease. J Neurol Neurosurg Psychiatry 1985; **48**: 413–421.

46. Ehrt U, Broich K, Larsen JP, et al. Use of drugs with anticholinergic effect and impact on cognition in Parkinson's disease: a cohort study. J Neurology Neurosurg Psychiatry 2010; **81**: 160–165.

47. Bohnen NI, Albin RL, Müller MLTM, et al. Frequency of cholinergic and caudate nucleus dopaminergic deficits across the predemented cognitive spectrum of Parkinson disease and evidence of interaction effects. JAMA Neurol 2015; **72**(2): 194–200.

48. Morrison C, Borod J, Brin M, et al. Effects of levodopa on cognitive functioning in moderate-to-severe Parkinson's disease (MSPD). J Neural Transm 2004; **111**: 1333–1341.

49. Stern Y, Richards M, Sano M, Mayeux R. Comparison of cognitive changes in patients with Alzheimer's and Parkinson's disease. Arch Neurol 1993; **50**(10): 1040–1045.

50. Levin BE, Llabre MM, Reisman S, et al. Visuospatial impairment in Parkinson's disease. Neurology 1991; **41**(3): 365.

51. Muslimović D, Post B, Speelman JD, Schmand B. Cognitive profile of patients with newly diagnosed Parkinson disease. Neurology 2005; **65**(8): 1239–1245.

52. Aarsland D, Brønnick K, Larsen JP, et al. Cognitive impairment in incident, untreated Parkinson disease. Neurology 2009; **72**(13): 1121–1126.

53. Pillon B, Deweer B, Agid Y, Dubois B. Explicit memory in Alzheimer's, Huntington's, and Parkinson's diseases. Arch Neurol 1993; **50**(4): 374–379.

54. Emre M, Aarsland D, Albanese A, et al. Rivastigmine for dementia associated with Parkinson's disease. N Engl J Med 2004; **351**: 2509–2518.

55. Tröster AI, Browner N. Movement disorders with dementia in older adults. In Ravdin LD and Katzen HL (eds.). *Handbook on the Neuropsychology of Aging and Dementia.* Springer Science + Business Media; 2013, 333–361.

56. Janvin CC, Larsen JP, Salmon DP, et al. Cognitive profiles of individual patients with Parkinson's disease and dementia: comparison with dementia with lewy bodies and Alzheimer's disease. Mov Disord 2006; **21**: 337–342.

57. Lewis SJG, Foltynie T, Blackwell AD, et al. Heterogeneity of Parkinson's disease in the early clinical stages using a data driven approach. J Neurol Neurosurg Psychiatry 2005; **76**: 343–348.

58. Aarsland D, Andersen K, Larsen JP, Lolk A. Prevalence and characteristics of dementia in Parkinson disease: an 8-year prospective study. Arch Neurol 2003; **60**(3): 387–392.

59. Fénelon G, Mahieux F, Huon R, Ziégler M. Hallucinations in Parkinson's disease: prevalence,

phenomenology and risk factors. Brain 2000; **123** (4): 733–745.

60. Aarsland D, Andersen K, Larsen JP, Lolk A. Prevalence and characteristics of dementia in Parkinson disease: an 8-year prospective study. Arch Neurol 2003; **60**(3): 387–392.

61. Aarsland D, Larsen JP, Tandberg E, Laake K. Predictors of nursing home placement in Parkinson's disease: a population-based, prospective study. J Am Geriatr Soc 2000; **48**: 938–942.

62. Emre M, Aarsland D, Brown R, et al. Clinical diagnostic criteria for dementia associated with Parkinson's disease. Mov Disord 2007; **22**: 1689–1707.

63. McKeith, IG, Burn D. Spectrum of Parkinson's disease, Parkinson's dementia, and Lewy body dementia. Neurolog Clin 2000; **18**(4): 865–883.

64. McKeith IG, Dickson DW, Lowe J, et al. Diagnosis and management of dementia with Lewy bodies. Neurology 2005; **65**(12): 1863–1872.

65. Noe E, Marder K, Bell KL, et al. Comparison of dementia with Lewy bodies to Alzheimer's disease and Parkinson's disease with dementia. Mov Disord 2004; **19**: 60–67.

66. Ballard CG, Aarsland D, McKeith I, et al. Fluctuations in attention. Neurology 2002; **59**(11): 1714–1720.

67. Pillon B, Deweer B, Agid Y, Dubois B. Explicit memory in Alzheimer's, Huntington's, and Parkinson's diseases. Arch Neurol 1993; **50**(4): 374–379.

68. Starkstein SE, Sabe L, Petracca G, et al. Neuropsychological and psychiatric differences between Alzheimer's disease and Parkinson's disease with dementia. J Neurol Neurosurg Psychiatry 1996; **61**: 381–387.

69. Cahn-Weiner DA, Williams K, Grace J, et al. Discrimination of dementia with Lewy bodies from Alzheimer disease and Parkinson disease using the Clock Drawing Test. Cog Behav Neurol 2003; **16**(2): 85–92.

70. Mosimann UP, Mather G, Wesnes KA, et al. Visual perception in Parkinson disease dementia and dementia with Lewy bodies. Neurology 2004; **63**(11): 2091–2096.

71. Fénelon G, Mahieux F, Huon R, Ziégler M. Hallucinations in Parkinson's disease: prevalence, phenomenology and risk factors. Brain 2000; **123** (4): 733–745.

72. Aarsland D, Ballard C, Larsen JP, McKeith I. A comparative study of psychiatric symptoms in dementia with Lewy bodies and Parkinson's disease with and without dementia. Int J Geriat Psychiatry 2001; **16**: 528–536.

73. Engelborghs S, Maertens K, Nagels G, et al. Neuropsychiatric symptoms of dementia: cross-sectional analysis from a prospective, longitudinal Belgian study. Int J Geriat Psychiatry 2005; **20**: 1028–1037.

74. Aarsland D, Brønnick K, Ehrt U, et al. Neuropsychiatric symptoms in patients with Parkinson's disease and dementia: frequency, profile and associated care giver stress. J Neurol Neurosurg Psychiatry 2007; **78**: 36–42.

75. Gjerstad MD, Aarsland D, Larsen JP. Development of daytime somnolence over time in Parkinson's disease. Neurology 2002; **58**(10): 1544–1546.

76. Emre M, Aarsland D, Albanese A, et al. Rivastigmine for dementia associated with Parkinson's disease. N Engl J Med 2004; **351**: 2509–2518.

77. Dubois B, Tolosa E, Katzenschlager R, et al. Donepezil in Parkinson's disease dementia: a randomized, double-blind efficacy and safety study. Mov Disord 2012; **27**: 1230–1238.

78. Aarsland D, Ballard B, Walker Z, et al. Memantine in patients with Parkinson's disease dementia or dementia with Lewy bodies: a double-blind, placebo-controlled, multicentre trial. Lancet Neurol 2009; **8**(7): 613–618.

Neuropsychiatric (Behavioral) Symptoms in Parkinson's Disease

Kasia Gustaw Rothenberg

Introduction – Neuropathological Correlates of Psychiatric Symptoms in Parkinson's Disease

Parkinson's disease (PD) has traditionally been considered a motor system disorder, but it is now widely recognized to be a complex one with diverse clinical features that include neuropsychiatric manifestations [1]. Psychiatric features of PD include but are not limited to cognitive impairment, psychosis, anxiety, depression, apathy, sleep disturbances, as well as fatigue. In a multicenter survey of over 1,000 patients with PD, virtually all (97%) of patients reported non-motor symptoms, with each patient experiencing an average of approximately eight different ones [2].

Certain non-motor features of PD (e.g. olfactory dysfunction, constipation, depression, anxiety, and REM sleep behavior disorder) may even precede manifestation of motor symptoms [3, 4]. Psychiatric symptoms, especially psychosis and/or dementia, may be even more disabling than motor features [5, 6].

Neuropathologically, PD is characterized by loss of dopaminergic neurons in the substantia nigra pars compacta (SNpc) and intracellular inclusions (Lewy bodies) and Lewy neurites, composed mostly of α-synuclein. α-synuclein aggregates in degeneration of SNpc dopamine neurons result in loss of striatal dopamine leading to classical motor symptoms of PD. Disruption of dopaminergic circuitry could also explain some psychiatric symptoms of PD. Dopaminergic pathways in the mesolimbic and mesocortical areas play important roles in the reward, affective, and impulse control. Disruptions of these circuits by cell loss or therapy, therefore, may have tremendous effects on behavior, mood, affect, and impulse control [7].

Little is known about the consequences of α-synuclein inclusions in these brain regions, or in neuronal subtypes other than dopamine neurons. Stoyka et al. [8] showed (based on a mice model) that bilateral injections of fibrils into the striatum results in robust bilateral α-synuclein inclusion formation in the cortex and amygdala. Fibril-injected mice show defects in a social dominance behavioral task and fear-conditioning, tasks that are associated with prefrontal cortex and amygdala function. Results of a study suggest that α-synuclein inclusion formation impairs behaviors associated with cortical and amygdala function, brain areas that play important roles in the complex cognitive and behavioral features of PD [8].

Cholinergic transmission deficit was proposed as a correlate of cognitive dysfunction in PD. Loss of cholinergic neurons in the nucleus basalis of Meynert and decreased cholinergic activity in the cortex appear to be at least as significant in PD as in Alzheimer's disease [9, 10]. Empirically, anti-cholinergic drugs often exacerbate cognitive deficits in PD patients [11] and cholinesterase inhibitors improve cognitive function in Parkinson's disease dementia (PDD) [12, 13].

By contrast, dopaminergic loss, while central to the pathogenesis of motor symptoms, is not consistently linked with the degree of cognitive dysfunction in patients with PD. While some neuroimaging studies have implicated frontostriatal dopaminergic pathways [14], dopaminergic medication has variable effects on cognitive performance; it may improve short-term memory early in the disease but not in more advanced patients [15, 16]. Even though dopaminergic influence on cognition varies, combined dopaminergic with cholinergic degenerations exhibit consistent influence on cognitive performance [17].

Other than acetylcholine or dopamine, neurotransmitter systems may be involved in psychiatric aspects of PD. Depression in PD is thought to implicate the noradrenergic, dopaminergic, and serotonergic pathways [17]. The pathophysiology of psychosis in PD is most likely multifactorial as well. Overstimulation of dopaminergic receptors, particularly in the mesocorticolimbic region, may occur in the context of chronic dopaminergic therapy and enhanced sensitivity of native receptors [18]. Imbalances between dopamine and acetylcholine also play a role, with compensatory increase in cholinergic activity in response to dopamine deprivation. Additionally, the use of dopaminergic medications may decrease intrinsic serotonin. This observation adds to an already growing body of evidence suggesting serotoninergic circuitry involvement in the phenomenon of PD psychosis. In autopsy studies of psychotic PD patients, abnormalities were found in 5HT-2A receptors (increased serotonin binding) especially in the inferior temporal cortex [19]. A positron emission tomography study found increased serotoninergic type 2A receptor binding in PD patients with visual hallucinations compared with those without [20]. Altered cortical visual processing and rapid eye movement (REM) sleep anomalies have been proposed as contributors to the process [4].

Evaluation of the patient with PD should start with a careful assessment of the patient's reported psychiatric symptoms and include complete mental status examination. Thorough cognitive evaluation should follow [21].

Some psychiatric symptoms may be associated with treatment of motor symptoms of PD: impulse control disorders, psychosis, irritability/agitation/dysphoria (i.e. "off" periods, treatment withdrawal, etc.). This has tremendous implications for the patient, as the treatment of psychiatric symptoms may result in poor control of motor performance, increased dysfunction, and poorer quality of life, particularly in late stages or phenotypically complicated disease.

Dramatic or unexpected worsening of motor control after the addition of psychotropics should prompt adjustment of the dose, consideration of an alternative, or optimization of antiparkinsonian medications.

Very few clinical studies look specifically at psychiatric symptoms in the course of Parkinson's disease, thus conclusions are extrapolated from clinical trials of psychotropic agents used in the treatment of idiopathic psychiatric disorders [22]. This extrapolation is based on the phenomenological similarities of the neuropsychiatric syndromes to psychiatric conditions and the absence of alternatives. The challenge remains that patients with PD are typically excluded from antipsychotic drug trials, as well as other groups of psychotropics (antidepressants, anxiolytics, stimulants, or hypnotics) [22].

The extension of these therapies to PD patients is based on many untested assumptions that may result in treating patients with agents that are ineffective or have safety and tolerability issues. Most patients with PD are elderly and this may affect the pharmacokinetics and the pharmacodynamics of an agent. The potential benefit of all psychotropics must thus be weighed against the significant risks, such as falls, cerebrovascular accidents or worse, mortality [23].

Cognitive Impairment in Parkinson's Disease

Extent of the Problem

While PD can coexist with other common neurodegenerative or vascular diseases, dementia is increasingly recognized as a common intrinsic feature of PD [21]. Clinical features can generally distinguish between PD and other movement disorders associated with dementia, such as dementia with Lewy bodies (DLB) where cognitive impairment precedes motor parkinsonism by at least a year [5, 6, 22].

Cognitive impairment in PD, based on the extent to which it interferes with daily activities, is generally divided into two major categories: mild cognitive impairment (MCI) in the course of PD and PDD [21].

Both MCI and dementia are clinical diagnoses in patients with firmly established PD of at least one year's duration. Subtle cognitive impairment, particularly with frontal lobe features in the executive functions and planning domains, is frequently associated with PD and may appear early. These may also include less severe (though clear) memory difficulties and visuo spatial difficulties [21]. Clinical criteria for the diagnosis of MCI in patients with PD were first proposed by an international consensus panel in 2012 [24] and have since been validated. In studies of patients with a new diagnosis of PD, the prevalence of mild cognitive impairment (MCI) ranges from approximately 10% to 35% [25].

Dementia should be suspected in patients with a decline in cognitive abilities that is interfering with daily function. The cognitive dysfunction of PDD is distinct from Alzheimer disease (AD). With PDD, memory impairment is less prominent early on, while executive dysfunction and visual spatial impairments are features that may be apparent and functionally limiting before the patient meets criteria for dementia [21].

Dementia syndrome with insidious onset and slow progression, developing in the context of established PD, is defined as: impairment in more than one cognitive domain (attention, executive function, visuospatial function, memory); decline from premorbid level, deficits severe enough to impair daily life (social, occupational, or personal care); independent of the impairment ascribable to motor or autonomic symptoms. Behavioral features such as apathy, changes in personality or mood, hallucinations, delusions, and excessive daytime sleepiness (EDS) are supportive of the diagnosis but not required [26].

Cross-sectional studies suggest that the mean prevalence of dementia is between 30% and 40% [27]. In prospective cohort studies, the incidence rate of dementia in patients with PD is consistently estimated at approximately 100 per 1,000 patient-years, a rate almost five- to six-fold higher than controls without PD [28]. It has been reported that approximately 30% of non-demented patients with PD developed dementia within 4 years; with almost 80% developing frank dementia after 8 years [29]. However, cumulative incidence rates of over 80% have been reported in patients followed for more than 20 years after onset of PD [30]. Dementia is thus not only common but nearly inevitable in patients with PD. Risk factors for developing PDD consist of: age at onset of PD ≥60 years, duration of PD, and severity of parkinsonism [31]. Additional risk factors for the development of more severe or early cognitive impairment in patients with PD include the presence of rapid eye movement sleep behavior disorder (RBD), autonomic dysfunction, hyposmia, abnormal visual color discrimination, slow resting electroencephalography (EEG) frequencies, and gait dysfunction [32].

Genetics may play a role in PD patients developing dementia. The majority of cases of PD appear to be sporadic and genetic risk factors for the development of dementia in those patients have been suggested [27]. Genetic forms of PD often involve early or severe cognitive changes. Examples include PD associated with mutations in the glucocerebrosidase (*GBA*) gene [33] and some forms of α-synuclein- (*SNCA*) associated PD [34]. Allelic variation in the gene encoding microtubule-associated protein tau (*MAPT*) appears to affect susceptibility as well [35, 36]. Similarly, a high catechol-O-methyl transferase (COMT) activity haplotype has been found to be associated with a higher risk of developing cognitive impairment in PD [37]. By contrast, dementia is an uncommon feature of PD associated with parkin (*PARK2*) mutations [38].

Apolipoprotein E (*APOE*) gene polymorphism (well established as a risk factor for AD) has been implicated as a potential risk for PDD. *APOE* was found to have a greater effect on the severity other than an onset of dementia syndrome [39]. In a prospective cohort study the presence of the ε4 allele was associated with rapid cognitive decline [36].

Cognitive impairment, associated with overall decline in mental status, could be complicated by psychosis. These are poor prognostic indicators and predict greater admission to nursing homes and early mortality. The presence of dementia and psychosis is the greatest limiting factor for the optimal use of anti-parkinsonian agents.

Rationale for Interventions and Pharmacotherapy

The development of cognitive impairment in patients being treated for PD should prompt careful evaluation of the medical status of the patient and any underlying factors (systemic and focal infections, respiratory insufficiency, metabolic factors, changes to the environment and offending medications, such as sedatives and anticholinergic agents). Anti-parkinsonian medications often require adjustment in this context as PD patients with cognitive decline are more sensitive to their side effects (i.e. anticholinergic agents; dopamine agonists). Every attempt should be made to simplify anti-PD medications by tapering off "adjunctive medications" (such as anticholinergics, MAO-B inhibitors, and amantadine; followed by dopamine agonists and COMT-inhibitors, if necessary) [11]. Ideally, PD patients with dementia should be on levodopa alone if at all possible [40].

Next steps should include a trial of cholinesterase inhibitors and/or memantine in a stepwise fashion. Most, but not all, studies of cholinesterase inhibitors in PDD have noted a mild to moderate benefit [41, 42]. Rivastigmine was evaluated in a 24-week, double-blind, placebo-controlled study of 501 patients with mild to moderate PDD and was found to result in moderate improvement in dementia (as assessed by ADAScog) [43]. Meta-analysis points to improvement in about 15% of patients [44]. Donepezil also appeared to be beneficial in some primary and secondary outcome measures, including measures of executive function and attention. Another potential benefit of cholinesterase inhibitors in PDD is improvement in neuropsychiatric symptoms, such as hallucinations [44].

Treatment is continued if improvement is noted either on testing or by the family. Taper is warranted if there has been no improvement or if there are intolerable side effects. When cholinesterase inhibitors are discontinued, they should not be abruptly terminated, if at all possible, but rather tapered to avoid sudden cognitive and behavioral worsening [45].

Memantine could be a treatment option. Several trials in which participants had either dementia with Lewy bodies (DLB) or PDD found that patients treated with memantine performed better on the primary outcome assessment measure, the clinical global impression of change. Memantine was well tolerated in these trials [46, 47]. Hallucinations and worsened neuropsychiatric symptoms however, have been anecdotally reported with the use of memantine for PDD [48].

Depression and Anxiety

Epidemiology and the Scope of the Problem

The incidence of depression and anxiety is greater in PD patients than in age-matched controls. It is the result of complex psychological and neurobiological factors [49]. The psychiatric burden doesn't solely come from functional decline associated with the threat of progressive motor dysfunction. Depression in PD follows a bi-modal distribution, with peaks of psychiatric burden around the time of onset of symptoms/diagnosis, as well as with loss of independence in late disease. There are several core and associated symptoms of depression (such as fatigue, apathy, sleep disruption, psychomotor retardation, weight loss) that are intrinsic to PD and confuse the assessment. Generalized anxiety disorder, panic disorder, social phobia, phobic disorder, agoraphobia, and obsessive-compulsive disorder have all been described in PD [41, 42].

Just like depression, anxiety can also be part of "pre-motor" manifestations of PD; and manifestation of wearing-off phenomena. In such cases, management focuses primarily on levodopa dosing adjustments and other strategies to mitigate fluctuations. Clinicians should also be aware that akathisia occurs in patients with PD and should be differentiated from anxiety, which may cause similar clinical manifestations.

Rationale for Treatment of Mood Symptoms as well as Anxiety in Parkinson's Disease

Depression in patients with PD should be a target of focused therapy as studies have shown that depression in this population is a major determinant of quality of life. The modality of treatment should be tailored to the severity of the depressive symptoms (Figure 8.1).

For mild depression associated with PD, nonpharmacological approaches may be indicated. These include supportive psychotherapy and cognitive behavioral therapy [5, 6]. CBT appears to be a particularly promising non-pharmacological approach [50].

In more advanced depression, pharmacotherapy is often indicated. Certain "off" phenomena, such as paroxysmal anxiety and panic, may not respond well to antidepressant and anxiolytic therapy but could respond to dopaminergic adjustments that minimize wearing-off periods.

In terms of pharmacotherapy, experts recommend dopamine agonists (DA) as a first step in the management of depression of PD assuming it is compatible with the management of the motor symptoms of PD. Pramipexole (range of doses 0.3–4.2 mg/day) and ropinirole (10 mg/day) have antidepressant properties in patients with PD. Regular monitoring to capture symptoms like pathologic gambling, hypersexuality, and overspending in the course of DA therapy is however crucial [51].

Strong evidence for the treatment of depression in PD has been reported with tricyclic

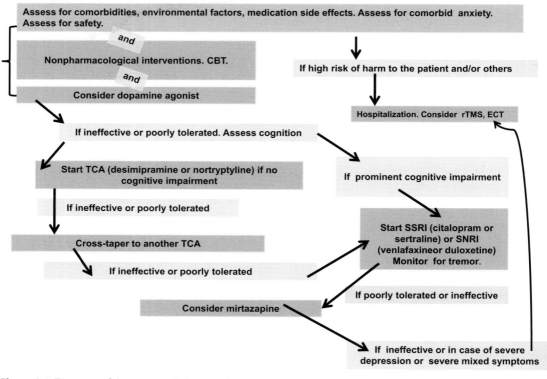

Figure 8.1 Treatment of depression in Parkinson's disease

antidepressants (TCAs) [22]. However, these agents may be poorly tolerated due to anticholinergic effects and arrhythmogenic properties, particularly at higher doses. Selective serotonin reuptake inhibitors (SSRIs) as well as serotonin noradrenaline reuptake inhibitors (SNRIs) may improve depressive and anxiety symptoms in patients with PD, with minimal worsening of movement symptoms [52]. Where pharmacotherapy has been ineffective or poorly tolerated, or where depression in PD is severe, electroconvulsive therapy (ECT) and transcranial magnetic stimulation (TMS) therapy may be helpful, though the evidence of efficacy for TMS in PD is still being gathered. It is important to mention that certain PD medications, such as dopamine agonists and MAO inhibitors, have demonstrated partial antidepressant effects in patients with PD, even when not being utilized for their pro-kinetic properties. These however are not typically used as sole treatment for the management of depression in PD. There is a remarkable paucity of randomized clinical trials for the pharmacological management of anxiety in PD. However, based on clinical experience, the agents that are effective in the treatment of primary

anxiety disorders (e.g. SSRIs), also appear to be effective in PD-related anxiety [49].

Apathy

Clinical Aspect of Apathy in Parkinson's Disease

Apathy can be defined as loss of or diminished motivation in comparison to the patient's previous level of functioning, which is not consistent with his age or culture. Symptoms in domains of behavior, cognition, and/or emotions should be consistently present for 4 weeks and cause clinically significant impairment in personal, social, occupational, or other important areas of functioning [53] (see Table 8.1). These changes in motivation may be reported by the patient himself or by the observations of others. Just as the symptoms of depression are sometimes hard to distinguish from those of PD itself (i.e. psychomotor slowing, lack of motivation, bradykinesia), differentiating between depression, the symptoms of PD, and apathy may also be challenging.

Table 8.1 Criteria for apathy in neurodegenerative disorders.

A: Loss of or diminished motivation in comparison to the patient's previous level of functioning and which is not consistent with his age or culture. These changes in motivation may be reported by the patient himself or by the observations of others.
B: Presence of at least one symptom in at least two of the three following domains for a period of at least four weeks and present most of the time.

    Domain B1—Behaviour: Loss of, or diminished, goal-directed behavior as evidenced by at least one of the following:
        Initiation symptom: loss of self-initiated behavior (for example: starting conversation, doing basic tasks of day-to-day living, seeking social activities, communicating choices)
        Responsiveness symptom: loss of environment-stimulated behavior (for example: responding to conversation, participating in social activities)
    Domain B2—Cognition: Loss of, or diminished, goal-directed cognitive activity as evidenced by at least one of the following:
        Initiation symptom: loss of spontaneous ideas and curiosity for routine and new events (i.e. challenging tasks, recent news, social opportunities, personal/family and social affairs).
        Responsiveness symptom: loss of environment-stimulated ideas and curiosity for routine and new events (i.e. in the person's residence, neighbourhood, or community).
    Domain B3— Emotion: Loss of, or diminished, emotion as evidenced by at least one of the following:
        Initiation symptom: loss of spontaneous emotion, observed or self-reported (for example, subjective feeling of weak or absent emotions, or observation by others of a blunted affect).
        Responsiveness symptom: loss of emotional responsiveness to positive or negative stimuli or events (for example, observer-reports of unchanging affect, or of little emotional reaction to exciting events, personal loss, serious illness, emotional-laden news).
C: These symptoms (A - B) cause clinically significant impairment in personal, social, occupational, or other important areas of functioning.
D: The symptoms (A - B) are not exclusively explained or due to physical disabilities (e.g. blindness and loss of hearing), to motor disabilities, to diminished level of consciousness or to the direct physiological effects of a substance (e.g. drug of abuse, a medication).

Adapted from: Mulin E, Leone E, Dujardin K, et al. Diagnostic criteria for apathy in clinical practice. Int J Geriatr Psychiatry 2011 Feb; 26(2):158-65.

Apathy appears to correlate well with greater severity of depression and functional impairment in PD, and may be a predictor of dementia in the absence of depression [54].

Apathy in Parkinson's Disease: Treatment

There are no standardized treatments for apathy or abulia in the absence of depression or for persistent apathy despite treatment of depression. Antidepressants commonly used to treat depression in PD, such as SSRIs, are generally ineffective treatment options for apathy and abulia. Often, optimization of motor symptoms with dopamine agonists and levodopa to induce "on-states" may alleviate apathy to some degree. Psychostimulants such as amphetamine salts and methylphenidate may be effective, though response is often incomplete and variable. Bupropion may also show some benefit with minimal risk of worsening movement symptoms [42]. Based on results of a single small trial, the cholinesterase inhibitor rivastigmine may be considered, even in those without depression or cognitive dysfunction

[12]. However, the clinical relevance and reproducibility of the changes observed in the trial are uncertain, and further studies are needed.

Fatigue in Parkinson's Disease: Assessment and Treatment

Fatigue was proposed as one of the symptoms on Parkinson's spectrum. Differentiating between bradykinesia, sleepiness, apathy, and fatigue may be difficult. Suboptimally treated bradykinesia sometimes presents as subjective fatigue. However, in some cases fatigue appears in patients with mild bradykinesia and its origin is poorly understood.

Treatment of fatigue in PD begins with an attempt to identify the cause. Excessive daytime sleepiness (EDS) and depression are both the most common and the most treatable identifiable causes. Potentially reversible causes, such as hypothyroidism and medication side effects, should be investigated as well [49].

Medications used for empiric treatment of fatigue, including amantadine and stimulants such as methylphenidate and pemoline, could be an option. However, the response to these is often insufficient. In one 6-week trial, 36 patients with PD were randomly assigned to treatment with either methylphenidate (10 mg three times daily) or placebo [55]. A significant reduction in two measures of self-reported fatigue for patients assigned to methylphenidate was reported. Following this trial, a practice parameter from the American Academy of Neurology (AAN) concluded that methylphenidate is "possibly useful" for treating fatigue in patients with PD [56]. However, it is unclear whether the benefit of methylphenidate for fatigue in this setting is clinically meaningful. Of note, modafinil was not effective for improving either EDS (the primary outcome measure) or fatigue (a secondary outcome measure) in the randomized controlled trial [57].

Psychosis in Parkinson's Disease

Definition of Psychosis and Psychosis of Parkinson's Disease

Psychosis is broadly defined as a loss of contact with reality. It defines syndromes that impair both thought content and thought process which can result from any number of diseases and disorders. Disturbances in thought content include perceptions that are not based in reality, whereas disturbances in thought process reflect thoughts that are disorganized and illogical in form. Psychosis may present as acute or chronic, primary psychiatric or secondary in the course of other medical conditions [58]. The term psychosis envelopes two phenomena: delusions and hallucinations. Delusions are persistent beliefs that are not accepted in the context of a person's cultural and religious background, whereas hallucinations are false sensory perceptions. A slightly broader definition of psychosis can include disorganized speech or behavior. Symptoms of psychosis are typically episodic and these episodes are generally precipitated or exacerbated by psychosocial stressors [5, 6, 58]. Psychosis is a debilitating symptom of PD. It is an independent risk factor for nursing home placement, increases caregiver distress and patient mortality [4]. Consensus diagnostic criteria were established for psychosis in PD [59]. National Institute of Neurological Disorders and Stroke and the National Institute of Mental Health (NINDS-NIMH) criteria require the presence of at least one of the following: hallucinations, delusions, illusions, or false sense of presence. Psychosis must occur within the setting of a clear sensorium and a chronic course (> 1 month), either recurrent or continuous. Other medical, neurologic, or psychiatric causes for the symptoms must be excluded [58].

Extent of the Problem, Pathogenesis, and Impact

The lifetime prevalence of psychosis in PD has been estimated at 50%, with a range of 25% to 60% depending on diagnostic criteria used [60, 61]. Criteria for PD psychosis include milder psychotic phenomena, such as visual illusions or sense of presence [58]. In one study of 116 PD patients, the cross-sectional prevalence of PD psychosis was 43% with the more traditional definition of psychosis, but with the more inclusive NINDS-NIMH criteria, increased to 60% [60, 61].

Visual hallucinations are the most common psychotic manifestation in PD. These hallucinations may be nonthreatening, brief, and well formed (reports of small children or animals are common). Hallucinations occur more frequently during times of decreased environmental stimulation, such as in the evening, low ambient lighting, or decreased sound levels. A false sense of presence or passage, as well as visual illusions, are considered minor psychotic phenomena but can affect anywhere from 17% to 72% of PD patients [61]. While auditory, olfactory, or tactile hallucinations are less common than their visual counterparts, they do occur; up to 20% of patients report auditory hallucinations. Nonvisual hallucinations or mixed hallucinations are more common in patients who develop psychotic symptoms at advanced ages [59]. Minor hallucinations such as presence and passage hallucinations may precede the structured visual hallucinations [61].

Delusions occur in about 5% of PD patients. Dopaminergic medications, cognitive dysfunction, depression, sleep disturbances, and longer duration of PD are risk factors for the emergence of psychosis in PD [62].

Rationale for Pharmacotherapy and Other Interventions

Tapering or elimination of antiparkinsonian medications, starting with the most recently added medications, is a first step, usually starting with those most likely to contribute to confusion (Figure 8.2). As mentioned before, if at all possible, psychotic PD

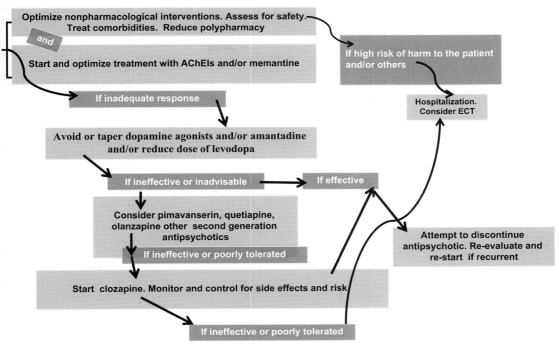

Figure 8.2 Treatment of psychosis in Parkinson's disease

patients should only be on levodopa for their motor symptoms [40].

Efforts to treat psychosis of PD with antipsychotics commonly used for primary psychotic disorders to date have been challenging and associated with significant deterioration of the motor symptoms [63]. Typical antipsychotics, particularly potent blockers of dopaminergic receptors, are usually contraindicated in PD.

Observational studies which targeted PDD found beneficial effects of olanzapine in addressing psychosis, especially delusions [63]. Worsening of motor function and overall psychiatric symptoms, however, have been reported in up to 80% of individuals with PDD following olanzapine treatment [64].

Risperidone was beneficial in managing psychotic symptoms of PDD. In the same group, treatment with risperidone improved levels of social, occupational, and psychological functioning. In practice, an unfavorable safety profile limits risperidone use [62].

Clozapine is efficacious in the treatment of PD psychosis as shown by randomized controlled trials even in relatively low dosing ranges (6.25 to 50 mg daily) [65]. Clozapine is a selective D1 mesolimbic receptor blocker without significant binding to striatal dopamine D2 receptors. This selectivity together with its greater serotoninergic 5HT-2A/2 C affinity, results in clozapine's favorable profile in managing PD psychosis. It is the antipsychotic medication that has consistently been found to be efficacious [62]. The risk of agranulocytosis and the necessity of blood monitoring with clozapine has led many experts to recommend a trial of other antipsychotics, mainly quetiapine (12.5 to 150 mg) before implementing use of clozapine. Clozapine should be immediately stopped when the absolute neutrophil count is below 2000 mm^3 and the white blood cell count is below 3.6 mm^3 [63, 65].

Quetiapine is the most frequently prescribed antipsychotic to target psychotic symptoms in PD. In its chemical structure, (dibenzothiazepine) quetiapine is similar to clozapine. Findings are, however, inconsistent and firm conclusions about quetiapine efficacy cannot be drawn. One open-label trial found a significant improvement in psychotic symptoms (as assessed by BPRS) in patients treated with quetiapine for 12 weeks. In this study the benefit of quetiapine (mean dose 91.5 mg/daily) was comparable with a benefit of clozapine (mean dose 26 mg/daily) [66]. A meta-analysis of data from different trials including a total of 241 participants randomized to either quetiapine or a comparator (placebo or clozapine) failed to show efficacy [67]. Several studies report improvement in the level of global clinical functioning of the PD patients with psychosis treated with quetiapine (as assessed by clinical global impression scales) [66, 67]. Most studies indicate that patients taking quetiapine experienced fewer side effects compared to other antipsychotics; however, quetiapine has yet to be proven to be more effective than placebo in the treatment of psychosis in this population.

In severe cases of PD psychosis, hospitalization should be considered in order to stabilize the patient. Somatic therapies may be an option in certain clinical situations. In PD, ECT was proved to be effective for depression and motor symptoms as well as for psychosis. It could then be considered to treat psychosis that has not responded to other interventions [68].

As noted earlier, the only pharmacological agent with FDA approval for treatment of Parkinson's disease psychosis (PDP) is pimavanserin, a selective-serotonin inverse agonist that preferentially targets 5-HT2A receptors, while avoiding activity at dopamine and other receptors commonly targeted by antipsychotics. The FDA's decision to approve pimavanserin was based on the results of a trial in which adults with PDP were randomly assigned to take 40 mg of pimavanserin or placebo daily for 6 weeks. Patients taking pimavanserin experienced fewer and less severe hallucinations and delusions without motor side effects, which is commonly seen in other antipsychotics that function through dopamine blockade. The most common adverse effects reported by patients taking pimavanserin included peripheral edema, nausea, and confusion [69].

Impulse Control Disorders and Dopamine Dysregulation Syndrome

Definition

The impulse control disorders (ICDs) are a family of neuropsychiatric conditions whose central feature is the uncontrollable need to engage in repetitive behaviors, often to a maladaptive degree. Due to their intimate relationship to dopamine agonist and replacement therapy, ICDs may represent a tremendous burden in and of themselves and may also limit optimal control of motor symptoms, leading to poorer functional outcomes and greater overall disease burden. The four most prominent

treatment-associated ICDs include compulsive gambling, hypersexuality, binge eating, and uncontrollable spending [58].

Impulse control disorders are found in almost 14% of patients being treated for PD, with pathological gambling and compulsive spending accounting for the largest percentage of cases [70]. ICDs are most prominent for patients taking dopamine agonists such as pramipexole and ropinirole, and may be enhanced when any of these are taken in conjunction with levodopa. Levodopa therapy alone is generally not associated with an increase in ICDs, except at very high dosages.

Levodopa, however, is commonly associated with the related dopamine dysregulation syndrome. Patients are often unlikely to volunteer information about the occurrence or increased urge to engage in impulsive behaviors such as hypersexuality and unrestrained gambling (though an attentive spouse or family member may bring it to the physician's attention). Certain ICDs may be idiosyncratic and specific to particular life-long tendencies (kleptomania, reckless generosity, and hoarding), and therefore difficult to uncover with general screening. This may be particularly true with "hobby-ism" and other dopamine dysregulation disorders [70].

Impulse control disorders in PD cluster with worse set-shifting and reward-related decision-making, and increased depression, anxiety, anhedonia, and impulsivity. All above have a negative impact on the quality of life of patients and their caregivers [71].

Rationale for Pharmacotherapy and Other Interventions

Patients with pre-existing or comorbid ICDs, as well as those with substance-use disorders, obsessive-compulsive disorder (OCD), or tic disorders are at a greater risk for the development of treatment-related ICDs and compulsive behaviors. Dopamine agonists should either be avoided in these patients if possible, or closely monitored to detect and avoid the occurrence of these disorders. In most patients, tapering and/or discontinuing dopamine agonist agents will improve or eliminate ICDs and compulsive behaviors. Generally, dopamine agonist therapy should be tapered slowly to reduce the risk of dopamine agonist withdrawal symptoms (DAWS) such as irritability, agitation, and dysphoria. Transition to levodopa is generally indicated in these situations.

In regards to symptomatic pharmacotherapy for ICD in PD patients – one randomized cross-over trial of 17 patients found that amantadine (target dose 100 mg twice daily), administered as add-on to baseline antiparkinsonian medications, reduced pathologic gambling in all treated patients [72]. Limited evidence favors active treatment with naltrexone [73].

Dopamine dysregulation syndrome may require transition from levodopa to dopamine agonist [62]. Where dysregulated behaviors (impulsive, compulsive, and/or addictive tendencies) persist despite elimination of dopaminergic agents, there is little evidence available for management. Anecdotal reports have demonstrated variable benefit from atypical antipsychotics, naltrexone, and/or mood stabilizers [74]. Moreover, deep brain stimulation of the subthalamic nucleus might be a potential method in controlling impulsive and compulsive behaviors in PD [74].

References

1. Gallagher DA, Schrag A. Psychosis, apathy, depression and anxiety in Parkinson's disease. Neurobiol Dis 2012; 46: 581–589.

2. Barone P, Antonini A, Colosimo C, et al. The PRIAMO study: a multicenter assessment of nonmotor symptoms and their impact on quality of life in Parkinson's disease. Mov Disord 2009; 24(11): 1641–1649.

3. Lin YQ, Chen SD. RBD: a red flag for cognitive impairment in Parkinson's disease? Sleep Med 2018; 44: 38.

4. Marsh L, Williams JR, Rocco M, et al. Psychiatric comorbidities in patients with Parkinson disease and psychosis. Neurology 2004; 63: 293–300.

5. Rothenberg KG. Assessment and management of psychiatric symptoms in neurodegenerative disorders (chapter 23) In: Babak T, Cummings J (eds.). Neuro-Geriatrics. Springer International Publishing AG; 2017.

6. Rothenberg KG, Rajaram R. Advances in management of psychosis in neurodegenerative diseases. Curr Treat Options Neurol 2019; 21(1): 3.

7. Blonder LX, Slevin JT. Emotional dysfunction in Parkinson's disease. Behav Neurol 2011; 24(3): 201–217.

8. Stoyka LE, Arrant AE, Thrasher DR, et al. Behavioral defects associated with amygdala and cortical dysfunction in mice with seeded α-synuclein inclusions. Neurobiol Dis 2020; 134: 104708: 1–11.

9. Bohnen NI, Kaufer DI, Hendrickson R, et al. Cognitive correlates of cortical cholinergic denervation in Parkinson's disease and parkinsonian dementia. J Neurol 2006; 253: 242.

10. Shimada H, Hirano S, Shinotoh H, et al. Mapping of brain acetylcholinesterase alterations in Lewy body disease by PET. Neurology 2009; 73: 273.

11. Ehrt U, Broich K, Larsen JP, et al. Use of drugs with anticholinergic effect and impact on cognition in Parkinson's disease: a cohort study. J Neurol Neurosurg Psychiatry 2010; 81: 160.

12. Devos D, Moreau C, Maltête D, et al. Rivastigmine in apathetic but dementia and depression-free patients with Parkinson's disease: a double-blind, placebo-controlled, randomised clinical trial. J Neurol Neurosurg Psychiatry 2014; 85(6): 668–674.

13. Dubois B, Tolosa E, Katzenschlager R, et al. Donepezil in Parkinson's disease dementia: a randomized, double-blind efficacy and safety study. Mov Disord 2012; 27: 1230–1238.

14. Ekman U, Eriksson J, Forsgren L, et al. Functional brain activity and presynaptic dopamine uptake in patients with Parkinson's disease and mild cognitive impairment: a cross-sectional study. Lancet Neurol 2012; 11: 679–687.

15. Marini P, Ramat S, Ginestroni A, Paganini M. Deficit of short-term memory in newly diagnosed untreated parkinsonian patients: reversal after L-dopa therapy. Neurol Sci 2003; 24: 184.

16. Morrison CE, Borod JC, Brin MF, et al. Effects of levodopa on cognitive functioning in moderate-to-severe Parkinson's disease (MSPD). J Neural Transm 2004; 111: 1333.

17. Bohnen NI, Albin RL, Müller ML, et al. Frequency of cholinergic and caudate nucleus dopaminergic deficits across the pre-demented cognitive spectrum of Parkinson disease and evidence of interaction effects. JAMA Neurol 2015; 72: 194.

18. Murai T, Muller U, Werheid K, et al. In vivo evidence for differential association of striatal dopamine and midbrain serotonin systems with neuropsychiatric symptoms in Parkinson's disease. J Neuropsychiatry Clin Neurosci 2001; 13: 222–228.

19. Huot P, Johnston TH, Darr T, et al. Increased 5-HT2A receptors in the temporal cortex of parkinsonian patients with visual hallucinations. Mov Disord 2010; 25: 1399–1408.

20. Ballanger B, Strafella AP, van Eimeren T, et al. Serotonin 2A receptors and visual hallucinations in Parkinson disease. Arch Neurol 2010; 67: 416.

21. Poletti M, Frosini D, Pagni C, et al. Mild cognitive impairment and cognitive-motor relationships in

newly diagnosed drug-naive patients with Parkinson's disease. J Neurol Neurosurg Psychiatry 2012; **83**: 601–606.

22. Cummings J, Ritter A, Rothenberg KG. Advances in management of neuropsychiatric syndromes in neurodegenerative diseases. Curr Psychiatry Rep 2019; **21**(8): 79.

23. Rothenberg KG, Wiechers IR. Antipsychotics for neuropsychiatric symptoms of dementia – safety and efficacy in the context of informed consent. Psychiatr Ann 2015; **45**(7): 348–353.

24. Litvan I, Goldman JG, Tröster AI, et al. Diagnostic criteria for mild cognitive impairment in Parkinson's disease: Movement Disorder Society Task Force guidelines. Mov Disord 2012; **27**(3): 349–356.

25. Weintraub D, Simuni T, Caspell-Garcia C, et al. Cognitive performance and neuropsychiatric symptoms in early, untreated Parkinson's disease. Mov Disord 2015; **30**: 919.

26. Emre M, Aarsland D, Brown R, et al. Clinical diagnostic criteria for dementia associated with Parkinson's disease. Mov Disord 2007; **22**: 1689–1707.

27. Svenningsson P, Westman E, Ballard C, Aarsland D. Cognitive impairment in patients with Parkinson's disease: diagnosis, biomarkers, and treatment. Lancet Neurol 2012; **11**: 697.

28. Aarsland D, Zaccai J, Brayne C. A systematic review of prevalence studies of dementia in Parkinson's disease. Mov Disord 2005; **20**: 1255.

29. Buter TC, van den Hout A, Matthews FE, et al. Dementia and survival in Parkinson disease: a 12-year population study. Neurology 2008; **70**(13): 1017–1022.

30. Hely MA, Reid WG, Adena MA, et al. The Sydney multicenter study of Parkinson's disease: the inevitability of dementia at 20 years. Mov Disord 2008; **23**: 837.

31. Levy G, Schupf N, Tang MX, et al. Combined effect of age and severity on the risk of dementia in Parkinson's disease. Ann Neurol 2002; **51**: 72.

32. Anang JB, Gagnon JF, Bertrand JA, et al. Predictors of dementia in Parkinson disease: a prospective cohort study. Neurology 2014; **83**(14): 1253–1260.

33. Liu G, Boot B, Locascio JJ, et al. Specifically neuropathic Gaucher's mutations accelerate cognitive decline in Parkinson's. Ann Neurol 2016; **80**: 674.

34. Obi T, Nishioka K, Ross OA, et al. Clinicopathologic study of a SNCA gene duplication patient with Parkinson disease and dementia. Neurology 2008; **70**: 238.

35. Williams-Gray CH, Evans JR, Goris A, et al. The distinct cognitive syndromes of Parkinson's disease: 5-year follow-up of the CamPaIGN cohort. Brain 2009; **132**: 2958–2969.

36. Morley JF, Xie SX, Hurtig HI, et al. Genetic influences on cognitive decline in Parkinson's disease. Mov Disord 2012; **27**: 512–518.

37. Lin CH, Fan JY, Lin HI, et al. Catechol-O-methyltransferase (COMT) genetic variants are associated with cognitive decline in patients with Parkinson's disease. Parkinsonism Relat Disord 2018; **50**: 48–53.

38. Grünewald A, Kasten M, Ziegler A, Klein C. Next-generation phenotyping using the parkin example: time to catch up with genetics. JAMA Neurol 2013; **70**: 1186.

39. Fang L, Tang BS, Fan K, et al. Alzheimer's disease susceptibility genes modify the risk of Parkinson disease and Parkinson's disease-associated cognitive impairment. Neurosci Lett 2018; **677**: 55–59.

40. Hindle JV. The practical management of cognitive impairment and psychosis in the older Parkinson's disease patient. J Neural Transm 2013; **120**: 649–653.

41. Seppi K, Weintraub D, Coelho M, et al. The Movement Disorder Society evidence-based medicine review update: treatments for the non-motor symptoms of Parkinson's disease. Mov Disord 2011; **26** Suppl 3: 42–80.

42. Connolly BS, Fox SH. Drug treatments for the neuropsychiatric complications of Parkinson's Disease. Expert Rev Neurother 2012; **12**: 1439–1449.

43. Emre M, Aarsland D, Albanese A, et al. Rivastigmine for dementia associated with Parkinson's disease. N Engl J Med 2004; **351**: 2509–2518.

44. Maidment I, Fox C, Boustani M. Cholinesterase inhibitors for Parkinson's disease dementia. Cochrane Database Syst Rev 2006; **25**(1): CD004747.

45. Minett TS, Thomas A, Wilkinson LM, et al. What happens when donepezil is suddenly withdrawn? An open label trial in dementia with Lewy bodies and Parkinson's disease with dementia. Int J Geriatr Psychiatry 2003; **18**: 988.

46. Aarsland D, Ballard C, Walker Z, et al. Memantine in patients with Parkinson's disease dementia or dementia with Lewy bodies: a double-blind, placebo-controlled, multicentre trial. Lancet Neurol 2009; **8**: 613–618.

47. Wang HF, Yu JT, Tang SW, et al. Efficacy and safety of cholinesterase inhibitors and memantine

in cognitive impairment in Parkinson's disease, Parkinson's disease dementia, and dementia with Lewy bodies: systematic review with meta-analysis and trial sequential analysis. J Neurol Neurosurg Psychiatry 2015; **86**: 135–143.

48. Monastero R, Camarda C, Pipia C, Camarda R. Visual hallucinations and agitation in Alzheimer's disease due to memantine: report of three cases. J Neurol Neurosurg Psychiatry 2007; **78**(5): 546.

49. Weintraub D, Burn D. Parkinson's disease: the quintessential neuropsychiatric disorder. Mov Disord 2011; **26**(6): 1022–1031.

50. Troeung L, Egan SJ, Gasson N. A meta-analysis of randomised placebo-controlled treatment trials for depression and anxiety in Parkinson's disease. PLoS One 2013; **8**(11): e79510.

51. Barone P, Scarzella L, Marconi R, et al. Depression/Parkinson Italian Study Group. Pramipexole versus sertraline in the treatment of depression in Parkinson's disease: a national multicenter parallel-group randomized study. J Neurol 2006; **253**(5): 601–607.

52. Richard IH, McDermott MP, Kurlan R, et al. A randomized, double-blind, placebo-controlled trial of antidepressants in Parkinson disease. Neurology 2012; **78**(16): 1229–1236.

53. Mulin E, Leone E, Dujardin K, et al. Diagnostic criteria for apathy in clinical practice. Int J Geriatr Psychiatry 2011; **26**(2): 158–165.

54. Dujardin K, Sockeel P, Delliaux M, et al. Apathy may herald cognitive decline and dementia in Parkinson's disease. Mov Disord 2009; **24**: 2391–2397.

55. Mendonça DA, Menezes K, Jog MS. Methylphenidate improves fatigue scores in Parkinson disease: a randomized controlled trial. Mov Disord 2007; **22**: 2070.

56. Zesiewicz TA, Sullivan KL, Arnulf I, et al. Practice parameter: treatment of nonmotor symptoms of Parkinson disease: report of the Quality Standards Subcommittee of the American Academy of Neurology. Neurology 2010; **74**: 924.

57. Ondo WG, Fayle R, Atassi F, Jankovic J. Modafinil for daytime somnolence in Parkinson's disease: double blind, placebo controlled parallel trial. J Neurol Neurosurg Psychiatry 2005; **76**: 1636.

58. *American Psychiatric Association Diagnostic and Statistical Manual of Mental Disorders*, 5th ed. American Psychiatric Association; 2013.

59. Ravina B, Marder K, Fernandez HH, et al. Diagnostic criteria for psychosis in Parkinson's disease: report of an NINDS, NIMH work group. Mov Disord 2007; **22**: 1061–1068.

60. Fenelon G, Soulas T, Zenasni F, de Langavant LC. The changing face of Parkinson's disease-associated psychosis: a cross-sectional study based on the new NINDS-NIMH criteria. Mov Disord 2010; **25**: 755–759.

61. Fenelon G, Alves G. Epidemiology of psychosis in Parkinson's disease. J Neurol Sci 2010; **289**: 12–17.

62. Goetz CG. New developments in depression, anxiety, compulsiveness, and hallucinations in Parkinson's disease. Mov Disord 2010; **25** Suppl 1: 104–109.

63. Goldman JG, Holden S. Treatment of psychosis and dementia in Parkinson's disease. Curr Treat Options Neurol 2014; **16**(3): 281–299.

64. Moretti R, Torre P, Antonello RM, et al. Olanzapine as a treatment of neuropsychiatric disorders of Alzheimer's disease and other dementias: a 24-month follow-up of 68 patients. Am J Alzheimers Dis Other Demen 2003; **18**: 205–214.

65. Pollak P, Tison F, Rascol O, et al. Clozapine in drug induced psychosis in Parkinson's disease: a randomised, placebo controlled study with open follow up. J Neurol Neurosurg Psychiatry 2004; **75** (5): 689–695.

66. Morgante L, Epifanio A, Spina E, et al. Quetiapine and clozapine in parkinsonian patients with dopaminergic psychosis. Clin Neuropharmacol 2004; **27**(4): 153–156.

67. Desmarais P, Massoud F, Filion J, Nguyen QD, Bajsarowicz P. Quetiapine for psychosis in Parkinson disease and neurodegenerative parkinsonian disorders: a systematic review. J Geriatr Psychiatry Neurol 2016; **29**(4): 227–236.

68. Hausner L, Damian M, Sartorius A, Frolich L. Efficacy and cognitive side effects of ECT in depressed elderly inpatients with co-existing mild cognitive impairment or dementia. J Clin Psychiatry 2011; **72**: 91–97.

69. Cummings J, Isaacson S, Mills R, et al. Pimavanserin for patients with Parkinson's disease psychosis: a randomised, placebo-controlled phase 3 trial. Lancet 2014; **383**(9916): 533–540.

70. Weintraub D, Claassen DO. Impulse control and related disorders in Parkinson's disease. Int Rev Neurobiol 2017; **133**: 679–717.

71. Martini A, Dal Lago D, Edelstyn NMJ, Grange JA, Tamburin S. Impulse control disorder in

Parkinson's disease: a meta-analysis of cognitive, affective, and motivational correlates. Front Neurol 2018; **28**(9): 654.

72. Thomas A, Bonanni L, Gambi F, Di Iorio A, Onofrj M. Pathological gambling in Parkinson disease is reduced by amantadine. Ann Neurol 2010; **68**(3): 400–404.

73. Papay K, Xie SX, Stern M, et al. Naltrexone for impulse control disorders in Parkinson disease: a placebo-controlled study. Neurology 2014; **83**(9): 826–833.

74. Zhang G, Zhang Z, Liu L, et al. Impulsive and compulsive behaviors in Parkinson's disease. Front Aging Neurosci 2014; **6**: 318.

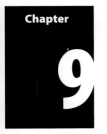

Mood Disorders in Parkinson's Disease

Po-Heng Tsai and Ganesh Gopalakrishna

Introduction

Parkinson's disease (PD) is traditionally characterized by its motor symptoms of tremors, bradykinesia, rigidity, and postural instability [1]. However, it is now recognized that non-motor symptoms including neuropsychiatric manifestations are frequently present in PD, and their onset not only could precede motor symptoms but is also associated with increased dysfunction and reduced quality of life [2–4]. This chapter focuses on depression, the most commonly seen mood disorder in PD, and provides an overview of the epidemiology, clinical symptoms, proposed pathophysiology, diagnostic tools, and treatment options available for depression in PD.

Epidemiology

Depression is common and could occur in any stage of PD from the prodromal phase (i.e. before the appearance of motor symptoms) [5, 6], early stage of diagnosis [7], and all the way until late in the course of the disease [8]. Reported prevalence rates of depression in PD ranged from 2.7% to 90%. The notable difference is likely related to several factors that include patient population studied, diagnostic method used, and types of depressive disorders included in the analysis. Generally, prevalence rates are lower in community-based cohorts and from studies where diagnosis was derived from structured or semi-structured interviews and diagnostic criteria while prevalence is higher in clinical settings such as outpatient and inpatient clinics and with self-reported measures.

A commonly quoted prevalence rate based on a systemic review of 36 studies indicated clinically significant depressive symptoms were present in 35% or around one-third of PD patients [9]. The presence of clinically relevant depressive symptoms was defined as either the patients who fulfilled depressive disorders criteria based on the *Diagnostic Statistical Manual* (DSM) or the patients who scored above the cut-off scores for depression rating scales. For those studies utilizing DSM criteria, the prevalence in PD patients for major depressive disorder was 17%, minor depression 22%, and dysthymia 13%.

Multiple prospective studies have investigated risk factors associated with the development of depression in PD patients [10, 11]. The most commonly identified risk factor is disease severity. Other factors that have been found to correlate with depression include female gender, more severe motor fluctuations, early onset of PD, occurrence of falls, autonomic and cognitive dysfunction, comorbid anxiety, presence of hallucinations, poorer nighttime sleep, and daytime sleepiness. For PD patients that have received deep brain stimulation, depression is a common complication when subthalamic nucleus was chosen as the site of stimulation [12].

Pathophysiology

Although the pathogenesis of depression in PD has not been completely elucidated, it is likely multifactorial in origin and involves anatomical and biochemical changes in PD, psychosocial issues associated with living with a chronic disease, genetic factors, and comorbid medical conditions [13].

Disturbances in the monoamine neurotransmitters (i.e. dopamine, serotonin, and norepinephrine) have been implicated as an important mechanism in depression in PD [14]. One of the most salient pathological changes in the brains of PD patients is the neuronal loss and gliosis of dopamine-containing cells in the substantia nigra and associated depletion of dopamine in the striatum. Increased nigral neuronal loss and decreased binding to dopamine transporters in the striatum have both been associated with depression in PD, possibly mediated through the frontostriatal and mesocorticolimbic dopaminergic circuits [15]. In addition to neuronal loss in the substantia nigra, cell loss of noradrenergic neurons in the locus ceruleus and less so with serotonergic neurons in the dorsal raphe nucleus have been associated with depression in PD as demonstrated in pathological, biochemical, structural, functional, and animal studies [16].

Besides the aforementioned neurobiological perspectives, psychosocial issues such as the stress associated with the presence of disability and its onset in relation to a patient's age and rate of progression have been suggested to contribute to depression in PD. Factors influencing a patient's ability to deal with such stress include personality, learned defense/coping mechanisms, social situations, and availability and quality of support are also important to consider [13]. Societal ableism resulting in stigmatizing attitudes and interactions could add to a PD patient's psychological difficulties as well [17].

Symptoms and Diagnosis

As noted above, depression is common among patients with PD and has a significant impact on quality of life for patients and caregivers. Patients, family, and often clinicians attribute feelings of sadness and associated depressive symptoms to emotional reactions. This could be in the context of being diagnosed with PD or other situational stressors. However, it is important to differentiate adjustment disorders from major depression among this cohort.

The DSM-5 does not have a distinct diagnosis for depression among PD patients. Depressive disorders in PD are diagnosed along the same diagnostic categories as with non-PD depression. Common symptoms include depressed mood, lack of interest in previously pleasurable activities (anhedonia), impaired sleep, disturbance in appetite, and fatigue. Patients may also develop death wishes and suicidal ideations. Major and minor depression are recognized based on the impact of depressive symptoms on the patient's functioning.

A substantial challenge in assessing for depression in PD is a significant overlap of symptoms, including somatic and neurocognitive symptoms, between the two disorders [18]. This is further complicated by the side effects from medications

to treat motor symptoms, comorbid psychosis, and cognitive decline. Hence, there is an emphasis on eliciting emotional depressive symptoms, such as depressed mood, guilt, feelings of hopelessness, negative ruminations, tearfulness, and self-harm thoughts, rather than neurovegetative symptoms, to assist in diagnosis and monitoring of symptoms [19]. An "inclusive approach" has been recommended in diagnosis and management of depression in PD [20]. Suicidal ideations are much more common in PD compared to the general population with rates as high as 30% in many studies. However, it is not clear if the completed suicide rates are different in this population [21].

Neurologists have demonstrated low sensitivity and high specificity in diagnosing depression among PD patients [22]. Direct inquiry with patients and their caregivers is important to detect depression early and treat accordingly. A clinical interview using DSM-5 diagnostic care is the standard practice in the clinical setting. Diagnostic rating scales can be useful in screening for various psychiatric symptoms, including depression and anxiety. They can also be instrumental in monitoring symptoms during longitudinal follow-up and assessing response to treatments. With the availability of multiple scales, it is important to choose a scale that suits the clinical or research need and is not significantly influenced by the overlap between symptoms of PD and depression. Among clinician-rated scales, Hamilton Depression Rating Scale-17 item (HAMD-17) has demonstrated very good reliability and discriminant validity for screening and measuring severity of depression in PD. Similarly, Montgomery-Asberg Depression Rating Scale (MADRS) has shown good validity and reliability. Abbreviated versions of these scales, which exclude somatic items, may be appropriate for screening purposes per Reijnders et al. [23]. The self-rated Geriatric Depression Scales (GDS-15 and GDS-30) are also appropriate for PD patients of all age groups. GDS-15, being self-rated with good validity and reliability, is an excellent tool for clinical care of depression in PD in ambulatory settings. Other scales to consider include Beck Depression Inventory (BDI), Patient Health Questionnaires (PHQ-2 and PHQ-9), Hospital Anxiety and Depression Scale-Depression Subscale (HADS-D), and Hamilton Depression Inventory (HDI). Patients with cognitive impairment may be screened with Cornell Scale for

Depression in Dementia (CSDD), which relies on observation and interviews with patient and informant. It is worth noting that the depression item of Unified Parkinson's Disease Rating Scale (UPDRS) does not appear to be valid based on the current evidence [24].

Management

Medications

See Table 9.1. The pharmacological treatment of depression in PD (dPD) is similar to management in non-PD patients. Most of the interventions aim to improve the monoamine depletion by various mechanisms. Denervation and subsequent derangement in the dopamine system has been postulated to distinguish the pathophysiology from non-PD depression [25, 26]. The variable definition and measurement of outcomes regarding depressive symptoms contributes to the heterogeneity among the studies. Overall, antidepressants across different classes are effective interventions with good tolerability. There has been evidence to the contrary as well. Selective serotonin reuptake inhibitors (SSRIs) and serotonin norepinephrine reuptake inhibitors (SNRIs) are often the first-line treatment due to better tolerability compared to tricyclic and tetracyclic antidepressants (TCAs) and monoamine oxidase inhibitors (MAOIs). TCAs are frequently associated with anticholinergic side effects, cognitive impairment, and sedation in elderly patients.

Several reviews and meta-analysis showed insufficient evidence to support the efficacy of antidepressants in dPD [27, 28]. Skapinakis et al. conducted a systemic review and meta-analysis of ten randomized controlled trials (RCTs) examining SSRIs in dPD [29]. They concluded lack of efficacy due to crude response rate being 36% with SSRIs and 34% in placebo arms. The authors acknowledged possible type II error due to the small number of studies but questioned the role of the serotonergic system in dPD. Based on three studies, the crude response rate also favored TCAs (57%) over SSRIs (41%). Later Liu et al. conducted a network meta-analysis of RCTS to compare efficacy among various therapeutics in dPD [30]. They used 11 RCTs from 1986 to 2013 in their meta-analysis. They found insufficient evidence to support SSRIs, pramipexole, pergolide, and SNRIs

and identified TCA as the best possible choice. TCAs were superior to SSRIs in response rates and tolerability. Troeung et al. included nine RCTs in their analysis to conclude non-significant pooled effects of antidepressant therapies for treatment of depression and anxiety [31].

In 2015, another systemic review and meta-analysis by Bomasang-Layno et al. examined 893 PD patients across 20 RCTs [32]. This group reported a significant aggregate effect of antidepressants on dPD. A statistically significant effect was noted with SSRIs and not with TCAs, thus contradicting previous similar analyses. Most recently, another group performing a systemic review and meta-analysis supported the efficacy of SSRIs, MAOIs, and TCAs compared to placebo in dPD [26]. The largest effect on depressive symptoms on their network meta-analysis was found with MAOIs.

There has been limited evidence for use of mirtazapine and bupropion in dPD [33]. There is limited evidence to compare SSRIs among themselves or with SNRIs [34]. There was concern about SSRIs worsening the motor symptoms of PD, which has not been substantiated thus far [34, 35].

Dopamine agonists have been evaluated for efficacy in treating dPD. Pramipexole, in particular, showed some efficacy in early studies [36–38]. A systemic review by Leentjens concluded insufficient evidence to support use of dopaminergic agents in treatment of dPD [39]. The most common side effect of dopamine agonists was nausea, followed by headache, dizziness and somnolence, aggravation of dyskinesia, hallucinations, and orthostatic hypotension [30]. Considering the risk of other side effects, the authors suggested using dopamine agonists for patients in early PD, or when depression is noted when dopamine agonists are reduced or discontinued. On a related note, patients on dopamine agonists may have depression-like symptoms during the "off periods" as the medication wears off [40]. It is important to recognize this phenomenon by eliciting the temporality of symptoms. In this case, adjusting the dosing regimen or addition of other medications, such as catechol-O-methyl transferase (COMT) inhibitors or MAO type B (MAOB) inhibitors, can be useful to reduce the hypodopaminergic periods.

Monoamine oxidase type B inhibitors are used as monotherapy and in combination with

Table 9.1 Antidepressants for use in depression in Parkinson's disease

Drug	Initial dose	Maximum dose	Special note
Selective Serotonin Reuptake Inhibitors (SSRIs)			
Fluoxetine	5–10 mg every morning	60 mg	Noted to be activating in elderly. Has a long half-life complicating the wash-out period. Has significant drug interactions.
Paroxetine	10 mg daily	40 mg	Has anticholinergic side effects like urinary retention, constipation, dry mouth, or drowsiness. Abrupt discontinuation or missed doses leads to serotonin withdrawal.
Sertraline	12.5–25 mg daily	200 mg	More gastrointestinal symptoms including diarrhea which may be persistent. Absorption influenced by food.
Citalopram	10 mg daily	20–40 mg	QT prolongation associated with doses more than 20 mg for patients older than 60, with significant hepatic impairment or on concurrent 2D6 inhibitors.
Escitalopram	5 mg every morning	20 mg	Mostly serotonergic action with fewer significant drug interactions.
Serotonin norepinephrine reuptake inhibitors (SNRIs)			
Venlafaxine	37.5 mg once daily	225 mg once daily for extended release. 150 mg twice daily for immediate release.	Available as immediate release or extended release. Stimulating medication apt for patients with low energy and apathy. Associated with dose-dependent increases in blood pressure. Abrupt discontinuation or missed doses leads to serotonin withdrawal.
Desvenlafaxine	50 mg daily	100 mg daily	Metabolite of venlafaxine. Renal dosing required in impairment.
Duloxetine	20 mg daily	60 mg once daily	Can be first choice in patients with co-morbid neuropathic pain.
Atypical antidepressants			
Mirtazapine	7.5 mg every evening	60 mg every evening	Hepatic and renal dosing required. Common side effects of sedation and weight gain. Can be used with poor appetite and poor sleep.
Bupropion	75 mg	450 mg	Available as immediate release, sustained release, and extended release. Activating medication apt for patients with lethargy and hypersomnia. Avoid in patients with seizure disorder.
Vilazodone	10 mg once daily with food	40 mg once daily with food	Absorption affected by food. Less weight gain and sexual side effects.
Tricyclic antidepressants (TCAs)			
Nortriptyline	10 mg every evening	100 mg every evening or in two divided doses.	Associated with anticholinergic side effects, cardiac conduction abnormalities, and orthostatic hypotension. Fatal in overdoses. Reserved for treatment of resistant depression. Therapeutic levels need to be monitored to prevent toxicity.
Desipramine	10 mg every morning	25 to 150 mg every morning or in two divided doses.	

dopamine agonists for treatment of motor symptoms. They are also considered as an option for treating resistant depression. Overall the evidence favors using seligiline or rasagiline in combination with levadopa to improve motor symptoms, activities of daily living, and mental outcome measured by UPDRS [41, 42]. The combination was well tolerated compared to placebo.

Psychotherapies

Psychotherapy is a process of treating psychopathology through communication between the patient and a trained professional in predetermined therapeutic sessions over a period of time. Various psychotherapeutic methods have shown efficacy treating depression among elderly [43]. It can also be an effective adjunctive treatment to antidepressants [44, 45].

Cognitive behavioral therapy (CBT) is a problem-focused intervention which aims to change maladaptive cognitive distortions and behaviors, and consequentially improve emotional adjustment. CBT is one of the most evidence-based psychological interventions for depression. A meta-analysis of longitudinal neuroimaging studies using fMRI, PET, SPECT, and MRS demonstrated a significant group by time effect in left rostral anterior cingulate with increased activity following CBT compared to controls [46]. There have been few studies demonstrating the effectiveness of CBT in PD [47, 48]. Recently, Dobkin et al. conducted an RCT of 80 depressed patients with PD comparing CBT plus clinical management, versus clinical management only. CBT showed significant improvements in several depressive symptoms with cognitive and behavioral (versus somatic) symptoms showing the greatest change [49]. A systemic review and meta-analysis of antidepressant treatments determined that CBT, along with antidepressants, improved depression [32].

Psychodynamic therapy is an intervention based on psychoanalysis, which focuses on influence of unconscious processes and its effects on current behaviors. The brief psychodynamic therapy is a briefer version where the therapist is more active in the session and focuses on a specific concern. A meta-analysis of brief psychotherapy found it to be probably effective in depression and amelioration of cognitive symptoms, albeit high clinical heterogeneity and low methodological validity of included trials [50].

Other Modalities of Treatment

Various other interventions have been explored for treatment of depression among patients with PD. Physical activity or exercise has demonstrated benefits in improving mobility, motor symptoms, balance, and gait in PD [51]. It is postulated that exercise can increase beta-endorphins, facilitated monoamine neurotransmission, and brain-derived neurotropic factor. A systemic review concluded that physical activity, particularly aerobic training, can improve depression and quality of life (QOL) for PD patients [51]. The authors recommend aerobic training including stretching-strengthening exercise, walking, stepping movement for 45–60 minutes, about two to three times a week lasting a total duration of 8 weeks to ameliorate depressive symptoms.

Specific exercise interventions like yoga, mindfulness, Tai Chi and Qigong (TCQ) have been studied for their role in improving mood among patients with depression in PD. Early pilot studies with adaptive yoga programs for PD patients showed improvements in depression scores and QOL [52, 53]. Recently, mindfulness yoga was shown to be superior compared to conventional stretching and resistance training in a multi-site, assessor masked RCT conducted in Hong Kong [54]. A small-scale study of 14 PD patients examined the effectiveness of an eight-week six-session mindfulness program on depression in PD patients [55]. At 6 months follow-up, compared to baseline, the intervention tailored for PD demonstrated reduced anxiety and depression with improved cognition and motor functioning. A systemic review about the effect of mindfulness-based stress reduction (MBSR) on stress and depression concluded limited and inconclusive evidence to support MBSR in PD [56]. A systemic review and meta-analysis by Song et al. evaluated the effects of TCQ on motor, non-motor functions, and QOL among patients with PD [57]. Based on five studies including four RCTs, TCQ showed significant reduction in depression scores compared to control groups with overall medium effect size and limited heterogeneity.

Neurostimulation

Depression, being a common comorbidity in PD, is also frequently resistant to treatment with antidepressants and other non-pharmacological interventions. This is compounded by the medication side effects and interactions with other medications.

This necessitates the use of neurostimulation such as electroconvulsive therapy (ECT) and transcranial magnetic stimulation (TMS).

Electroconvulsive therapy is the procedure of administering electrical current through the brain with an objective to induce a seizure under general anesthesia and muscle relaxation. ECT has demonstrated excellent efficacy in treating depression in general, especially among geriatric patients [58]. The cognitive adverse effects are usually transient and not typically severe. The use of ECT has been restricted due to concerns about cognitive side effects, especially post-ictal delirium, among PD patients [59, 60]. Recently, use of modified ECT delivery methods, such as right unilateral ultra-brief pulse-width ECT, has mitigated the cognitive adverse events while maintaining the efficacy [61]. These results were replicated by Williams et al. in a small open-label study (n=6) among PD patients with treatment-resistant depression or psychosis [60]. A significant improvement in depression as measured by HSRD compared to baseline was noted immediately after treatment and at one-month follow-up. No deficits in cognition were noted and significant improvements were also noted in apathy, motor symptoms, and psychosis.

Transcranial magnetic stimulation is a non-invasive application of an electromagnetic stimulus to the cortex to modify cortical activity in a specific location [62]. It posits upon the hypothesis of left-right imbalance in prefrontal cortical activity with negative impact on prefrontal-limbic networks [63]. TMS involves office-based treatments, without anesthesia, daily for four to six weeks. A meta-analysis evaluating the efficacy of repetitive transcranial magnetic stimulation (rTMS) examined eight RCTs comparing rTMS to either sham treatment or SSRIs. rTMS was noted to be superior to sham-rTMS but had similar efficacy compared to SSRIs. rTMS also demonstrated some improvement in motor functions compared to the other intervention groups. Another meta-analysis investigated the effects of rTMS over prefrontal cortex by examining nine studies with about 137 PD patients [64]. rTMS showed a significant positive effect on depression comparing the pre and post scores, especially using 5.0 Hz frequency with 90% resting motor threshold (RMT). However, this effect was not noted when studies compared rTMS to placebo.

Deep brain stimulation (DBS) is a treatment modality, involving placement of electrodes and stimulation of specific loci on the brain. Despite DBS being used for treatment-resistant depression and PD, it is important to note that the locus of electrode placement is different for the indications. DBS used for PD is commonly placed in the subthalamic nucleus (STN) or globus pallidus internus (GPI). Initial findings of better mood outcomes related to GPI stimulation, compared to STN, has not been substantiated in subsequent studies [65, 66].

References

1. Jankovic J. Parkinson's disease: clinical features and diagnosis. J Neurol Neurosurg Psychiatry 2008; **79**(4): 368–376.

2. Barone P, et al. The PRIAMO study: a multicenter assessment of nonmotor symptoms and their impact on quality of life in Parkinson's disease. Mov Disord 2009; **24**(11): 1641–1649.

3. Weintraub D, et al. Effect of psychiatric and other nonmotor symptoms on disability in Parkinson's disease. J Am Geriatr Soc 2004; **52**(5): 784–788.

4. Schrag A, Jahanshahi M, Quinn N. What contributes to quality of life in patients with Parkinson's disease? J Neurol Neurosurg Psychiatry 2000; **69**(3): 308–312.

5. Ishihara L, Brayne C. A systematic review of depression and mental illness preceding Parkinson's disease. Acta Neurol Scand 2006; **113**(4): 211–220.

6. Shiba M, et al. Anxiety disorders and depressive disorders preceding Parkinson's disease: a case-control study. Mov Disord 2000; **15**(4): 669–677.

7. Ravina B, et al. The impact of depressive symptoms in early Parkinson disease. Neurology 2007; **69**(4): 342–347.

8. Starkstein SE, et al. Depression in Parkinson's disease. J Nerv Ment Dis 1990; **178**(1): 27–31.

9. Reijnders JS, et al. A systematic review of prevalence studies of depression in Parkinson's disease. Mov Disord 2008; **23**(2): 183–189; quiz 313.

10. Dissanayaka NN, et al. Factors associated with depression in Parkinson's disease. J Affect Disord 2011; **132**(1–2): 82–88.

11. Schrag A, Jahanshahi M, Quinn NP. What contributes to depression in Parkinson's disease? Psychol Med 2001; **31**(1): 65–73.

12. Kleiner-Fisman G, et al. Subthalamic nucleus deep brain stimulation: summary and meta-analysis of outcomes. Mov Disord 2006; **21** (Suppl 14): S290–304.

13. Aarsland D, et al. Depression in Parkinson disease–epidemiology, mechanisms and management. Nat Rev Neurol 2011; **8**(1): 35–47.

14. Ehgoetz Martens KA, Lewis SJ. Pathology of behavior in PD: what is known and what is not? J Neurol Sci 2017; **374**: 9–16.

15. Ikemoto S, Yang C, Tan A. Basal ganglia circuit loops, dopamine and motivation: a review and enquiry. Behav Brain Res 2015; **290**: 17–31.

16. Schapira AHV, Chaudhuri KR, Jenner P. Non-motor features of Parkinson disease. Nat Rev Neurosci 2017; **18**(7): 435–450.

17. Simpson J, McMillan H, Reeve D. Reformulating psychological difficulties in people with Parkinson's disease: the potential of a social relational approach to disablism. Parkinsons Dis 2013; **2013**: 608562.

18. Gallagher DA, Schrag A. Psychosis, apathy, depression and anxiety in Parkinson's disease. Neurobiol Dis 2012; **46**(3): 581–589.

19. Marsh L. Depression and Parkinson's disease: current knowledge. Curr Neurol Neurosci Rep 2013; **13**(12): 409.

20. Marsh L, et al. Provisional diagnostic criteria for depression in Parkinson's disease: report of an NINDS/NIMH Work Group. Mov Disord 2006; **21**(2): 148–158.

21. Shepard MD, et al. Suicide in Parkinson's disease. J Neurol Neurosurg Psychiatry 2019; **90**(7): 822–829.

22. Bouwmans AE, Weber WE. Neurologists' diagnostic accuracy of depression and cognitive problems in patients with parkinsonism. BMC Neurol 2012; **12**: 37.

23. Reijnders JS, Lousberg R, Leentjens AF. Assessment of depression in Parkinson's disease: the contribution of somatic symptoms to the clinimetric performance of the Hamilton and Montgomery-Asberg rating scales. J Psychosom Res 2010; **68**(6): 561–565.

24. Torbey E, Pachana NA, Dissanayaka NN. Depression rating scales in Parkinson's disease: a critical review updating recent literature. J Affect Disord 2015; **184**: 216–224.

25. Thobois S, et al. Non-motor dopamine withdrawal syndrome after surgery for Parkinson's disease: predictors and underlying mesolimbic denervation. Brain 2010; **133**(Pt 4): 1111–1127.

26. Mills KA, et al. Efficacy and tolerability of antidepressants in Parkinson's disease: a systematic review and network meta-analysis. Int J Geriatr Psychiatry 2018; **33**(4): 642–651.

27. Weintraub D, et al. Antidepressant studies in Parkinson's disease: a review and meta-analysis. Mov Disord 2005; **20**(9): 1161–1169.

28. Miyasaki JM, et al. Practice parameter: evaluation and treatment of depression, psychosis, and dementia in Parkinson disease (an evidence-based review): report of the Quality Standards Subcommittee of the American Academy of Neurology. Neurology 2006; **66**(7): 996–1002.

29. Skapinakis P, et al. Efficacy and acceptability of selective serotonin reuptake inhibitors for the treatment of depression in Parkinson's disease: a systematic review and meta-analysis of randomized controlled trials. BMC Neurol 2010; **10**: 49.

30. Liu J, et al. Comparative efficacy and acceptability of antidepressants in Parkinson's disease: a network meta-analysis. PLoS One 2013; **8**(10): e76651.

31. Troeung L, Egan SJ, Gasson N. A meta-analysis of randomised placebo-controlled treatment trials for depression and anxiety in Parkinson's disease. PLoS One 2013; **8**(11): e79510.

32. Bomasang-Layno E, et al. Antidepressive treatments for Parkinson's disease: a systematic review and meta-analysis. Parkinsonism Relat Disord 2015; **21**(8): 833–842; discussion 833.

33. Connolly B, Fox SH. Treatment of cognitive, psychiatric, and affective disorders associated with Parkinson's disease. Neurotherapeutics 2014; **11**(1): 78–91.

34. Richard IH, et al. A randomized, double-blind, placebo-controlled trial of antidepressants in Parkinson disease. Neurology 2012; **78**(16): 1229–1236.

35. Arbouw ME, et al. Influence of initial use of serotonergic antidepressants on antiparkinsonian drug use in levodopa-using patients. Eur J Clin Pharmacol 2007; **63**(2): 181–187.

36. Barone P, et al. Pramipexole for the treatment of depressive symptoms in patients with Parkinson's disease: a randomised, double-blind, placebo-controlled trial. Lancet Neurol 2010; **9**(6): 573–580.

37. Rektorova I, et al. Pramipexole and pergolide in the treatment of depression in Parkinson's disease: a national multicentre prospective randomized study. Eur J Neurol 2003; **10**(4): 399–406.

38. Barone P, et al. Pramipexole versus sertraline in the treatment of depression in Parkinson's disease: a national multicenter parallel-group randomized study. J Neurol 2006; **253**(5): 601–607.

39. Leentjens AF. The role of dopamine agonists in the treatment of depression in patients with Parkinson's disease: a systematic review. Drugs 2011; **71**(3): 273–286.

40. Storch A, et al. Nonmotor fluctuations in Parkinson disease: severity and correlation with motor complications. Neurology 2013; **80**(9): 800–809.

41. Jiang DQ, et al. Comparison of selegiline and levodopa combination therapy versus levodopa monotherapy in the treatment of Parkinson's disease: a meta-analysis. Aging Clin Exp Res 2019; **32**: 769–779.

42. Jiang DQ, et al. Rasagiline combined with levodopa therapy versus levodopa monotherapy for patients with Parkinson's disease: a systematic review. Neurol Sci 2020; **41**(1): 101–109.

43. Jonsson U, et al. Psychological treatment of depression in people aged 65 years and over: a systematic review of efficacy, safety, and cost-effectiveness. PLoS One 2016; **11**(8): e0160859.

44. Harter M, et al. Psychotherapy of depressive disorders: evidence in chronic depression and comorbidities. Nervenarzt 2018; **89**(3): 252–262.

45. Meister R, et al. Psychotherapy of depressive disorders: procedures, evidence and perspectives. Nervenarzt 2018; **89**(3): 241–251.

46. Sankar A, et al. A systematic review and meta-analysis of the neural correlates of psychological therapies in major depression. Psychiatry Res Neuroimaging 2018; **279**: 31–39.

47. Farabaugh A, et al. Cognitive-behavioral therapy for patients with Parkinson's disease and comorbid major depressive disorder. Psychosomatics 2010; **51**(2): 124–129.

48. Dobkin RD, et al. Cognitive-behavioral therapy for depression in Parkinson's disease: a randomized, controlled trial. Am J Psychiatry 2011; **168**(10): 1066–1074.

49. Dobkin RD, et al. Cognitive behavioral therapy improves diverse profiles of depressive symptoms in Parkinson's disease. Int J Geriatr Psychiatry 2019; **34**(5): 722–729.

50. Xie CL, et al. A systematic review and meta-analysis of cognitive behavioral and psychodynamic therapy for depression in Parkinson's disease patients. Neurol Sci 2015; **36**(6): 833–843.

51. van der Kolk NM, King LA. Effects of exercise on mobility in people with Parkinson's disease. Mov Disord 2013; **28**(11): 1587–1596.

52. Sharma NK, et al. A randomized controlled pilot study of the therapeutic effects of yoga in people with Parkinson's disease. Int J Yoga 2015; **8**(1): 74–79.

53. Boulgarides LK, Barakatt E, Coleman-Salgado B. Measuring the effect of an eight-week adaptive yoga program on the physical and psychological status of individuals with Parkinson's disease. A pilot study. Int J Yoga Therap 2014; **24**: 31–41.

54. Kwok JYY, et al. Effects of mindfulness yoga vs stretching and resistance training exercises on anxiety and depression for people with Parkinson disease: a randomized clinical trial. JAMA Neurol 2019; **76**(7): 755–763.

55. Dissanayaka NN, et al. Mindfulness for motor and nonmotor dysfunctions in Parkinson's disease. Parkinsons Dis 2016; **2016**: 7109052.

56. McLean G, et al. Mindfulness-based stress reduction in Parkinson's disease: a systematic review. BMC Neurol 2017; **17**(1): 92.

57. Song R, et al. The impact of Tai Chi and Qigong mind-body exercises on motor and non-motor function and quality of life in Parkinson's disease: a systematic review and meta-analysis. Parkinsonism Relat Disord 2017; **41**: 3–13.

58. Geduldig ET, Kellner CH. Electroconvulsive therapy in the elderly: new findings in geriatric depression. Curr Psychiatry Rep 2016; **18**(4): 40.

59. Figiel GS, et al. ECT-induced delirium in depressed patients with Parkinson's disease. J Neuropsychiatry Clin Neurosci 1991; **3**(4): 405–411.

60. Williams NR, et al. Unilateral ultra-brief pulse electroconvulsive therapy for depression in Parkinson's disease. Acta Neurol Scand 2017; **135**(4): 407–411.

61. Sackeim HA, et al. Effects of pulse width and electrode placement on the efficacy and cognitive effects of electroconvulsive therapy. Brain Stimul 2008; **1**(2): 71–83.

62. Rossi S, et al. Safety, ethical considerations, and application guidelines for the use of transcranial magnetic stimulation in clinical practice and research. Clin Neurophysiol 2009; **120**(12): 2008–2039.

63. D'Ostilio K, Garraux G. The network model of depression as a basis for new therapeutic strategies for treating major depressive disorder in Parkinson's disease. Front Hum Neurosci 2016; **10**: 161.

64. Zhou L, et al. Antidepressant effects of repetitive transcranial magnetic stimulation over prefrontal cortex of Parkinson's disease patients with depression: a meta-analysis. Front Psychiatry 2018; **9**: 769.

65. Xu H, et al. Subthalamic nucleus and globus pallidus internus stimulation for the treatment of Parkinson's disease: a systematic review. J Int Med Res 2017; **45**(5): 1602–1612.

66. Wang JW, et al. Cognitive and psychiatric effects of STN versus GPi deep brain stimulation in Parkinson's disease: a meta-analysis of randomized controlled trials. *PLoS One* 2016; **11**(6): e0156721.

Olfactory Dysfunction in Parkinson's Disease and Related Disorders

Richard L. Doty and Christopher H. Hawkes

Introduction

Smell dysfunction is among the earliest and most salient non-motor signs of Parkinson's disease (PD), occurring in an estimated 90% of so-called sporadic cases years before the onset of the classic motor symptoms. Until olfaction is tested formally, the vast majority of PD patients are unaware of their loss, which is usually less than total. The smell problem is rarely identified by neurologists, reflecting, in part, their failure to enquire about smell function let alone testing the olfactory nerve formally. The Quality Standards Committee of the American Academy of Neurology has designated olfactory dysfunction as one of the key diagnostic criteria for PD [1] and the Movement Disorder Society has recommended olfactory testing in the diagnosis of PD [2] and in the identification of prodromal PD [3].

Apart from representing a harbinger of PD, it is underappreciated that smell dysfunction, per se, is debilitating to PD patients. It impacts multiple aspects of their lives, including personal safety, hygiene, nutrition, and enjoyment from nature, foods, and beverages. In one international multicenter survey of PD non-motor symptoms, 26.0% complained of problems tasting or smelling, compared to 7.3% of a control group [4]. This was higher than complaints of bowel incontinence (4.9%), hallucinations (19.5%), sweating (25.2%), and diplopia (21.9%). Smell loss is particularly problematic for patients whose food intake is already compromised and whose mobility limits their ability to react to fire or leaking natural gas. Although statistics are not available for PD, per se, it is well known that those with smell loss are more likely to experience dangerous situations associated with spoiled food, fire, or leaking natural gas [5]. For example, a disproportionate number of otherwise healthy elderly die in accidental gas poisonings due, in part, to age-related smell deterioration [6, 7].

This chapter reviews what is known about the smell loss in various forms of PD, as well as essential tremor (ET), a disorder often confused with PD, and idiopathic rapid eye movement sleep behavior disorder (RBD), a disease that commonly leads to PD.

Classic Parkinson's Disease

Olfactory Phenotype

As reviewed elsewhere [8], the olfactory deficit of sporadic (classical) PD is marked, bilateral, and unresponsive to dopamine-related therapies. It is discernible by all types of standardized olfactory tests, is less severe in smokers or previous smokers than in never smokers, is greater in men than in women, and usually appears, as noted above, long before the onset of the motor dysfunction. The deficit is surprisingly stable over time and in most cases appears to be unrelated to disease stage or duration, although exceptions may occur. It is not confined to any specific set of odorants and exhibits high sensitivity and specificity in differentiating PD from normal controls (0.91 and 0.88, respectively, in males ≤ 60 years of age) [9] and from several diseases commonly confused with PD (e.g. progressive supranuclear palsy (PSP), multiple system atrophy (MSA), and ET). Remarkably, the olfactory deficit of PD is largely indistinguishable from that of mild Alzheimer's disease (AD), regardless of whether odor identification or detection threshold test scores are assessed (Figure 10.1). This is of particular interest, since a) PD patients with olfactory dysfunction are at a much higher risk for subsequent development of dementia and b) PD-related olfactory test scores are correlated, albeit not strongly, with cognitive measures such as verbal memory and executive function [10–12].

There have been several endeavors to identify a short-list of PD-specific odors, principally to help reduce olfactory screening times. Initially pizza and oil of wintergreen from the University

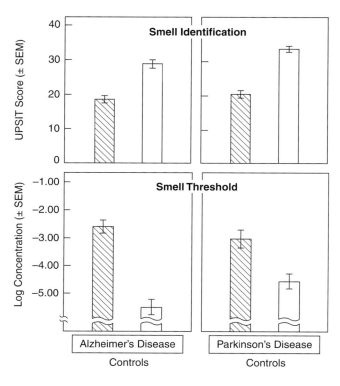

Figure 10.1 Mean (SEM) scores on the University of Pennsylvania Smell Identification Test (UPSIT) and a single ascending staircase detection threshold test using phenyl ethyl alcohol for patients with mild AD (n = 34) or PD (n = 81) and equivalent numbers of age-, gender-, and race-matched controls. All subjects had to score 35 or greater on the Picture Identification Test, a test analogous to the UPSIT except that pictures, rather than smells, are to be identified, thereby controlling for inability of subjects to understand the odorant concepts. Data from [16] and [128].

Copyright © 2017 Richard L. Doty.

of Pennsylvania Smell Identification Test (UPSIT) were found to be significant discriminators by Hawkes and Shephard [13], but subsequent evaluations have yielded variable findings without a consistent pattern. Joseph et al. [14] describe the largest of such studies. This study evaluated the sensitivity and specificity of 23,231,378 combinations of 1–7 UPSIT odorant items to identify subsets of items that optimized sensitivity and specificity in differentiating PD patients from controls. The best seven-item subset produced essentially the same sensitivity and specificity as 12-item B-SIT version B, a test that incorporated the optimal stimuli of Hawkes (respective sensitivities/specificities: 87.3/83.0% versus 88.2/85.4%). Based on their research, the authors ultimately employed a six-odorant screening test for their ongoing PREDICT-PD study comprised of menthol, coconut, onion, clove, orange, and cherry odorants.

There is evidence that asymptomatic first-degree relatives of PD patients with olfactory dysfunction are at higher risk for future development of PD than those with no such impairment. In one study, olfaction was measured in 361 asymptomatic relatives of PD patients [15]. [123I]ß-CIT labeled DA transporter uptake was measured in patients whose test scores fell within the top and bottom

10% of the group. Two years later, none of the 38 relatives who scored in the top 10% had developed clinically defined PD or exhibited DA transporter dysfunction. All of those in the bottom 10% showed reduced DA transporter uptake and four developed clinically defined PD.

It is important to emphasize that hyposmia, not anosmia, is the norm for PD patients, with average UPSIT scores of around 20/40, a score that falls within the severe microsmic range. In one study, only 38% of 81 PD patients were totally anosmic whereas 87% reliably perceived the highest concentration of phenyl ethanol in an odor-detection threshold test [16]. In another study, 40 of 41 PD patients reported that 35 or more of the odorants on the 40-item UPSIT had some type of odor, even though the odors were not clearly discernible or did not correspond to any of the response alternatives [17].

Olfactory System Pathology in Classic Parkinson's Disease

The basis of the smell disturbance of classic PD is enigmatic, since multiple interacting factors, both genetic and environmental, are likely involved. From a pathologic perspective, one hypothesis is that the smell loss reflects early deposition of misfolded α-synuclein primarily within the olfactory bulbs and anterior olfactory nucleus, in accord with the developmental stages of disease progression [18]. This hypothesis accords well with the concept that some environmental agents may enter the brain via the olfactory neuroepithelium to induce or catalyze olfactory dysfunction and other elements of the disease – the so-called Olfactory Vector Hypothesis.

Another theory suggests that smell loss precedes α-synuclein-related pathology, possibly reflecting damage to neurotrophic, neuromodulator, or neurotransmitter systems associated with olfactory function [19]. Such damage may subsequently facilitate prion-like progression of α-synuclein-related pathology throughout the brain. Described below is what is generally known about the olfactory pathology of PD.

Olfactory Neuroepithelium

The hallmark neuropathology of PD is the presence of Lewy neurites and Lewy bodies (LBs). Dystrophic neurites and fragments of amyloid precursor protein analogous to those observed in AD have been demonstrated in the olfactory neuroepithelium [20]. Moreover, all types of synuclein (α, β, γ) are expressed in olfactory receptor neurons, particularly α-synuclein. Importantly, the expression of abnormal α-synuclein within the PD olfactory mucosa does not appear to differ from that of healthy older controls and patients with AD, MSA, and Lewy body disease [21], conditions which are all associated with smell dysfunction. In a study of olfactory epithelial biopsies from seven PD patients (nine of whom had smell dysfunction) and 16 controls, Witt et al. [22] found no clear differences in the relative expression of antibodies against α-synuclein, β-tubulin (BT), cytokeratin, olfactory marker protein (OMP), p75NGFr, protein gene product 9.5 (PGP 9.5), proliferation-associated antigen (Ki 67), and the stem cell marker nestin. They concluded that the olfactory loss of PD is more likely due to central than peripheral olfactory system damage. More recent studies have shown Lewy neurites, but not LBs, within the lamina propria – the basal layer of the olfactory epithelium [23]. Another investigation demonstrated Lewy pathology in the olfactory epithelium of six out of eight PD patients and one with incidental Lewy body disease [24]. Provisionally,

these two recent observations lend support to the concept of the olfactory epithelium as an initiation site for PD.

Central Olfactory Structures

Lewy body and other PD-related pathology is common within the olfactory bulbs and tracts of patients with PD. In a pioneering study, the olfactory bulbs of eight PD patients, but not those of eight controls, exhibited LBs within the mitral cells and cells of anterior olfactory nucleus (AON) [25]. The LB morphology resembled that seen in the cortex, although classic tri-laminar inclusions were rare. Neuronal loss within the AON correlated with disease duration and the number of LBs [26]. In a study by Beach et al. [27], 55 of 58 PD olfactory bulbs contained LBs, resulting in 95% sensitivity and 91% specificity in differentiating PD from controls. A similar finding was noted earlier in a smaller study by Jellinger [28]. The density of α-synucleinopathy within the bulbs correlated strongly with that in other brain regions, as well as with scores on the Mini-Mental State Examination (MMSE) and Unified Parkinson's Disease Rating Scale (UPDRS). More recently, a quantitative assessment of post-mortem olfactory bulb glomeruli revealed a predominantly ventral deficit in the glomerular layers [29], consistent with spread from the underlying nasal olfactory epithelium. In keeping with Braak et al. staging [30], Ubeda-Banon and colleagues demonstrated abnormal α-synuclein expression within the temporal division of the piriform cortex, olfactory tubercle, and the anterior entorhinal cortex [31]. In homozygous transgenic mice that overexpressed the human A53 T variant of α-synuclein (equivalent to the human disease, PARK 1/4), this group also showed that the olfactory bulb and piriform cortex were both affected early on, that is, at 2 months of age. This was earlier than that seen in the anterior olfactory nucleus, olfactory tubercle, posterolateral cortical amygdala, and lateral entorhinal cortex [32]. No changes were observed in the substantia nigra (up to age 8 months). These changes are consistent with the concept of olfactory damage preceding motor involvement.

Deficits in smell function, as measured behaviorally, have also been documented in Thy1-aSyn transgenic mice that overexpress α-synuclein [33]. Such mice have high levels of α-synuclein expression throughout the brain, but nigrostriatal dopamine neurons are intact up to 8 months.

Although not totally anosmic, such mice were found to have impairment on tests designed to find an exposed or hidden odorant, a block test involving exposure to self and non-self odors, and a habituation/dishabituation test based on exposure to non-social odors.

Neurotransmitter/Neuromodulator Systems

It is possible that PD-related olfactory deficits reflect the altered function of specific neurotransmitters or neuromodulators (NT/NM) that shape or modulate the olfactory percept [19]. NT/NM decrements may precede obvious neuronal degeneration, although the process may be circular in that the degeneration may, in turn, alter NT/NM function. Such effects could occur anywhere in the olfactory pathway. It is noteworthy that the human olfactory bulb itself contains at least 20 different neurotransmitters, including dopamine, although in some cases the cell bodies for some NT/NM fall outside the bulbs themselves [e.g. the nucleus basalis supplies olfactory bulb acetylcholine (ACh) as well as much of forebrain ACh].

Acetylcholine

Acetylcholine plays an important role in the innate immune system. Anti-inflammatory pathways within the basal forebrain are regulated by nicotinic ACh receptors found on macrophages and microglia [34]. When cholinergic cells are damaged, resistance to pathogens decreases [35]. The differentiation of myelin-forming oligodendrocytes is enhanced in the CNS by ACh via increased myelin gene expression, an important point given that myelinated nerves are less susceptible to PD pathology. Basal forebrain cholinergic neurons appear to be more sensitive than other neurons to pathogenic agents and ischemic damage [36]. Acetylcholinesterase (AChE) inhibitors such as donepezil and galanatamine protect neuronal cells from glutamate neurotoxicity [37]. Positron emission tomography (PET) studies demonstrate depressed AChE activity within the ascending cholinergic pathways of PD, but not PSP, which has relatively little olfactory dysfunction [38]. In PD, strong correlations have been demonstrated between UPSIT scores and PET-measured AChE within the hippocampal formation ($r = 0.63$, $p = 0.0001$, amygdala $r = 0.55$, $p = 0.0001$), and neocortex ($r = 0.57$, $p = 0.0003$) [10]. [1] Like most studies of olfactory function, the

cholinergic dysfunction measured by PET does not appear to progress with disease severity [39].

Dopamine

Although there are correlations between olfactory test scores and dopamine (DA) transporter uptake in the caudate and putamen, such relationships are not strong. Moreover, olfactory test scores are not influenced by L-DOPA and DA agonists. Thus, if DA is involved, the DA-related receptors in the olfactory pathways may be too dysfunctional or severely depleted to respond. At autopsy, DA deficiency is not evident in the olfactory bulbs of PD patients. In fact, an *increase* in the number of bulbar periglomerular dopaminergic neurons, as well as up regulation of tyrosine hydroxylase (TH), was found in one study [40]. Since TH is the precursor of DA synthesis, DA upregulation was proposed as the reason for the microsmia. Although a subsequent study failed to replicate these findings, a trend was still apparent [41]. A similar elevation of TH expression was observed in the olfactory bulbs of three Macaca monkeys who had been injected with proneurotoxin methyl-phenyl-tetrahydropyridine (MPTP) [42]. Increased bulbar TH expression has also been found in transgenic rats and mice bearing the PD α-synuclein mutations, *A30P* and *A53 T* [43, 44]. In the MPTP mouse model of PD, a four-fold increase of DA in the olfactory bulb has also been reported [45]. This may reflect compensation for loss of a DA-responsive substrate, possibly from increased migration of DA-secreting cells into the olfactory bulb from the sub-ventricular zone/rostral migratory stream.

Norepinephrine and Serotonin

A major influence of alterations in CNS norepinephrine (NE) and serotonin (5-HT) on olfactory function of PD patients seems unlikely. Patients

---

[1] $ Based on data after scores on the University of Pennsylvania Smell Identification Test (UPSIT) of 0 were omitted. Because the UPSIT is a four-alternative 40-odorant forced-choice test, chance performance would be around 10, not 0, which the authors used in a few cases where clear anosmia was evident (Nicolas Bohnen, personal communication, August 30, 2011). The original cholinergic correlations with UPSIT scores were 0.56 for the hippocampus, 0.50 for the amygdala, and 0.46 for the neocortex. After the 0 omissions, dopamine-related associations, as measured by monoamine transporter type 2, became non-significant (ps > 0.05).

with depression, which is often accompanied by decreased levels of NE and 5-HT, do not exhibit much if any olfactory dysfunction. The same is the case for patients with dopamine β-hydroxylase deficiency, an inherited recessive autosomal disorder with diminished NE synthesis [46]. Interestingly, such patients are also spared cognitive dysfunction [47]. Although pharmacologic block of α- and β-adrenergic receptors alters learning of an odor discrimination task in rats, such disruption has no effect once the task is learned [48]. This is also true when bulbar NE is locally depleted by 6-hydroxydopamine [49].

Drug-Induced Parkinsonism

Wide-spectrum DA antagonists such as haloperidol (Serenace) and trifluoperazine (Stelazine) can produce motor dysfunction largely indistinguishable from PD, a phenomenon called drug-induced parkinsonism (DIP). Population-based epidemiological studies suggest that after PD, DIP is the most common cause of parkinsonism. In recent years, the prevalence of DIP has declined following the introduction of selective D_2 DA receptor antagonists such as clozapine (Clozaril), olanzepine (Zyprexa), quetiapine (Seroquel), and risperidone (Risperdal). In 2000, Hensiek et al. [50] administered the UPSIT to ten non-demented DIP patients (MMSE scores >26). Their parkinsonism was due to at least two weeks of treatment with phenothiazine preparations. Five performed abnormally on the UPSIT and none completely recovered their smell function or the parkinsonian symptoms even after stopping or changing the offending medication. Of the remaining five who did regain motor function after their treatment was altered, all but one had normal smell function. Some of these patients had prior psychotic disorders which may have caused or contributed to their smell problem. It should be emphasized that some patients with DIP may be predisposed to develop PD, such that exposure to a dopamine-depleting drug unmasks underlying PD and the associated olfactory dysfunction. Given that around 50% of patients with classical PD have depression at some stage of their illness, it is not surprising that exposure to broad-spectrum dopamine blockers would uncover PD especially in a non-neurological environment.

More recent DIP studies have observed similar effects. In one study, 15 depressed patients treated with selective or non-selective dopamine-blocking medications (haloperidol, flupenthixol, and risperidone) exhibited, relative to controls, lower odor test scores for identification and detection threshold, but not discrimination [51]. Unmedicated depressed patients and depressed patients who received similar medications without developing DIP had normal olfactory test scores, suggesting depression, per se, was not the cause of the olfactory dysfunction. Another study divided 16 DIP patients into those with normal (n = 9) and abnormal (n = 7) DA transporter SPECT imaging [52]. Only those with pathologic putamen uptake had abnormal olfactory test scores. These scores were correlated with the putamen uptake values, suggesting that the olfactory deficit is more closely associated with central DA damage than with drug-induced DA receptor blockade.

The impact of DIP on olfactory function is, however, variable and likely depends upon a range of idiosyncratic factors, including the duration and dosage of drug administration. Lee et al. [53] assessed B-SIT scores of 15 DIP and 15 matched normal controls. The DIP followed use of levosulpiride, haloperidol, flunarizine, perphenazine, metoclopramide, or risperidone. The B-SIT scores of the DIP patients did not differ from those of their 15 controls and were significantly higher than 24 patients with sporadic PD (6.9 versus 4.4; p < 0.001). Nevertheless, Morley et al. [54] found, in a study of 30 DIP patients, that six of seven (86%) of those with abnormal DA transporter SPECT imaging evidenced abnormal UPSIT scores (age and sex adjusted), whereas only two of 23 (9%) of those with normal DA imaging did so. This suggests olfactory testing of DIP patients may aid in identifying dopaminergic denervation consistent with incipient PD.

In 1992, the UPSIT and an odor-detection threshold test were administered to six of the original young California drug users who had inadvertently injected an illegal pethidine analogue methyl-phenyl-tetrahydropyridine (MPTP) [55]. Although UPSIT and detection threshold test scores were within normal limits, there was a non-significant trend towards higher thresholds in the exposed group (Figure 10.2). Whether systemic MPTP administration can induce smell loss is controversial. Miwa et al. [56] reported that MPTP injections caused three marmosets to have difficulty locating bananas by smell. Moreover, they would eat bananas odorized with skatole

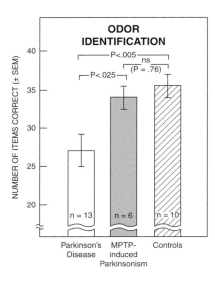

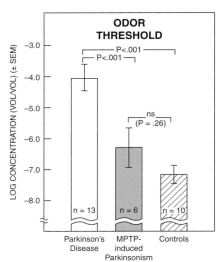

Figure 10.2 Mean (SEM) UPSIT and phenyl ethyl alcohol detection threshold test scores for persons with MPTP-induced parkinsonism, young patients with idiopathic PD, and matched normal controls. From [55] with permission.

Copyright © 1992 American Neurological Association.

(putrid, fecal) or isovaleric acid (dirty socks, rancid cheese). This was not the case for two controls or to these animals prior to the MPTP treatment. However, smell function is normal in mouse models of PD in which MPTP is injected intraperitoneally [57], whether measured behaviorally or by summated odor-induced potentials on the olfactory epithelia. Conversely, intranasal infusion of MPTP has an adverse effect on olfaction in both mouse and rat models of PD [57–59].

Essential Tremor

Essential tremor (ET), unlike PD, is characterized by tremor on voluntary movement rather than at rest and affects the arms, voice, and head. Unlike PD, ET is not accompanied by slowness of movement, a stooped posture, or a shuffling gait. Nonetheless, ET can be confused with benign tremulous PD especially when there is no evidence of muscle rigidity. ET patients are at higher risk than persons in the general population for future development of AD and PD [60, 61]. A family history is often evident in keeping with autosomal dominant inheritance, although onset is bimodal with peaks in young and late adult life.

In contrast to PD, ET is not associated with meaningful olfactory dysfunction, making smell testing of value in the differential diagnosis of these two disorders. Busenbark and colleagues were first to report that patients with ET scored normally on the UPSIT [62]. More recently, Shah et al. [63] compared UPSIT scores of 59 ET patients, 64 tremor-dominant PD patients, and

245 healthy controls. The scores of the ET patients were indistinguishable from those of the controls. A surprising finding was that those who had a first-degree relative with tremor actually scored significantly *better* than age- and gender-matched controls. Djaldetti et al. [64] did not find a correlation with the extent of dopaminergic loss as measured by DaTScan, and ET patients with and without rest tremor did not have abnormal smell tests. Finally, Louis et al. [65], in a study examining the relationship in ET patients between UPSIT scores and the cerebellar neurotoxin Harmane (methylpyridoindole), found no difference in the mean UPSIT scores between the ET patients and controls. There have been no detailed pathological studies of the olfactory pathways in ET, and only a few on the rest of the brain [66]. The major pathology is in the cerebellum, where Purkinje cell axonal swelling ("torpedoes") are found more frequently than in control brains [67].

Familial Parkinson's Disease

There are several monogenetic inherited forms of PD, although they account for a relatively small number of PD cases. Although the frequency and severity of the olfactory dysfunction often appears analogous to that of classic PD in some forms, considerable heterogeneity is evident. Table 10.1 summarizes the primary olfactory findings from familial monogenic cases of PD [8].

The impact familial PD has on olfactory function is perhaps best exemplified by studies of

Table 10.1 Currently proposed genetic forms of parkinsonism with some associated pathological features and olfactory deficits where known

Park Number	Gene and Common Mutations	Inheritance Pattern & Locus	Age of Onset	Function or Effect of Mutation	Lewy Bodies	Olfactory Deficit	Comment
1 & 4	asynuclein (SNCA). G209A. Missense mutations: A53 T, A30P and E46 K. Also duplications and triplications.	AD 4q21.3-q22	30–40	Dopamine transmission	++	+++	Early onset. + response to levodopa. Impaired olfaction in one case [112]. Abnormal in two of seven Greek cases [113] and in six Japanese [114]. Severe olfactory defect in two cases from Germany [73]. Abnormal identification in 14 or 16 cases [115]. Duplications resemble classic PD. Dementia prominent in duplications and triplications. No evidence of smell loss was observed by in an asymptomatic carrier of the E46 K substitution in the α-synuclein gene.
2	Parkin Over 200 mutations	AR 6q26	<40	Mitochondrial disorder. UPS, E3-ubiquitin ligase.	+?	+	Early onset, slow progression. Good response to levodopa. No dementia. Normal/mild impairment of olfaction in manifesting and non-manifesting carriers, heterozygotes but not compound heterozygotes [116, 117]. Susceptibility to glioma, lung cancer, possibly leprosy and TB.
3 & 5	**Not confirmed**						
6	PINK1 Over 60 mutations	AR 1p36.12	20–50	Mitochondrial kinase. Defective mitophagy	+	++	Early onset and slow progression. Good response to levodopa. Dementia. Moderate impairment of olfaction in all cases and some asymptomatic heterozygotes [118, 119]. One autopsy showed LB but sparing of locus ceruleus and amygdala. Olfactory bulbs (OB) not examined [120].
7	DJ-1 10 mutations.	AR 1p36	20–40	Oxidative stress. Defective mitophagy	?	0?	Good response to levodopa. Normal olfaction based on one patient [121].
8	LRRK2 / Dardarin	AD	40–60		++	+++	

Table 10.1 (cont.)

Park Number	Gene and Common Mutations	Inheritance Pattern & Locus	Age of Onset	Function or Effect of Mutation	Lewy Bodies	Olfactory Deficit	Comment
	G2019S; N1437 H	12q12		Membrane trafficking, Kinase.			Moderate–severe olfactory impairment in manifesting patients from London, New York, Lisbon, Brazil, and Germany [72, 73, 122–125]. Variable or no impairment in non-manifesting carriers [70, 77, 122]. Dementia and tremor common. Good response to levodopa. Susceptibility to leprosy and TB.
9	ATP13A2 10 mutations	AR 1p36	11–16	Lysosome ATPase	?	++	Kufor-Rakeb disease. Based on four subjects [73]. Similar to Hallervorden-Spatz disease. Levodopa-responsive PD with pyramidal signs, supranuclear gaze palsy, and dementia [126].
10–13	**Not confirmed**						
14	PLA2G6 Karak syndrome	AR 22q13.1	20–25	Phospho-lipase enzyme	+++	?	Karak syndrome. Adult-onset dystonia-parkinsonism. Temporary response to levodopa. Dementia. Cortical LB in four autopsies. No OB data but hippocampus involved in some [127]
15	FBOX7 AR	AR 22q11.2	10–19	Ubiquitin protein ligase	?	?	Early-onset levodopa-responsive parkinsonism with dystonia and spasticity
16	**Not confirmed**						
17	Heterozygous mutation (D620 N) in VPS35 gene	AD 16q12	40–60	Membrane trafficking.	0 One limited autopsy	?	Indistinguishable from tremor-dominant PD. Dementia uncommon. Good response to levodopa

GBA = glucocerebrosidase mutation. POLG1 = mitochondrial DNA polymerase subunit gamma one. LB = Lewy bodies. OLF = olfactory defect. AD = autosomal dominant. AR = autosomal recessive.

patients with PARK 8, one of the most prevalent causes of familial PD. The leucine-rich repeat kinase 2 gene (*LRRK2*) on chromosome 12p11.2-q13.1 is one of the most prevalent causes of familial PD. While only around 1% of North American PD patients carry this mutation, it is present in over 40% of Arab-Berbers of North Africa [68]. This condition gives rise to late-onset benign tremor and may be indistinguishable from sporadic PD. Penetrance of the most common *LRRK2* mutation (G2019S) is incomplete and age-dependent. Limited pathologic studies show Lewy and tau pathology within the olfactory pathways [69].

UPSIT scores typical of classic PD were found in five PARK 8 patients with the G2019S mutation from London [70] and sixteen from Lisbon [71]. Unaffected relatives at 50% risk of PARK 8 were not affected. In another preliminary study from Brazil, impaired olfaction using Sniffin' Sticks (SS) was found in 22 LRRK2 patients carrying the G2019S mutation but it was less severe than those with classic PD [72]. In a German study, seven PARK 8 patients, three of whom were symptomatic and four of whom were non-symptomatic, exhibited low UPSIT scores relative to controls [73]. Less clear-cut results were documented in a large French pedigree that carried the G2019S mutation [74].

A large UPSIT study of 126 G2019S mutation carriers found no significant olfactory dysfunction in non-manifesting carriers, suggesting that microsmia is not predictive of LRRK2-related parkinsonism [75]. Another investigation from Spain assessed UPSIT scores in a) 29 subjects with PARK8 due to the G2019S mutation, b) 49 asymptomatic mutation carriers, c) 47 non-carrier relatives, d) 50 subjects with idiopathic PD, and e) 50 community-based controls [76]. In the G2019S manifesting carrier group, 50% were hyposmic compared to 82% in the IPD group and there was no significant difference between these two. Hyposmia was less frequent in the asymptomatic carrier group (26%) and asymptomatic non-carriers (28%), suggesting that olfactory dysfunction is not found in asymptomatic carriers of G2019S. Normal B-SIT scores were found in a Norwegian study of 47 non-symptomatic family members of LRRK2 PD patients, of whom 32 were positive and 15 negative for either the G2019S or the N1437 H mutation [77].

In summary, PD patients with *LRRK2* mutations on average appear to have a decreased sense of smell, but the severity is less than that of idiopathic PD. Non-manifesting carriers appear to have no olfactory impairment but before it is concluded that hyposmia is not a premotor feature for PARK8, larger populations need to be tested.

Glucocerebrosidase-Related Parkinsonism

Parkinsonism can be a presenting feature of Gaucher's disease (GD), the most prevalent autosomal recessive lysosomal disorder. Other distinguishing features of this disorder are bone, hematologic, and pulmonary abnormalities [78]. GD is caused by mutations in the glucocerebrosidase (*GBA*) gene. In one study of six carriers of the *GBA* mutation, three were anosmic, two severely microsmic, and one moderately microsmic, with the mean UPSIT score falling within the range expected for patients with sporadic PD [79]. In another study, borderline lower scores (p = 0.08) on a 12-item odor identification test were observed in 20 PD patients heterozygous for one of the two *GBA* mutations (N370S, L444P) [80]. In still another study, one of two *GBA* cases, both of whom were anosmic, was a 54-year-old man who reported that his smell sense declined as a teenager [78]. Only when he reached the age of 48 years did he notice a hand tremor. Shortly thereafter other symptoms emerged such as anxiety, depression, low blood pressure, urinary urgency, and medication sensitivity.

McNeill and colleagues studied 30 patients with Gaucher parkinsonism, their heterozygous GBA mutation carriers, and 30 mutation negative controls matched for age, gender, and race [81]. UPSIT scores were significantly lower in the Gaucher patients and heterozygous carriers. In a subsequent study, such scores declined slightly from baseline over a two-year period (respective UPSIT means = 31.85 versus 30.71) [82]. It is not clear whether any carriers free of clinical evidence of parkinsonism, as measured by the Unified Parkinson's Disease Rating Scale (UPDRS), had abnormal UPSIT scores or whether any carrier with normal olfaction had an abnormal UPDRS score.

Idiopathic Rapid Eye Movement Sleep Behavior Disorder

Rapid eye movement sleep behavior disorder is a progressive disorder characterized by loss of muscle tone and the acting out of dream-related behavior during REM sleep. Often it is considered a prodromal form of PD and other synucleinopathies (e.g. MSA, Lewy Body Disease (LBD)), although its pathology is unclear. There is evidence of pontine and medullary degeneration, affecting the sublaterodorsal nuclei, and their glutaminergic projections to the medullary or magnocellular reticular formation [83]. Recently, punch biopsies from the leg skin of RBD patients revealed a reduction in intraepidermal nerve fiber density reflecting small fiber neuropathy [84]. Since small fiber neuropathy is associated with nicotinic cholinergic processes [85], this association could be a marker for cholinergic dysfunction associated with smell loss reflecting the impaired sural nerve latencies in ALS [86]. In PD, PET studies have found that the symptoms of RBD are closely associated with cholinergic denervation within cortical, limbic, and thalamic brain regions [87].

In a five-year prospective follow-up study of 62 patients with idiopathic RBD, impaired olfaction at baseline was related to a 65% five-year risk of developing a defined neurodegenerative disease, compared to a 14% risk for those with normal olfaction [88]. The olfactory loss is similar to that of PD and some other neurodegenerative diseases (e.g. AD), with mean UPSIT scores falling around 20 [89]. Commonly the olfactory dysfunction appears up to five years before the RBD diagnosis. It is of interest that independent of RBD, acute sleep deprivation per se has a specific but mild adverse effect on the ability to identify odors – an influence that cannot be explained on the basis of task difficulty [90]. As yet, it is not clear whether this phenomenon is a cause or just an association of RBD.

Multiple System Atrophy

Multiple system atrophy (MSA) is a rapidly progressive type of parkinsonism accompanied by autonomic and cerebellar dysfunction in varying proportions. MSA-Parkinsonism (MSA-P), the most common form of MSA (~80% of cases), is defined by akinesia and rigidity. In the rarer MSA-Cerebellar (MSA-C) variety cerebellar ataxia is dominant. Typical clinical features are dysarthria, stridor, contractures, dystonia, orthostatic hypotension, constipation, bladder control issues, sexual dysfunction, and rapid eye movement sleep

behavior disorder (RBD) [91]. Typical pathology (glial cytoplasmic inclusions, GCIs) is located within the basal ganglia, cortex, spinal cord, and olfactory bulbs, but peripheral autonomic neurons are spared [92]. The discovery of GCAs in MSA brains confirmed beliefs that striatonigral degeneration, sporadic olivopontocerebellar atrophy, and the Shy-Drager syndrome are different clinical expressions of MSA [93].

In a pioneering study, the UPSIT was administered to 29 patients with MSA and 123 controls [94]. Moderate dysfunction was evident in the MSA patients relative to the controls (respective means = 26.7 and 33.5). The test scores of the MSA-P and MSA-C types did not differ. Others have observed similar olfactory deficits in MSA patients [46, 95–97]. Unlike PD, no meaningful correlations have been detected between UPSIT scores and measures of cardiac ^{123}I-metaiodobenzylguanidine (MIBG) uptake [98].

Parkinson Dementia Complex of Guam

The Guam PD–dementia complex (PDC) is characterized, alone or in combination, by Alzheimer-type dementia, parkinsonism, and ALS. Pathologically, it is classed as a tauopathy with neurofibrillary tangles and no Lewy bodies, unlike idiopathic PD. Like PD, the number of cells within the AON are significantly decreased [99]. Interestingly, a significant number of PDC patients, as well as some non-symptomatic relatives, exhibit a retinopathy with an appearance similar to larval migration [100–102]. This unique retinopathy has not been found in any other part of the world or in any other neurodegenerative disease. It resembles the well-documented "snail-track" degeneration of the retina. No larva has ever been found.

The Guam PD–dementia complex is most evident in the Chamorro population on the Pacific Island of Guam, although it has also been found in individuals in the Mariana islands, the Kii peninsula of Japan, and the coastal plain of West New Guinea. This disease accounted for at least 15% of adult deaths in the indigenous Chamorro population of Guam between 1957 and 1965 [103, 104]. Since that time, its prevalence has markedly decreased. By 1999, its ALS component has been absent [105], suggesting the potential etiologic involvement of such environmental toxins as

Cycad nut toxins or high aluminium, or low calcium and magnesium levels in drinking water – conditions that no longer remain [106]. Administration of the UPSIT to 24 patients with PDC revealed severe olfactory dysfunction similar to that of idiopathic PD, although a few exhibited additional cognitive impairment which could have lowered the scores slightly [107].

Vascular Parkinsonism

Vascular parkinsonism (VP), unlike PD, is not considered a progressive neurodegenerative disease even though it mimics many features of PD. It is usually caused by small strokes and is most common in patients with extensive cerebrovascular disease involving the basal ganglia. Unlike PD, it is rarely accompanied by resting tremor or abnormal PET or SPECT striatal dopamine transporter imaging deficits [108]. It exhibits more variable responses to L-DOPA than PD. Insidious onset cases tend to have more diffusely distributed abnormalities than acute onset cases, who have comparatively more lesions in the subcortical gray nuclei (thalamus, striatum, globus pallidus) [109].

Katzenschlager et al. [110] administered the UPSIT to 14 VP patients, 18 PD patients, and 27 normal controls of similar age. The UPSIT scores of the VP patients did not differ significantly from those of healthy controls (respective means = 26.1 and 27.6), both of which differed from the scores of the PD patients (mean = 17.1; ps < 0.0001). In contrast, Navarro-Otano [111], in a study of 15 cases of clinically diagnosed VP, found severe impairment of odor identification (mean UPSIT = 18.3) that did not differ from the mean of their PD patients (mean = 15.3). Both were much lower than the mean of the control subjects (30.7). In light of such discrepant findings, it is clear that more research is needed to evaluate VP and how it may be differentiated from PD on the basis of olfactory tests.

In summary, smell dysfunction is common in classical PD as well as in a number of related disorders. The basis of the dysfunction remains elusive, although presently multiple non-mutually exclusive factors appear to be involved, including complex interactions between genetics and environment. Future studies are needed to better define the relative contributions of such factors.

References

1. Suchowersky O, Reich S, Perlmutter J, et al. Practice parameter: diagnosis and prognosis of new onset Parkinson disease (an evidence-based review). Report of the Quality Standards Subcommittee of the American Academy of Neurology. Neurology 2006; **66**: 968–975.

2. Postuma RB, Berg D, Stern M, et al. MDS clinical diagnostic criteria for Parkinson's disease. Mov Disord 2015; **30**: 1591–1601.

3. Berg D, Postuma RB, Adler CH, et al. MDS research criteria for prodromal Parkinson's disease. Mov Disord 2015; **30**: 1600–1611.

4. Chaudhuri KR, Martinez-Martin P, Schapira AHV, et al. International multicenter pilot study of the first comprehensive self-completed nonmotor symptoms questionnaire for Parkinson's disease: The NMSQuest study. Mov Disord 2006; **21**: 916–923.

5. Pence TS, Reiter ER, DiNardo LJ, Costanzo RM. Risk factors for hazardous events in olfactory-impaired patients. JAMA Otolaryngol Head Neck Surg 2014; **140**: 951–955.

6. Chalke HD, Dewhurst JR, Ward CW. Loss of smell in old people. Pub Health 1958; **72**: 223–230.

7. Doty RL, Shaman P, Applebaum SL, et al. Smell identification ability: changes with age. Science 1984; **226**: 1441–1443.

8. Hawkes CH, Doty RL. *Smell and Taste Disorders*. Cambridge University Press; 2018.

9. Doty RL, Bromley SM, Stern MB. Olfactory testing as an aid in the diagnosis of Parkinson's disease: development of optimal discrimination criteria. Neurodegeneration 1995; **4**: 93–97.

10. Bohnen NI, Muller ML, Kotagal V, et al. Olfactory dysfunction, central cholinergic integrity and cognitive impairment in Parkinson's disease. Brain 2010; **133**: 1747–1754.

11. Parrao T, Chana P, Venegas P, et al. Olfactory deficits and cognitive dysfunction in Parkinson's disease. Neurodegener Dis 2012; **10**: 179–182.

12. Doty RL, Riklan M, Deems DA, Reynolds C, Stellar S. The olfactory and cognitive deficits of Parkinson's disease: evidence for independence. Ann Neurol 1989; **25**: 166–171.

13. Hawkes CH, Shephard BC. Selective anosmia in Parkinson's disease? Lancet 1993; **341**: 435–436.

14. Joseph T, Auger SD, Peress L, et al. Screening performance of abbreviated versions of the UPSIT smell test. J Neurol 2019; **266**: 1897–1906.

15. Ponsen MM, Stoffers D, Booij J, et al. Idiopathic hyposmia as a preclinical sign of Parkinson's disease. Ann Neurol 2004; **56**: 173–181.

16. Doty RL, Deems DA, Stellar S. Olfactory dysfunction in parkinsonism: a general deficit unrelated to neurologic signs, disease stage, or disease duration. Neurology 1988; **38**: 1237–1244.

17. Doty RL, Stern MB, Pfeiffer C, Gollomp SM, Hurtig HI. Bilateral olfactory dysfunction in early stage treated and untreated idiopathic Parkinson's disease. J Neurol Neurosurg Psychiat 1992; **55**: 138–142.

18. Braak H, Del TK, Rub U, et al. Staging of brain pathology related to sporadic Parkinson's disease. Neurobiol Aging 2003; **24**: 197–211.

19. Doty RL. Olfactory dysfunction in neurodegenerative diseases: is there a common pathological substrate? Lancet Neurol 2017; **16**: 478–488.

20. Crino PB, Martin JA, Hill WD, et al. Beta-Amyloid peptide and amyloid precursor proteins in olfactory mucosa of patients with Alzheimer's disease, Parkinson's disease, and Down syndrome. Ann Otol Rhinol Laryngol 1995; **104**: 655–661.

21. Duda JE, Shah U, Arnold SE, Lee VM, Trojanowski JQ. The expression of alpha-, beta-, and gamma-synucleins in olfactory mucosa from patients with and without neurodegenerative diseases. Exp Neurol 1999; **160**: 515–522.

22. Witt M, Bormann K, Gudziol V, et al. Biopsies of olfactory epithelium in patients with Parkinson's disease. Mov Disord 2009; **24**: 906–914.

23. Funabe S, Takao M, Saito Y, et al. Neuropathologic analysis of Lewy-related alpha-synucleinopathy in olfactory mucosa. Neuropathology 2013; **33**: 47–58.

24. Saito Y, Shioya A, Sano T, et al. Lewy body pathology involves the olfactory cells in Parkinson's disease and related disorders. Mov Disord 2016; **31**: 135–138.

25. Daniel SE, Hawkes CH. Preliminary diagnosis of Parkinson's disease by olfactory bulb pathology [letter]. Lancet 1992; **340**: 186.

26. Pearce RK, Hawkes CH, Daniel SE. The anterior olfactory nucleus in Parkinson's disease. Mov Disord 1995; **10**: 283–287.

27. Beach TG, White CL, III, Hladik CL, et al. Olfactory bulb alpha-synucleinopathy has high specificity and sensitivity for Lewy body disorders. Acta Neuropathol 2009; **117**: 169–174.

28. Jellinger KA. Olfactory bulb alpha-synucleinopathy has high specificity and sensitivity for Lewy body disorders. Acta Neuropathol 2009; **117**: 215–216.

29. Zapiec B, Dieriks BV, Tan S, et al. A ventral glomerular deficit in Parkinson's disease revealed by whole olfactory bulb reconstruction. Brain 2017; **140**: 2722–2736.

30. Braak H, Ghebremedhin E, Rub U, Bratzke H, Del TK. Stages in the development of Parkinson's disease-related pathology. Cell Tissue Res 2004; **318**: 121–134.

31. Ubeda-Banon I, Saiz-Sanchez D, Rosa-Prieto C, et al. Alpha-Synucleinopathy in the human olfactory system in Parkinson's disease: involvement of calcium-binding protein- and substance P-positive cells. Acta Neuropathol 2010; **119**: 723–735.

32. Ubeda-Banon I, Saiz-Sanchez D, Rosa-Prieto C, Martinez-Marcos A. Alpha-Synuclein in the olfactory system of a mouse model of Parkinson's disease: correlation with olfactory projections. Brain Struct Funct 2012; **217**: 447–458.

33. Chesselet MF, Richter F, Zhu C, et al. A progressive mouse model of Parkinson's disease: the Thy1-aSyn ("Line 61") mice. Neurotherapeutics 2012; **9**: 297–314.

34. Egea J, Buendia I, Parada E, et al. Anti-inflammatory role of microglial alpha7 nAChRs and its role in neuroprotection. Biochem Pharmacol 2015; **97**: 463–472.

35. Boeckxstaens G. The clinical importance of the anti-inflammatory vagovagal reflex. Handb Clin Neurol 2013; **117**: 119–134.

36. McKinney M, Jacksonville MC. Brain cholinergic vulnerability: relevance to behavior and disease. Biochem Pharmacol 2005; **70**: 1115–1124.

37. Takada-Takatori Y, Kume T, Sugimoto M, et al. Acetylcholinesterase inhibitors used in treatment of Alzheimer's disease prevent glutamate neurotoxicity via nicotinic acetylcholine receptors and phosphatidylinositol 3-kinase cascade. Neuropharmacology 2006; **51**: 474–486.

38. Shinotoh H, Namba H, Yamaguchi M, et al. Positron emission tomographic measurement of acetylcholinesterase activity reveals differential loss of ascending cholinergic systems in Parkinson's disease and progressive supranuclear palsy. Ann Neurol 1999; **46**: 62–69.

39. Shimada H, Hirano S, Shinotoh H, et al. Mapping of brain acetylcholinesterase alterations in Lewy body disease by PET. Neurology 2009; **73**: 273–278.

40. Huisman E, Uylings HBM, Hoogland PV. A 100% increase of 687 dopaminergic cells in the olfactory bulb may explain hyposmia in Parkinson's disease. Mov Disord 2004; **19**: 687–692.

41. Huisman E, Uylings HBM, Hoogland PV. Gender-related changes in increase of dopaminergic

neurons in the olfactory bulb of Parkinson's disease patients. Mov Disord 2008; **23**: 1407–1413.

42. Belzunegui S, Sebastian WS, Garrido-Gil P, et al. The number of dopaminergic cells is increased in the olfactory bulb of monkeys chronically exposed to MPTP. Synapse 2007; **61**: 1006–1012.

43. Lelan F, Boyer C, Thinard R, et al. Effects of human alpha-synuclein A53T-A30P mutations on SVZ and local olfactory bulb cell proliferation in a transgenic rat model of Parkinson disease. Parkinsons Dis 2011; **2011**: 987084.

44. Ubeda-Banon I, Saiz-Sanchez D, Rosa-Prieto C, et al. Staging of alpha-synuclein in the olfactory bulb in a model of Parkinson's disease: cell types involved. Mov Disord 2010; **25**: 1701–1707.

45. Yamada M, Onodera M, Mizuno Y, Mochizuki H. Neurogenesis in olfactory bulb identified by retroviral labeling in normal and 1-methyl-4-phenyl-1,2,3,6-tetrahydropyridine-treated adult mice. Neuroscience 2004; **124**(1): 173–181.

46. Garland EM, Raj SR, Peltier AC, Robertson D, Biaggioni I. A cross-sectional study contrasting olfactory function in autonomic disorders. Neurology 2011; **76**: 456–460.

47. Jepma M, Deinum J, Asplund CL, et al. Neurocognitive function in dopamine-beta-hydroxylase deficiency. Neuropsychopharmacology 2011; **36**: 1608–1619.

48. Doucette W, Milder J, Restrepo D. Adrenergic modulation of olfactory bulb circuitry affects odor discrimination. Learn Mem 2007; **14**: 539–547.

49. Doty RL, Ferguson-Segall M, Lucki I, Kreider M. Effects of intrabulbar injections of 6-hydroxydopamine on ethyl acetate odor detection in castrate and non-castrate male rats. Brain Res 1988; **444**: 95–103.

50. Hensiek AE, Bhatia K, Hawkes CH. Olfactory function in drug-induced parkinsonism. J Neurol 2000; **247**(Suppl 3): 82.

51. Kruger S, Haehner A, Thiem C, Hummel T. Neuroleptic-induced parkinsonism is associated with olfactory dysfunction. J Neurol 2008; **255**: 1574–1579.

52. Bovi T, Antonini A, Ottaviani S, et al. The status of olfactory function and the striatal dopaminergic system in drug-induced parkinsonism. J Neurol 2010; **257**: 1882–1889.

53. Lee PH, Yeo SH, Yong SW, Kim YJ. Odour identification test and its relation to cardiac I-123-metaiodobenzylguanidine in patients with drug induced parkinsonism. J Neurol Neurosurg Psychiatry 2007; **78**: 1250–1252.

54. Morley JF, Cheng G, Dubroff JG, et al. Olfactory impairment predicts underlying dopaminergic deficit in presumed drug-induced parkinsonism. Mov Disord Clin Pract 2017; **4**: 603–606.

55. Doty RL, Singh A, Tetrud J, Langston JW. Lack of major olfactory dysfunction in MPTP-induced parkinsonism. Ann Neurol 1992; **32**: 97–100.

56. Miwa T, Watanabe A, Mitsumoto Y, et al. Olfactory impairment and Parkinson's disease-like symptoms observed in the common marmoset following administration of 1-methyl-4-phenyl-1,2,3,6-tetrahydropyridine. Acta Oto-Laryngologica 2004; **124**: 80–84.

57. Kurtenbach S, Wewering S, Hatt H, Neuhaus EM, Lubbert H. Olfaction in three genetic and two MPTP-induced Parkinson's disease mouse models. PLoS One 2013; **8**: e77509.

58. Prediger RD, Aguiar AS, Jr., Rojas-Mayorquin AE, et al. Single intranasal administration of 1-methyl-4-phenyl-1,2,3,6-tetrahydropyridine in C57BL/6 mice models early preclinical phase of Parkinson's disease. Neurotox Res 2010; **17**: 114–129.

59. Prediger RDS, Batista LC, Medeiros R, et al. The risk is in the air: intranasal administration of MPTP to rats reproducing clinical features of Parkinson's disease. Exp Neurol 2006; **202**: 391–403.

60. Louis ED. Essential tremors: a family of neurodegenerative disorders? Arch Neurol 2009; **66**: 1202–1208.

61. Laroia H, Louis ED. Association between essential tremor and other neurodegenerative diseases: what is the epidemiological evidence? Neuroepidemiology 2011; **37**: 1–10.

62. Busenbark KL, Huber SI, Greer G, Pahwa R, Koller WC. Olfactory function in essential tremor. Neurology 1992; **42**: 1631–1632.

63. Shah M, Muhammed N, Findley LJ, Hawkes CH. Olfactory tests in the diagnosis of essential tremor. Parkinsonism Relat Disord 2008; **14**: 563–568.

64. Djaldetti R, Nageris BI, Lorberboym M, et al. [I-123]-FP-CIT SPECT and olfaction test in patients with combined postural and rest tremor. J Neural Transm 2008; **115**: 469–472.

65. Louis ED, Rios E, Pellegrino KM, et al. Higher blood harmane (1-methyl-9H-pyrido[3,4-b] indole) concentrations correlate with lower olfactory scores in essential tremor. Neurotoxicology 2008; **29**: 460–465.

66. Louis ED, Vonsattel JPG, Honig LS, et al. Neuropathologic findings in essential tremor. Neurology 2006; **66**: 1756–1759.

67. Louis ED, Vonsattel JP, Honig LS, et al. Essential tremor associated with pathologic changes in the cerebellum. Arch Neurol 2006; **63**: 1189–1193.

68. Lesage S, Ibanez P, Lohmann E, et al. G2019S LRRK2 mutation in French and North African families with Parkinson's disease. Ann Neurol 2005; **58**: 784–787.

69. Silveira-Moriyama L, Holton JL, Kingsbury A, et al. Regional differences in the severity of Lewy body pathology across the olfactory cortex. Neurosci Lett 2009; **453**: 77–80.

70. Silveira-Moriyama L, Guedes LC, Kingsbury A, et al. Hyposmia in G2019S LRRK2-related parkinsonism: clinical and pathologic data. Neurology 2008; **71**: 1021–1026.

71. Ferreira JJ, Guedes LC, Rosa MM, et al. High prevalence of LRRK2 mutations in familial and sporadic Parkinson's disease in Portugal. Mov Disord 2007; **22**: 1194–1201.

72. Silveira-Moriyama L, Munhoz RP, de JC, Raskin S et al. Olfactory heterogeneity in LRRK2 related Parkinsonism. Mov Disord 2010; **25**: 2879–2883.

73. Kertelge L, Bruggemann N, Schmidt A, et al. Impaired sense of smell and color discrimination in monogenic and idiopathic Parkinson's disease. Mov Disord 2010; **25**: 2665–2669.

74. Lohmann E, Leclere L, De AF, et al. A clinical, neuropsychological and olfactory evaluation of a large family with LRRK2 mutations. Parkinsonism Relat Disord 2009; **15**: 273–276.

75. Saunders-Pullman R, Mirelman A, Wang C, et al. Olfactory identification in LRRK2 G2019S mutation carriers: a relevant marker? Ann Clin Transl Neurol 2014; **1**: 670–678.

76. Sierra M, Sanchez-Juan P, Martinez-Rodriguez MI, et al. Olfaction and imaging biomarkers in premotor LRRK2 G2019S-associated Parkinson disease. Neurology 2013; **80**: 621–626.

77. Johansen KK, White LR, Farrer MJ, Aasly JO. Subclinical signs in LRRK2 mutation carriers. Parkinsonism Relat Disord 2011; **17**: 528–532.

78. Saunders-Pullman R, Hagenah J, Dhawan V, et al. Gaucher disease ascertained through a Parkinson's center: imaging and clinical characterization. Mov Disord 2010; **25**: 1364–1372.

79. Goker-Alpan O, Lopez G, Vithayathil J, et al. The spectrum of parkinsonian manifestations associated with glucocerebrosidase mutations. Arch Neurol 2008; **65**: 1353–1357.

80. Brockmann K, Srulijes K, Hauser AK, et al. GBA-associated PD presents with nonmotor characteristics. Neurology 2011; **77**: 276–280.

81. McNeill A, Duran R, Proukakis C, et al. Hyposmia and cognitive impairment in Gaucher disease patients and carriers. Mov Disord 2012; **27**: 526–532.

82. Beavan M, McNeill A, Proukakis C, et al. Evolution of prodromal clinical markers of Parkinson disease in a GBA mutation-positive cohort. JAMA Neurol 2015; **72**: 201–208.

83. Iranzo A. The REM sleep circuit and how its impairment leads to REM sleep behavior disorder. Cell Tissue Res 2018; **373**: 245–266.

84. Schrempf W, Katona I, Dogan I, et al. Reduced intraepidermal nerve fiber density in patients with REM sleep behavior disorder. Parkinsonism Relat Disord 2016; **29**: 10–16.

85. Kyte SL, Toma W, Bagdas D, et al. Nicotine prevents and reverses paclitaxel-induced mechanical allodynia in a mouse model of CIPN. J Pharmacol Exp Ther 2018; **364**: 110–119.

86. Sajjadian A, Doty RL, Gutnick DN, et al. Olfactory dysfunction in amyotrophic lateral sclerosis. Neurodegeneration 1994; **3**: 153–157.

87. Kotagal V, Albin RL, Muller ML, et al. Symptoms of rapid eye movement sleep behavior disorder are associated with cholinergic denervation in Parkinson disease. Ann Neurol 2012; **71**: 560–568.

88. Postuma RB, Gagnon JF, Vendette M, Desjardins C, Montplaisir JY. Olfaction and color vision identify impending neurodegeneration in rapid eye movement sleep behavior disorder. Ann Neurol 2011; **69**: 811–818.

89. Aguirre-Mardones C, Iranzo A, Vilas D, et al. Prevalence and timeline of nonmotor symptoms in idiopathic rapid eye movement sleep behavior disorder. J Neurol 2015; **262**: 1568–1578.

90. Killgore WD, McBride SA. Odor identification accuracy declines following 24 h of sleep deprivation. J Sleep Res 2006; **15**: 111–116.

91. Kaufmann H, Biaggioni I. Autonomic failure in neurodegenerative disorders. Semin Neurol 2003; **23**: 351–363.

92. Kovacs T, Papp MI, Cairns NJ, Khan MN, Lantos PL. Olfactory bulb in multiple system atrophy. Mov Disord 2003; **18**: 938–942.

93. Papp MI, Kahn JE, Lantos PL. Glial cytoplasmic inclusions in the CNS of patients with multiple system atrophy (striatonigral degeneration, olivopontocerebellar atrophy and Shy-Drager syndrome). J Neurol Sci 1989; **94**: 79–100.

94. Wenning GK, Shephard B, Hawkes C, et al. Olfactory function in atypical parkinsonian syndromes. Acta Neurol Scand 1995; **91**: 247–250.

95. Muller A, Mungersdorf M, Reichmann H, Strehle G, Hummel T. Olfactory function in Parkinsonian syndromes. J Clin Neurosci 2002; **9**: 521–524.

96. Abele M, Riet A, Hummel T, Klockgether T, Wullner U. Olfactory dysfunction in cerebellar

ataxia and multiple system atrophy. J Neurol 2003; 250: 1453–1455.

97. Goldstein DS, Holmes C, Bentho O, et al. Biomarkers to detect central dopamine deficiency and distinguish Parkinson disease from multiple system atrophy. Parkinsonism Relat Disord 2008; 14: 600–607.

98. Lee PH, Yeo SH, Kim HJ, Youm HY. Correlation between cardiac 123I-MIBG and odor identification in patients with Parkinson's disease and multiple system atrophy. Mov Disord 2006; 21: 1975–1977.

99. Doty RL. Olfactory dysfunction in neurogenerative disorders. In Getchell TV, Doty RL, Bartoshuk LM, Snow JBJ (eds.). *Smell and Taste in Health and Disease*. Raven Press; 1991: 735–751.

100. Cox TA, McDarby JV, Lavine L, Steele JC, Calne DB. A retinopathy on Guam with high prevalence in Lytico-Bodig. Ophthalmology 1989; 96: 1731–1735.

101. Kato S, Hirano A, Llena JF, Ito H, Yen SH. Ultrastructural identification of neurofibrillary tangles in the spinal cords in Guamanian amyotrophic lateral sclerosis and parkinsonism-dementia complex on Guam. Acta Neuropathol 1992; 83: 277–282.

102. Kokubo Y, Ito K, Fukunaga T, Matsubara H, Kuzuhara S. Pigmentary retinopathy of ALS/PDC in Kii. Ophthalmology 2006; 113: 2111–2112.

103. Reed D, Plato C, Elizan T, Kurland LT. The amyotrophic lateral sclerosis/parkinsonism-dementia complex – A ten-year follow-up on Guam. I. Epidemiological studies. Amer J Epidemiol 1966; 83: 54–73.

104. Reed DM, Brody JA. Amyotrophic lateral sclerosis and parkinsonism-dementia on Guam 1945–1972. I. Descriptive epidemiology. Amer J Epidemiol 1975; 101: 287–301.

105. Plato CC, Garruto RM, Galasko D, et al. Amyotrophic lateral sclerosis and parkinsonism-dementia complex of Guam: changing incidence rates during the past 60 years. Am J Epidemiol 2003; 157: 149–157.

106. Oyanagi K. The nature of the parkinsonism-dementia complex and amyotrophic lateral sclerosis of Guam and magnesium deficiency. Parkinsonism Relat Disord 2005; 11(Suppl 1): S17–S23.

107. Doty RL, Perl DP, Steele JC, et al. Odor identification deficit of the parkinsonism-dementia complex of Guam: equivalence to that of Alzheimer's and idiopathic Parkinson's disease. Neurology 1991; 41: 77–80.

108. Tzen KY, Lu CS, Yen TC, Wey SP, Ting C. Differential diagnosis of Parkinson's disease and vascular parkinsonism by Tc-99m-TRODAT-1. J Nuclear Med 2001; 42: 408–413.

109. Zijlmans JCM, Thijssen HOM, Vogels OJM, et al. MRI in patients with suspected vascular parkinsonism. Neurology 1995; 45: 2183–2188.

110. Katzenschlager R, Zijlmans J, Evans A, Watt H, Lees AJ. Olfactory function distinguishes vascular parkinsonism from Parkinson's disease. J Neurol Neurosurg Psychiatry 2004; 75: 1749–1752.

111. Navarro-Otano J, Gaig C, Muxi A, et al. (123) I-MIBG cardiac uptake, smell identification and (123)I-FP-CIT SPECT in the differential diagnosis between vascular parkinsonism and Parkinson's disease. Parkinsonism Relat Disord 2014; 20: 192–197.

112. Markopoulou K, Larsen KW, Wszolek EK, et al. Olfactory dysfunction in familial parkinsonism. Neurology 1997; 49: 1262–1267.

113. Bostantjopoulou S, Katsarou Z, Papadimitriou A, et al. Clinical features of parkinsonian patients with the alpha-synuclein (G209A) mutation. Mov Disord 2001; 16: 1007–1013.

114. Nishioka K, Ross OA, Ishii K, et al. Expanding the clinical phenotype of SNCA duplication carriers. Mov Disord 2009; 24: 1811–1819.

115. Koros C, Stamelou M, Simitsi A, et al. Selective cognitive impairment and hyposmia in p.A53T SNCA PD vs typical PD. Neurology 2018; 90: e864–e869.

116. Khan NL, Katzenschlager R, Watt H, et al. Olfaction differentiates parkin disease from early-onset parkinsonism and Parkinson disease. Neurology 2004; 62: 1224–1226.

117. Alcalay RN, Siderowf A, Ottman R, et al. Olfaction in Parkin heterozygotes and compound heterozygotes: the CORE-PD study. Neurology 2011; 76: 319–326.

118. Ferraris A, Ialongo T, Passali GC, et al. Olfactory dysfunction in Parkinsonism caused by *PINK1* mutations. Mov Disord 2009; 24: 2350–2357.

119. Eggers C, Schmidt A, Hagenah J, et al. Progression of subtle motor signs in PINK1 mutation carriers with mild dopaminergic deficit. Neurology 2010; 74: 1798–1805.

120. Samaranch L, Lorenzo-Betancor O, Arbelo JM, et al. PINK1-linked parkinsonism is associated with Lewy body pathology. Brain 2010; 133: 1128–1142.

121. Verbaan D, Boesveldt S, van Rooden SM, et al. Is olfactory impairment in Parkinson disease

related to phenotypic or genotypic characteristics? Neurology 2008; **71**: 1877–1882.

122. Saunders-Pullman R, Stanley K, Wang C, et al. Olfactory dysfunction in LRRK2 G2019S mutation carriers. Neurology 2011; **77**: 319–324.

123. Khan NL, Jain S, Lynch JM, et al. Mutations in the gene LRRK2 encoding dardarin (PARK8) cause familial Parkinson's disease: clinical, pathological, olfactory and functional imaging and genetic data. Brain 2005; **128**: 2786–2796.

124. Berg D, Schweitzer K, Leitner P, et al. Type and frequency of mutations in the *LRRK2* gene in familial and sporadic Parkinson's disease. Brain 2005; **128**: 3000–3011.

125. Lin CH, Tzen KY, Yu CY, et al. LRRK2 mutation in familial Parkinson's disease in a Taiwanese population: clinical, PET, and functional studies. J Biomed Sci 2008; **15**: 661–667.

126. Klein C, Schneider SA, Lang AE. Hereditary parkinsonism: Parkinson disease look-alikes– an algorithm for clinicians to "PARK" genes and beyond. Mov Disord 2009; **24**: 2042–2058.

127. Paisan-Ruiz C, Li A, Schneider SA, et al. Widespread Lewy body and tau accumulation in childhood and adult-onset dystonia-parkinsonism cases with PLA2G6 mutations. Neurobiol Aging 2012; **33**: 814–823.

128. Doty RL, Reyes PF, Gregor T. Presence of both odor identification and detection deficits in Alzheimer's disease. Brain Res Bull 1987; **18**: 597–600.

Oculomotor and Visual-Vestibular Disturbances in Parkinson's Disease

Adolfo M. Bronstein, Tim Anderson, Diego Kaski, Michael MacAskill, Aasef Shaikh

In this chapter we will describe how Parkinson's disease (PD) affects patients' eye movements, both bedside and laboratory, preceded by brief review of the anatomo-physiological substrate of eye movements. We will provide a practical summary of how to use the eye movement examination to aid the differential diagnosis of the parkinsonian syndromes, in particular, idiopathic PD from multiple system atrophy (MSA), progressive supranuclear palsy (PSP), and corticobasal syndrome (CBS). A sub-section will describe how deep brain stimulation (DBS) also influences eye movements in PD. Despite a plethora of eye movement laboratory studies in PD it is still relatively unknown what the eye movements of these patients are like in real life. Given that the eyes move in order to see better, does the akinesia of PD impose visual deprivation or delays during ecological whole-body movements? Finally, because the visual, vestibular, and oculomotor systems are tightly coupled, we will review this interaction which has bearing on the decades-long question of the contribution of central vestibular dysfunction to abnormalities of postural balance in PD. A practical implication of visuo-vestibular interactions in PD is that an observation of mini-ocular tremor in PD, with huge potential implications as a disease marker, has now been shown to be an artefact. Most authors agree that minute head oscillations, primary or transmitted from other body tremor, in these patients induce a compensatory eye movement response via the vestibulo-ocular reflex (VOR), which, on eye movement recordings but not clinically, looks like an ocular tremor.

Underlying Neural Mechanisms Involved in Eye Movements

Eye movements fall into two general classes. The first acts to stabilize the fovea in the face of motion of the head or objects of interest in the external world (the vestibulo-ocular reflex (VOR), fixation, smooth pursuit (SP), and optokinetic nystagmus (OKN)). The second, saccades, quickly bring the fovea with its superior acuity to bear upon salient objects. The first are largely automatic or reflexive responses whilst the second, saccades, are an inherent component of the continuously active cycle of perception, action, and cognition. In PD, the most apparent clinical and laboratory impairments are with saccades. Their tight link with attentional processes indicates that they are likely to reflect not only motor function but especially cognitive impairment in PD.

Saccades

Saccades are generated to support a variety of behavioral tasks. These range from the simple (reflexively glancing at the location of a suddenly occurring visual or auditory event) to complex and volitionally planned (looking at the remembered location of an object for a specific purpose, such as a clock on the wall in order to tell the time). Some tasks are laboratory specific, such as anti-saccades (looking in the *opposite* direction to a suddenly appearing target) and devised to layer cognitive requirements on top of the final oculomotor execution. Anti-saccade production requires suppression of the competing reflexive saccade to the visual target while concurrently planning a saccade in the opposite direction to a calculated, non-visual target location. Although all saccades share a final common pathway, differing task demands can result in differential recruitment of higher-level control areas (see Figure 11.1).

Cerebral Control of Saccades

The functional areas controlling saccades are depicted and described in Figures 11.1 and 11.2.

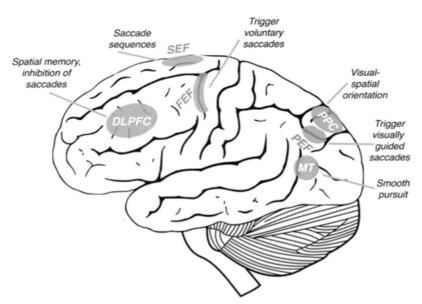

Figure 11.1 Selected cortical areas involved in oculomotor control. These include the dorsolateral prefrontal cortex (DLPFC), frontal, supplementary, and parietal eye fields (FEF, SEF, PEF), posterior parietal cortex (PPC), and the middle temporal visual area (MT). An additional region not shown is the cingulate eye field (CEF) in the anterior cingulate [14]. (For the color version, please refer to the plate section.)

These cortical regions, all with reciprocal connections, project caudally primarily to the superior colliculus (SC). In addition, frontal areas project to SC via an indirect basal ganglia pathway and also directly to pontine nuclei, especially the nucleus reticularis tegmenti pontis (NRTP), which in turn projects to dorsal vermis and fastigial nucleus in the cerebellum. There are minor direct projections from the frontal eye fields (FEF) to the paramedian pontine reticular formation (PPRF) [1]. The basal ganglia (BG) oculomotor pathway is concerned most with eye movements related to reward and initiation of remembered, predictive, and self-paced voluntary saccades (Figure 11.2). The net result of these various connections for the SNpr, the main output of the BG for eye movements, is that the indirect pathway is excitatory and the direct pathway inhibitory [2, 3]. In this manner the BG pathway regulates voluntary saccades by maintaining, enhancing, or releasing the SNpr tonic inhibition of the SC. Thus, the production of saccades is a consequence of the various cortical and subcortical excitatory and inhibitory influences upon the brainstem generating structures.

Smooth Pursuit

Smooth pursuit (SP) eye movements, in concert with fixation, stabilize the fovea in relation to movement of objects in the surrounding environment. During head movement the smooth pursuit system combines with the vestibulo-ocular reflex (VOR), fixation, and optokinetic system to maintain clear and stable vision. Visual information for smooth pursuit initiation and maintenance is processed by the extrastriate cortical regions MT (V5, in the middle temporal visual area) and MST (medial superior temporal visual area) and thence PPC, FEF, and SEF. Projections caudally from these regions descend ipsilaterally to pontine nuclei, then to the cerebellum (dorsal vermis, paraflocculus, and flocculus). These cerebellar regions then project via fastigial nucleus, vestibular nuclei, and Y-group to the oculomotor nuclei [1, 4]. The long and widespread nature of these pathways explains that smooth pursuit abnormalities are a sensitive albeit non-specific marker of CNS dysfunction.

Clinical Oculomotor Examination Findings in Parkinson's Disease

Decreased saccade amplitude can be detected even in clinical examination of PD patients by observing saccades made in response to verbal commands to look repeatedly between two of the examiner's fingers in the horizontal and vertical directions (Figure 11.3). The amplitude of saccades is visibly reduced when the patient is then asked to execute the same movements repetitively at their own volition (e.g. self-paced saccades), especially for

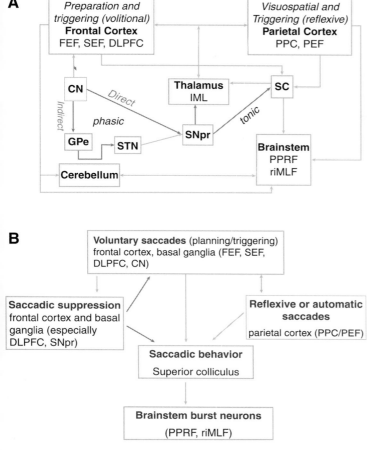

A

Figure 11.2 Schema for the cerebral control of saccades. (A, top) The posterior parietal cortex (PPC) or parietal eye field (PEF) is particularly involved in target selection (where and what to look at) and triggering reflexive (automatic) saccades. The frontal cortex (FEF, DLPFC, SEF) is particularly concerned with willed saccadic behavior (if, when, and how to look) and performance of voluntary saccades. The basal ganglia pathway is particularly concerned with volitional and not reflexive saccades. There is tonic inhibition of the SC by SNpr. There is also phasic release, or increase of inhibition, depending on the balance of activity in the direct and indirect pathways. (B, bottom) Saccade production is the result of interplay between cortical and subcortical excitatory and inhibitory influences. Red arrows denote inhibitory connections; green arrows denote excitatory connections. DLPFC: dorsolateral prefrontal cortex; FEF: frontal eye fields; GPe: globus pallidus externa; IML: intramedullary lamina; PPRF: parapontine reticular formation; riMLF: rostral interstitial nucleus of the medial longitudinal fasciculus; SC: superior colliculus; SEF: supplementary eye fields; SNpr: substantia nigra pars reticulate; STN: subthalamic nucleus. (For the color version, please refer to the plate section.)

Adapted and modified from [94].

upwards saccades, with a series of several saccades needed to reach the target. In patients with PD, reduced saccade amplitude is detectable early in the disease course, presumably reflecting neurodegeneration (Figure 11.4). The bedside anti-saccade (BAS) task has been employed in the assessment of executive dysfunction in persons with mild cognitive impairment (MCI) and dementia due to a variety of disorders including some with PD but there has been no study of the BAS task specifically in PD [5]. Other deficits on clinical examination are increased number of square wave jerks (SWJs) and impairment in smooth pursuit, VOR suppression, and OKN (optokinetic nystagmus) but these are mild and difficult to distinguish from age-related changes.

Convergence insufficiency is present in some 40% of PD patients and may present as diplopia in a proportion (16%) during near vision (e.g. reading) [6]. It has commonly been thought that there

is mild restriction of conjugate upgaze in PD but confirmatory studies with age-matched controls have been lacking. Many PD patients exhibit reduced blink rate and some a degree of lid retraction and lid lag though these latter features are more commonly seen in PSP [7]. Other ocular problems encountered in PD include dry eyes (exacerbated by antiparkinsonian drugs with anticholinergic activity), amantadine-induced corneal oedema and keratitis, decreased contrast sensitivity and reduced color discrimination, visuospatial impairments, and misperceptual disorders (illusions and hallucinations; see Chapter 8) [8].

Laboratory Eye Movement Findings in Parkinson's Disease

Starting with the landmark observations by DeJong and Jones [9], laboratory studies have

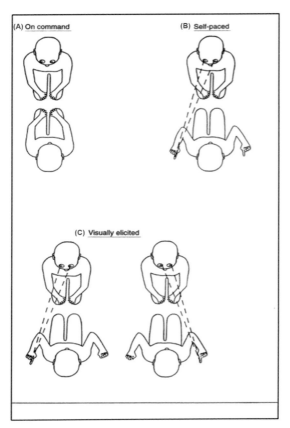

Figure 11.3 Different ways of examining saccades. (A) Without any specific visual target the patient is instructed to look right, left, up, or down, sometimes repetitively e.g. right-left-right-left-right etc. (B) Self-paced saccades whereby the patient is instructed to look as many times as possible between two static visual targets (fingers, in the figure) without further verbal encouragement. (C) Conventionally, saccades are elicited with the aid of a suddenly appearing visual target with or without simultaneous verbal reinforcement ("right," "left" as the fingers flick as in the picture). Saccades elicited this way are usually within normal limits for age in patients with PD. In (A) and (B), PD patients may start off with normometric saccades but within a couple of cycles begin to exhibit considerable hypometria and sometimes "freezing" of saccades, namely the eyes remain jammed on a target for a few seconds before being able to shift them again.

(With kind permission of Bronstein et al. [95].)

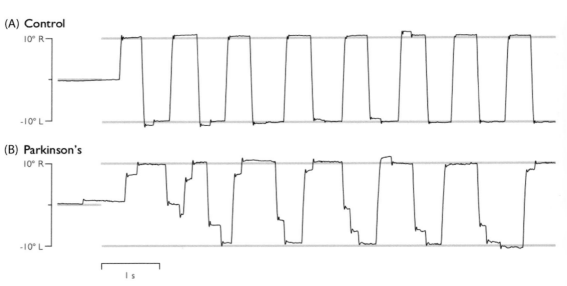

Figure 11.4 Laboratory recordings of horizontal self-paced saccades in a control (A) and PD patient (B) as they are asked to refixate back and forth between the two targets set 20 degrees apart, 10 degrees either side of center. Controls sometimes overshoot with a corrective saccade back to the target. PD patients frequently undershoot, requiring one or more corrective saccades in the same direction to acquire the target (i.e. hypometria).

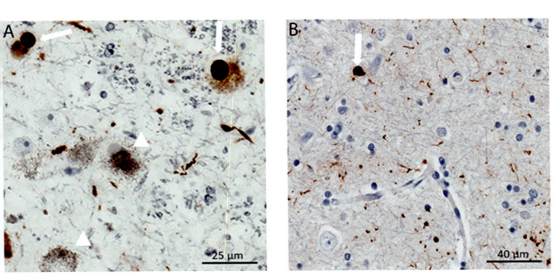

Figure 4.1 Histological slides of a case with Lewy body dementia immunostained for α-synuclein. (A) shows the substantia nigra; (B) the amygdala. Note the large number of Lewy neurites (in brown). Arrows point to Lewy bodies and arrow heads to neuromelanin-containing neurons.

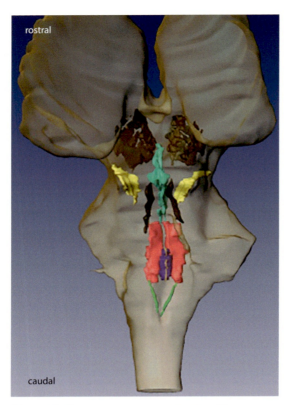

Figure 4.2 Three-dimensional reconstruction of key brainstem nuclei involved in early Lewy body disease. Braak stage 1: dorsal motor nucleus of the vagus (lower green); Braak stage 2: gigantocellular nucleus of the reticular formation (red), raphe magnus (purple) and locus coeruleus (lower black); Braak stage 3: dorsal raphe (upper green), pedunculopontine tegmental nucleus (yellow), and substantia nigra (upper black).

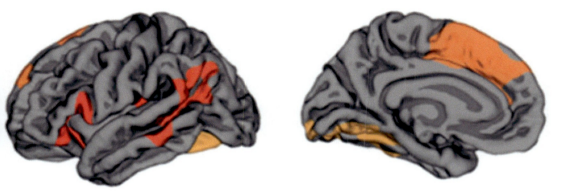

Figure 5.1 A cortical surface map showing where there is a significant correlation between gray matter thickness and MoCA cognitive ratings in Parkinson's disease [12].

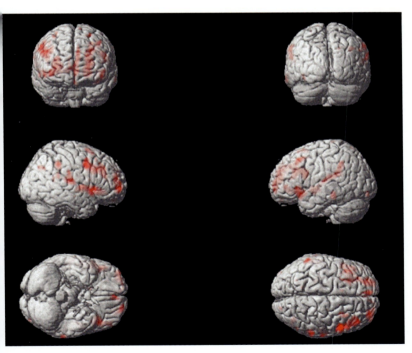

Figure 5.2 A cortical surface map showing areas of significantly reduced glucose metabolism in non-demented Parkinson's disease patients [14].

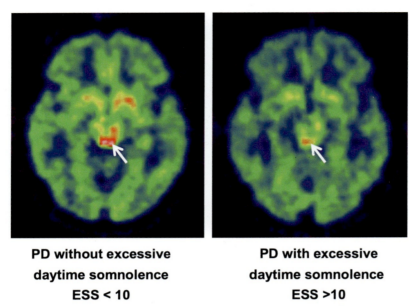

**PD without excessive
daytime somnolence
ESS < 10**

**PD with excessive
daytime somnolence
ESS >10**

Figure 5.3 Reduced ^{11}C-DASB binding in the thalamus and median raphe of PD patients with excessive daytime somnolence. Picture courtesy of N. Pavese.

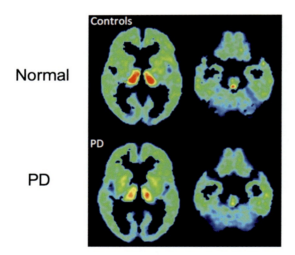

Figure 5.4 Reduced ^{11}C-MeNER binding in the thalamus and locus ceruleus of PD patients with REM sleep behavior disorder. Picture courtesy of M. Sommerauer.

Figure 5.5 Reduced [11] C-donepezil uptake in the intestine and myocardium of a PD patient relative to a healthy control. Picture courtesy of P. Borghammer.

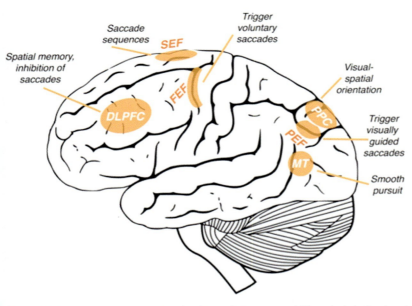

Figure 11.1 Selected cortical areas involved in oculomotor control. These include the dorsolateral prefrontal cortex (DLPFC), frontal, supplementary, and parietal eye fields (FEF, SEF, PEF), posterior parietal cortex (PPC), and the middle temporal visual area (MT). An additional region not shown is the cingulate eye field (CEF) in the anterior cingulate [14].

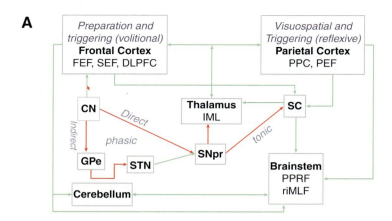

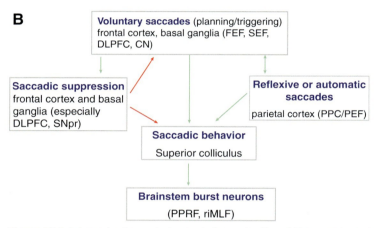

Figure 11.2 Schema for the cerebral control of saccades. (A, top) The posterior parietal cortex (PPC) or parietal eye field (PEF) is particularly involved in target selection (where and what to look at) and triggering reflexive (automatic) saccades. The frontal cortex (FEF, DLPFC, SEF) is particularly concerned with willed saccadic behavior (if, when, and how to look) and performance of voluntary saccades. The basal ganglia pathway is particularly concerned with volitional and not reflexive saccades. There is tonic inhibition of the SC by SNpr. There is also phasic release, or increase of inhibition, depending on the balance of activity in the direct and indirect pathways. (B, bottom) Saccade production is the result of interplay between cortical and subcortical excitatory and inhibitory influences. Red arrows denote inhibitory connections; green arrows denote excitatory connections. DLPFC: dorsolateral prefrontal cortex; FEF: frontal eye fields; GPe: globus pallidus externa; IML: intramedullary lamina; PPRF: parapontine reticular formation; riMLF: rostral interstitial nucleus of the medial longitudinal fasciculus; SC: superior colliculus; SEF: supplementary eye fields; SNpr: substantia nigra pars reticulate; STN: subthalamic nucleus. Adapted and modified from [94].

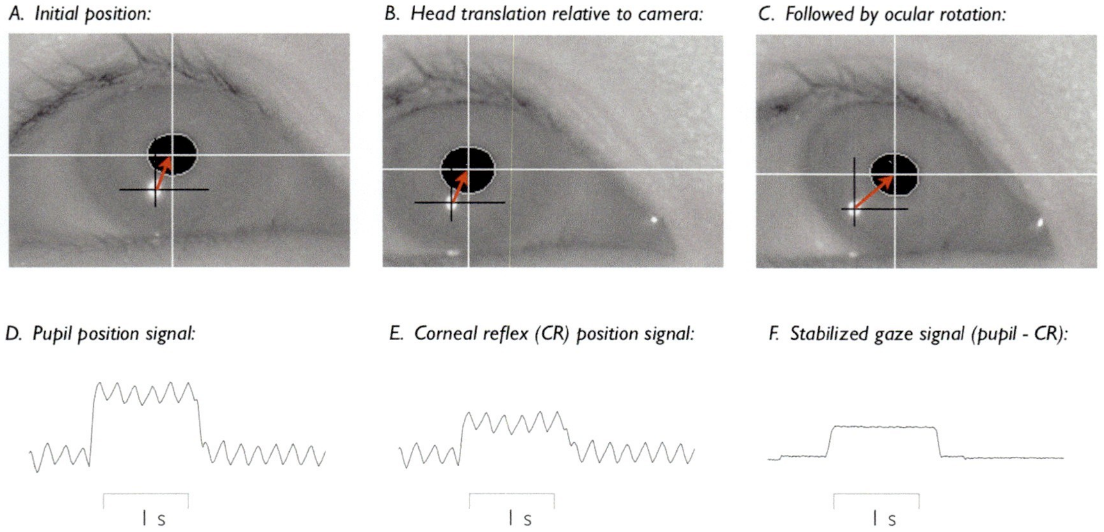

A. *Initial position:*

B. *Head translation relative to camera:*

C. *Followed by ocular rotation:*

D. *Pupil position signal:*

E. *Corneal reflex (CR) position signal:*

F. *Stabilized gaze signal (pupil - CR):*

I s

I s

I s

Figure 11.6 Here we illustrate the principles of pupil center-corneal reflex video-oculography and how it can remove artefacts due to somatomotor tremor in PD. (A) A PD patient with tremor. The pupil is centered in the camera field of view. The red arrow is the vector showing the relative position of the corneal reflex and the pupil center. (B) The head has moved substantially relative to the camera while the eye maintains a constant gaze direction in space. The relative positions of the pupil and corneal reflex within the image are unchanged. (C) The eye after a saccade, making a pure rotation within a stationary head. The pupil center and the corneal reflection have moved differentially within the image. (D) The horizontal pupil center position of a person with PD and substantial somatomotor tremor, showing a substantial oscillation due to head movement. The patient is tracking a target stepping 20 degrees rightwards and then leftwards. (E) The corneal reflex signal shares the same oscillation. (F) Simply subtracting the corneal reflex signal from the pupil position reveals a stabilized gaze signal, showing that the patient was actually maintaining steady fixations upon fixed targets, interrupted only by saccades and micro saccades. That is, the substantial oscillations are solely due to head motion, with no residual ocular tremor.

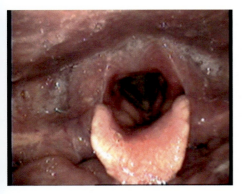

Figure 13.1 Fiber optic endoscopy in a patient with PD.

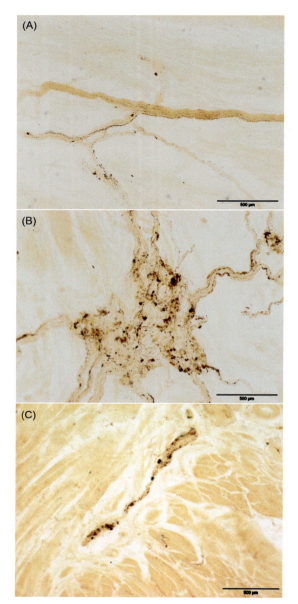

Figure 13.3 Lewy pathology in the Auerbach (intramural) plexus of the ENS in sporadic PD. (A) Aggregated α-synuclein in single axons within fiber bundles interconnecting the ganglia of the gastric cardia: 65-year-old male, Hoehn & Yahr 3, with stage 3 brain pathology. (B) Severe lesions in the gastric cardia: 78-year-old female with disease duration of 11 years, Hoehn & Yahr 4, stage 5 brain pathology. (C) Lewy bodies in the distal esophagus (*at left*, longitudinal musculature; *at right*, circular musculature): 71-year-old female with disease duration of 10 years, Hoehn & Yahr 5, stage 5 brain pathology. Syn-1 (1:2000; Clone number 42; BD Biosciences, Eysins, Switzerland) immunoreactions in tangential (A, B) and transversal (C) cryosections of 100 μm thickness.

(Reproduced with kind permission of Dr. Kelly Del Tredici-Braak, Ulm, Germany) dealt predominantly with saccades and less so smooth pursuit. Voluntary saccades (endogenously generated) have exhibited greater abnormalities than reflexive (exogenously induced) saccades. In reflexive tasks the sudden onset of a stimulus automatically determines the saccade target, but in voluntary saccade tasks some cognitive operation is required to select the saccade target [10]. In most voluntary saccade tasks participants must shift attention to a visual stimulus without making a saccade to that stimulus, and either initiate a saccade in the opposite direction (antisaccades), or wait for a further cue (delayed or memory-guided saccades). People with PD consistently make more unintended saccades to the visual stimulus (hyper-reflexivity), and they make the correct voluntary saccades at longer latencies and with smaller amplitudes (hypometria) than controls [11]. Oculomotor hypometria is present early in the disease, while more cognitively driven impairments (prolonged latencies and reduced inability to inhibit saccades in antisaccade and delayed-response tasks) become evident as non-dopaminergic cortical-level degeneration occurs [12, 13]. Saccadic latency and velocities in cognitively normal PD patients, especially for reflexive saccades, have generally been normal [14] or minimally abnormal [15] with minor hypometria the commonest feature of reflexive saccades [3, 12, 16].

Mild impairment of smooth pursuit (SP) is a consistent finding [17]. Interestingly there does not seem to be an underlying abnormality in the SP pathway itself. Rather, there is a saccadic abnormality whereby anticipatory saccades take the eyes ahead of the moving target perhaps again reflecting deficits in inhibition as already discussed [18].

Saccades and Cognitive Impairment in Parkinson's Disease

There have been no published systematic studies of confrontational eye movement examination in those with cognitive impairment and dementia in PD though supranuclear vertical gaze palsy may be observed in a minority of dementia with Lewy bodies (DLB) patients [19]. PD patients with mild cognitive impairment (PD-MCI) exhibit mild prolongation of reflexive visually guided saccade latency compared to those with normal cognition, but no difference in amplitude [12]. Those with

PD and dementia (PDD) exhibit prolonged latency and reduced amplitude of reflexive and voluntary saccades, impaired predictive behavior, and reduced saccadic inhibition, compared to those with normal cognition and controls [11, 12]. Thus, saccadic latency correlates with cognitive status in PD, suggesting that eye movement recordings could provide useful objective markers for cognitive decline.

Ocular Dyskinesia and Other Levodopa Effects on Eye Movements

Up to 16% of advanced PD patients with levodopa-induced dyskinesias (LID) of limbs and trunk may also exhibit simultaneous ocular dyskinesia – stereotyped upward and/or horizontal conjugate gaze movements [20]. We have observed similar dyskinesia but in a smaller percentage of patients with LID, with the dominant deviation being upwards, and not appreciated by the patients themselves.

The effects of levodopa on eye movements in PD are not well established. Improvement in convergence insufficiency [21] and pursuit performance [22] has been reported but it is the influence of levodopa on saccades in PD that has been the most explored. No consistent effect has emerged and this accords with the authors' experience that dopaminergic therapy has little effect on saccadic performance, suggesting that non-dopaminergic pathways are more influential in PD saccadic dysfunction.

Eye Movements in the Atypical Parkinsonian Disorders

The careful clinical eye movement examination is most helpful in distinguishing PD (mild and nonspecific deficits) from the atypical parkinsonian disorders, which have both shared and characteristic oculomotor abnormalities.

Eye Movements in Multiple System Atrophy

Patients with MSA-C (cerebellar type) usually present with symptoms that suggest a late-onset cerebellar syndrome associated with typical cerebellar eye signs such as gaze-evoked, downbeat and rebound nystagmus, and impaired smooth pursuit [23]. Eye movements in early MSA-P (parkinsonian type) may initially be similar to those in PD, but

Adolfo M. Bronstein, Tim Anderson, Diego Kaski, Michael MacAskill, Aasef Shaikh

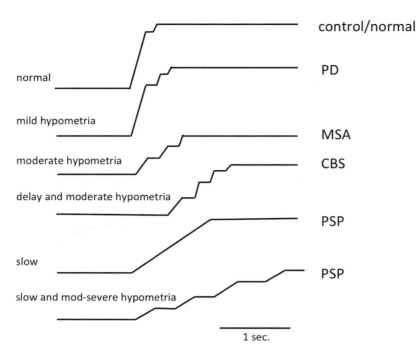

Figure 11.5 Schematic of typical saccade abnormalities in PD and the atypical parkinsonian disorders. It is common for healthy individuals to slightly undershoot the target and use a small secondary saccade to achieve the target. PD patients commonly show mild hypometria (undershooting) requiring two or more corrective saccades to reach the target. In MSA and CBS the degree of saccadic hypometria is often greater than in PD with delayed launching of saccades (saccadic apraxia) an additional feature of CBS. In PSP the hallmark is early saccadic slowing with considerable hypometria developing over time. CBS: corticobasal syndrome; MSA: multiple system atrophy; PD: Parkinson's disease; PSP: progressive supranuclear palsy. Figure by Bronstein & Anderson (2021), distributed at https://doi.org/10.6084/m9.figshare.14390951 under an open CC-BY 4.0 license.

a combination of increased square wave jerks, mild or moderate saccade hypometria and impaired VOR suppression and smooth pursuit indicate that the patient is unlikely to have PD [24]. Saccade velocities are normal in patients with MSA and only a minority have a vertical supranuclear gaze palsy which if present is mild [24]. Positional downbeat nystagmus or perverted head-shaking nystagmus (vertical nystagmus on horizontal head oscillation) is present in about one-third of patients with MSA-P [24, 25]. Slow saccades or significant supranuclear gaze palsy indicate an alternative diagnosis, particularly PSP (Figure 11.5).

Eye Movements in Progressive Supranuclear Palsy

The earliest and most diagnostically important eye movement abnormality in patients with PSP-RS (Richardson syndrome) is slowing of vertical saccades; slowing of horizontal saccades appears later [26]. Though slowing of downward saccades was considered a hallmark of PSP-RS [27], upward saccade velocity is as slow as, or sometimes even slower, than downward saccades, and upgaze palsy occurs more frequently than downgaze palsy [26] perhaps, in part, related to the upgaze limitation

commonly present in the elderly. Vertical and horizontal saccades become very hypometric which, when added to the low velocity of each saccadic segment, can make the eyes take more than one to two seconds to travel from one end of the orbit to the opposite. Smooth pursuit is at least moderately impaired [28]. Small-amplitude horizontal SWJs on fixation are more prominent than in other parkinsonian disorders [29]. In addition, reduced blink rate, eye-opening and eye-closing apraxia – observed as slowness of eye opening and closing – are frequently present, and blepharospasm in some. Eye movements in patients with PSP-P (PSP-parkinsonism and PSP-PAGF (PSP-pure akinesia with gait freezing) are less well studied. Supranuclear gaze palsy is usually absent during early PSP-P but develops late in the disease course in 70% of patients [30]. By definition, supranuclear gaze palsy is not evident in the first five years after disease onset in patients with PSP-PAGF, but can appear as a late feature [31].

Eye Movements in Corticobasal Syndrome

The oculomotor characteristic of clinically diagnosed CBS is saccadic apraxia [32], evidenced clinically as delay in the initiation of saccades to command or towards a target, especially towards the side of the apraxic limbs, and in the laboratory as a marked increase in saccade latency [33]. This difficulty in launching saccades is often accompanied and signaled by the patient using an auxiliary head movement in the same direction. In contrast to PSP, saccade velocities in patients with CBS are normal [34]. Smooth pursuit may be moderately impaired, but not as much as in patients with PSP. Antisaccade errors in CBS are similar in extent to those encountered in PSP [33, 34].

In summary, in the differential diagnosis of parkinsonism, slowed vertical saccades can suggest a diagnosis of PSP (and help rule out PD, MSA, or CBS), cerebellar eye signs (especially gaze-evoked, headshaking, or positional downbeat nystagmus) suggest MSA, and saccadic apraxia suggests CBS (Figure 11.4).

Effects of Deep Brain Stimulation on Eye Movements and Vestibular Function

There is a paucity of understanding how DBS affects oculomotor and balance deficits that are common in PD and lead to problems in navigation, walking, and to falls. DBS can improve, worsen, or have no effect on these functions. The focus of this section is to understand typical clinical oculomotor or balance deficits that are seen in PD with DBS, and how to manage them.

Effects of Deep Brain Stimulation on Eye Movements

Subthalamic nucleus (STN) DBS can cause ocular dysconjugacy with adduction and depression of the eye ipsilateral to the side of STN DBS [35]. Such ocular misalignment, if mild, leads to blurred vision but if moderate or severe, to diplopia. The basis of this deficit is the strategic location of the oculomotor nerve fascicles emerging from the oculomotor nucleus. The oculomotor nerve passes medially, ventrally, and posteriorly to the STN. If the active DBS electrode within the STN is in proximity to the oculomotor nerve fibers, the electrical charge may activate the ipsilateral nerve fibers causing monocular medial and downward deviation and on some occasions, tonic counter-clockwise torsion and lid retraction of the

ipsilateral eye [35]. These oculomotor signs can be used to guide localization of the DBS electrode. Another oculomotor side effect is conjugate gaze deviation away from the side of STN DBS due to activation of the fronto-pontine fibers within the internal capsule by a lead that is too lateral. Treatment of any of such stimulation-dependent DBS side effects usually requires moving the location of the active electrode to an alternate contact. Alternative strategies include minimizing the electric spread to the oculomotor fibers that can be accomplished by constricting the volume of tissue activation by reducing the voltage or pulse-width, switching to bipolar montage, or current steering with contemporary directional electrode leads.

Subthalamic nucleus DBS does not necessarily lead to negative visual consequences. Some who have existing visuomotor deficits may even experience benefits. There is sparse literature examining effects of STN DBS on visuomotor function [36]. It is however likely that STN DBS mediates any visuomotor benefits by modulating abnormal basal ganglia outflow that would otherwise adversely affect the superior colliculus, precerebellar pontine nuclei, or the cerebellum [2]. More studies are required to examine the mechanistic underpinning of beneficial and adverse effects of DBS on visuomotor deficits in PD. Combined PPD and STN stimulation seems to add further benefit on antisaccadic task performance, suggesting a DBS ascending effect on frontal lobe processing [37].

Effects of Deep Brain Stimulation on Vestibular Function and Balance

The effects of STN DBS on balance function are unpredictable, improving it in some patients but worsening it in others [38, 39]. These conflicting observations suggest that STN DBS affects multiple neuronal pathways. One important nearby pathway that can be modulated by the electrical field generated by STN DBS is the cerebello-thalamic pathway, a major output from the deep cerebellar nuclei [40]. This probably explains stimulation-dependent increase in vertigo and other complex self-motion illusions [41]. STN DBS can also modulate vestibular activity via activation of the precerebellar nuclei and thereby the subthalamo-pontocerebellar projections [40]. Although these different mechanisms can describe diverse effects of STN

DBS on vestibular function, such hypotheses need further experimental support.

In summary, there are various effects of DBS on oculomotor and vestibular function, depending, in part, on the location of the stimulation. Diplopia and blurred vision that is commonly seen in DBS patients is usually due to direct activation of the oculomotor nerve fascicles, with tonic conjugate deviation of the eyes secondary to activation of cortico-bulbar fibers. Vestibular effects of the STN DBS may be caused by activation of cerebello-thalamic fibers projecting to the cerebral cortex responsible for motion perception. The approach to addressing these DBS-induced vestibular or visual side effects is to constrict the volume of tissue activation by delivering less electrical charge or orientating the current away from the relevant anatomical target.

Eye Movements in the Real World

Evolving technology has made it feasible to record gaze in naturalistic settings. A systematic review of studies of real-world eye movements in PD concluded that eye movement strategies were used to compensate for the more severe somatomotor symptoms despite presence of typical oculomotor impairments [42]. These studies show that oculomotor performance in real-world tasks is closely linked to visual and cognitive impairments. Of note, PD can add massive delays upon visual target acquisition – up to half a second for large gaze re-orientations [43].

Impaired or even frozen gait in PD can be facilitated by strong visual cues [44]. Although striking, the mechanism remains unclear. For example, do stripes on the floor act directly as a visual target to drive the feet toward them, or indirectly, by shifting attention downward toward the lower limbs themselves? When external visual cues (e.g. floor stripes) are provided, with or without the view of the lower limbs being occluded, gaze tracking indicates that both those with PD and controls fixate the cues one or more steps ahead of the current foot position. Such external cues are sufficient to improve parkinsonian gait, with direct visualization of the limbs unnecessary [45]. Freezing-of-gait (FOG) can be induced by changing gait direction. Body turns ideally consist of an orderly sequence of rotations, commencing with saccades and followed in order by the head, trunk, and feet. In PD however, *en bloc* turning is

common, and with parkinsonian saccades being hypometric, more saccades are needed, leading, in part, to a longer duration of the entire turn [43, 46].

Cognitive decline in PD is common so it is relevant to consider how much impairment might constrain neuropsychological test performance, independent of cognitive decline. Gaze recordings of images from neuropsychological tests (e.g. the Rey complex figure and interlocking pentagons), show that saccadic hypometria leads to a restricted range of areas being fixated [47]. Meanwhile, gaze strategies in neuropsychological tasks are relatively normal in PD with normal cognition but become progressively worse in PD-MCI and then PDD [48]. Surprisingly, there has been little investigation of eye movements during reading in PD, although reading speed correlates with gait performance [49, 50].

Eye tracking during completion of the Symbol-Digits Modalities Test (SDMT), which requires decoding of symbols on a page by referring to a "key" at the top of the page, was able to identify the time point when people had learned the symbol-digit associations sufficiently to write responses without continually needing to look up the key [51]. Poorer performance in PD participants with mild cognitive impairment was not due to impaired oculomotor control, validating the SDMT as a cognitively specific assessment tool in PD.

Visuo-Vestibular Interaction in Parkinson's Disease

Parkinson's disease patients suffer from prominent postural problems and it is therefore reasonable to ask whether vestibular dysfunction may be partly responsible for these. Here, however, we will not review gait and postural control in PD as a whole because this topic is vast, reviewed often, and lies outside the remit of this visuo-vestibular-oculomotor chapter [52–54].

Vestibulo-Ocular Reflex and Otolith Function

Despite decades of study, whether the VOR is affected in PD still remains somewhat controversial. In 1982 Reichert et al. reported reduced or absent nystagmus in 36 PD patients to a bithermal caloric stimulation, a finding that was associated with postural instability, suggesting perhaps a link between impaired vestibular function and postural control in PD [55]. Abnormal caloric-induced nystagmus was later reported in over 80% of PD patients but the response was heightened not reduced in over half and was not related to clinical PD motor symptoms [56]. A recent study with well-selected PD patients did not report abnormalities in the caloric vestibular test [57]. By contrast, in two small studies in patients with Pisa syndrome (lateral trunk flexion), one found unilateral vestibular hypofunction in each case and the other, greater subjective visual vertical errors than those without Pisa syndrome, consistent with otolith dysfunction [58, 59]. Notably however, the subjective visual vertical is preserved in non-selected PD patients [57, 60].

The VOR assessed with rotating chairs in the dark is challenging in PD. Reduced rotational function in the dark with paradoxical enhancement during fixation-mediated VOR suppression in early reports was likely due to drowsiness [61]. The advent of easily available computerized measures of the VOR has led to further work, with modestly elevated VOR gains in PD than controls using the video head impulse test (vHIT; i.e. 1.20 versus 0.99, respectively) [62]. Whilst this result may be consistent with the increased caloric nystagmus reported by Cipparrone et al. [56], subtle differences in VOR gains observed may be due to the technical challenge of utilizing the vHIT in patients with neck rigidity/stiffness. Besides, the *increased* vHIT gain in PD patients runs counter to the initial papers reporting *reduced* vestibular caloric responses. Furthermore, the normal interplay between VOR activation and suppression required during ecological head-eye coordination tasks is essentially preserved in PD, again indicating preserved vestibular function [43, 63, 64].

There has been interest in exploring neurophysiological brainstem function in PD, not least following reports that noisy galvanic vestibular stimulation (nGVS) or caloric vestibular stimulation can reduce severity of some PD symptoms (see Cronin et al. for a comprehensive review [65]). The vestibular-startle, elicited by free-fall, is preserved in PD but abnormal in atypical parkinsonism [66] as the latter is known to have brainstem reticular formation pathology. Reduced or absent vestibular-evoked myogenic potential (VEMP) responses in PD patients correlate with contralateral rigidity, bradykinesia score, ipsilateral dyskinesia score, as well as sleep, mood, and memory impairment [67]. The cVEMP (a loud click-evoked vestibulo-collic reflex thought to be otolith mediated) in PD has been reported as frequently abnormal (although not unanimously [68]), despite group latency values being preserved [57, 67, 69–73].

Otolith dysfunction in PD could theoretically arise from degeneration in the vestibular nuclei of PD patients, disrupting connections between vestibular nuclei and the dorsal raphe nuclei, and reducing the effect of dopamine on the excitability of vestibular nuclei. Nevertheless, in routine clinical practice, peripheral vestibular function is usually normal in PD patients.

It is important that in PD patients with complaints of vertigo or recent falls, not only should orthostatic blood pressure be measured but also a Dix-Hallpike maneuver undertaken to exclude benign positional paroxysmal vertigo (BPPV), the commonest cause of episodic vertigo regardless of any co-existing neurological disorder.

Multi-sensory Integration and the Vestibular System

Early experiments in the motor, ocular-motor, and postural systems indicated that PD patients were visually "dependent" [63, 74, 75]. Specifically, postural responses elicited by a large moving visual display were larger and less susceptible to adaptation in PD patients than controls [74]. Such findings can be interpreted either as an upregulated visuo-motor postural loop or a downregulated vestibulo-proprioceptive loop. The latter is in agreement with Purdon Martin's classical experiments on postural responses in post-encephalitic Parkinsonian patients where, based on similar postural responses to a tilting support surface in Parkinsonian patients and subjects with bilaterally absent vestibular function, he concluded that the main cause of instability in Parkinsonism was central vestibular dysfunction [76]. However, any investigation of postural responses in Parkinsonism could be confounded by the severe global motor difficulties these patients experience. For this reason researchers switched to perceptual rather than motor assessments of vestibular function.

Nakamura et al. investigated the perception of head rotation (vestibular, cervical, or combined) in PD with a remembered saccade paradigm [77, 78]. The confound introduced by the motor system (in this case the oculomotor system) was confirmed by the finding that, despite remembered saccades being hypometric, the actual perception of head rotation was preserved in PD patients, indicating preserved vestibular function. In further perceptual experiments measuring the relative strength of visual-vestibular inputs, again bypassing any motor influence, PD patients were normal [60].

Galvanic (DC electrical) vestibular stimulation in PD patients elicits normal or even increased postural responses [79], a finding incompatible with vestibular dysfunction being the cause of the postural disturbance in PD. Similarly, the long latency component of the stretch reflex to limb displacement is also enhanced in PD [80]. Taken together these results indicate that any sensory channel – visual, vestibular, or proprioceptive – when individually (experimentally) stimulated induces normal or large postural responses in PD patients. Therefore, PD does not disrupt simple, mono-sensory, reflex responses. Rather, the underlying problem responsible for instability and ultimately falls is hypokinetic (small) and slow (bradykinetic) postural responses, which are not scaled to the magnitude of the perturbation [81, 82]. It seems that any sensory processing contribution to the postural problem in PD is negligible compared to the central disruption of integrative motor programs.

Perceiving the direction of self-motion – heading – is a type of multi-sensory integration that depends on visual and vestibular information. Precision of heading perception is typically assessed in a heading discrimination task where subjects are presented with a whole-body linear translation (leftward/rightward), of varying intensity, and are asked to indicate the perceived direction of motion to derive a threshold. Such paradigms have been used in PD patients using linear translations on a motion platform. One study found increased vestibular thresholds in PD [83], but another that used the same method reported no impairment [84]. Patients with normal performance were less severely affected so it has been proposed that heading discrimination may only be impaired in later stages of the disease. PD

patients also appear to be less accurate in judging forward tilt but only in a multi-cue condition such as combining tilt movements with translations [85].

Sensory paradigms in the fMRI scanner may help understand central sensory-motor integration without motor interference by PD. One study has used fMRI in PD patients to study cortical activation in areas involved in visual motion processing [86]. PD patients exhibited significantly reduced activity in the medial temporal area and cingulate sulcus visual areas in response to simulated optic flow. Activation of the cingulate sulcus visual area was inversely correlated with disease severity, suggesting that impaired visuospatial performance in PD may be a result of impaired neural processing within visual motion and visuo-vestibular regions [87].

Is the So-Called Pervasive Ocular Tremor in Parkinson's Disease the Result of a Normal Visuo-Vestibular Interaction?

In 2012 Gitchel and colleagues reported "pervasive ocular tremor" that was universally present in a cohort of 112 PD patients, and mostly absent in healthy controls [88]. The presence, or not, of "ocular tremor" in PD has been the object of recent controversy [88]. The eye oscillations described had an average fundamental frequency of 5.7 Hz (i.e. within the range of the limb tremor in PD: 4–7 Hz), a mean horizontal amplitude of 0.27 degrees, and mean vertical amplitude of 0.33 degrees. The tremor persisted for the duration of the recording, although the waveform characteristics were variable. The authors did not use head restraint but recorded head movements using a magnetic tracker in a subset of patients and controls; no head oscillation was detected in any subject implying that the observable ocular tremor was independent of head motion. Nevertheless, given the lack of other reports of ocular fixation instability across decades of eye movement recordings in patients with parkinsonism, the possible origin of the pervasive ocular tremor generated significant discussion and controversy.

A subsequent study reported ocular oscillations during oculography in two consecutive PD patients attending a balance clinic. These were accompanied by a recordable head tremor that had the same fundamental frequency and high coherence with both the eye oscillations and a recordable limb tremor [89]. The eye oscillations were in the opposite direction (anti-phase) to the head oscillation and dampened by physically restraining the head. This suggests that the ocular tremor is a compensatory eye movement secondary perhaps to a head tremor transmitted from the limbs. Indeed, despite extensive oculographic recordings in PD, ocular tremor had not previously been described [90]. Further, during fundoscopy of many hundreds of PD patients over decades we (personal observations) and others have not observed such tremor of the globes [90].

It transpires that the existence of "ocular tremor" depends on the technique and equipment used to record the eye movements in a person with PD (see Kaski and Bronstein for a review [91]). In our experience, when recording eye movements with video-oculography – the almost universal technique nowadays – in PD patients it is very common to see the eye image oscillating considerably within the field of view of the camera, due to tremor of the limbs being transmitted mechanically to the head. The recorded gaze signal, however, can be completely steady. This reflects that, despite the head motion, with an intact VOR, the patient's eyes remain steady in space, which is what an eye tracker using corneal reflection stabilization measures. In the original report of the phenomenon, corneal reflection stabilization was not applied [88]. We subsequently analyzed 681 recordings from 188 patients and 66 controls and indeed observed a tremulous pupil signal in many, though not all, patients at around 4 Hz frequency, matching the characteristics reported by Gitchel et al. Crucially, a near-identical signal existed in the corneal reflection signal. The Fast Fourier Transform power of both oscillations was strongly correlated with clinical UPDRS tremor ratings. When the two signals were subtracted, the oscillation disappeared (Figure 11.6) [92]. This indicates that so-called ocular tremor is indeed a consequence of head motion, secondary to somatomotor tremor.

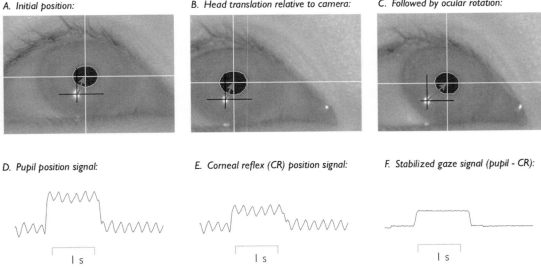

Figure 11.6 Here we illustrate the principles of pupil center-corneal reflex video-oculography and how it can remove artefacts due to somatomotor tremor in PD. (A) A PD patient with tremor. The pupil is centered in the camera field of view. The red arrow is the vector showing the relative position of the corneal reflex and the pupil center. (B) The head has moved substantially relative to the camera while the eye maintains a constant gaze direction in space. The relative positions of the pupil and corneal reflex within the image are unchanged. (C) The eye after a saccade, making a pure rotation within a stationary head. The pupil center and the corneal reflection have moved differentially within the image. (D) The horizontal pupil center position of a person with PD and substantial somatomotor tremor, showing a substantial oscillation due to head movement. The patient is tracking a target stepping 20 degrees rightwards and then leftwards. (E) The corneal reflex signal shares the same oscillation. (F) Simply subtracting the corneal reflex signal from the pupil position reveals a stabilized gaze signal, showing that the patient was actually maintaining steady fixations upon fixed targets, interrupted only by saccades and micro saccades. That is, the substantial oscillations are solely due to head motion, with no residual ocular tremor.

What are the clinical implications of these observations? It seems that ocular tremor in PD does not exist. Rather, the observations are indicative of a head tremor, either transmitted to the neck muscles from the trunk or limbs, or even from the neck muscles themselves [93] in the presence of an intact VOR and manifest as an ocular tremor if the head is not fixed.

References

1. Leigh RJ, Zee DS. *The Neurology of Eye Movements*, 5th Ed. Oxford University Press; 2015, xx, 1109.

2. Hikosaka O, Takikawa Y, Kawagoe R. Role of the basal ganglia in the control of purposive saccadic eye movements. Physiol Rev 2000; **80**(3): 953–978.

3. Terao Y, Fukuda H, Ugawa Y, Hikosaka O. New perspectives on the pathophysiology of Parkinson's disease as assessed by saccade performance: a clinical review. Clin Neurophysiol 2013; **124**(8): 1491–1506.

4. Buttner U, Buttner-Ennever JA. Present concepts of oculomotor organization. Prog Brain Res 2006; **151**: 1–42.

5. Hellmuth J, Mirsky J, Heuer HW, et al. Multicenter validation of a bedside antisaccade task as a measure of executive function. Neurology 2012; **78**(23): 1824–1831.

6. Schindlbeck KA, Schonfeld S, Naumann W, et al. Characterization of diplopia in non-demented patients with Parkinson's disease. Parkinsonism Relat Disord 2017; **45**: 1–6.

7. Corin MS, Elizan TS, Bender MB. Oculomotor function in patients with Parkinson's disease. J Neurol Sci 1972/3; **15**(3): 251–265.

8. Weil RS, Schrag AE, Warren JD, et al. Visual dysfunction in Parkinson's disease. Brain 2016; **139**(11): 2827–2843.

9. DeJong JD, Jones GM. Akinesia, hypokinesia, and bradykinesia in the oculomotor system of patients with Parkinson's disease. Exp Neurol 1971; **32**(1): 58–68.

10. Walker R, Walker DG, Husain M, Kennard C. Control of voluntary and reflexive saccades. Exp Brain Res 2000; **130**(4): 540–544.

11. Mosimann UP, Müri RM, Burn DJ, et al. Saccadic eye movement changes in Parkinson's disease dementia and dementia with Lewy bodies. Brain 2005; **128**: 1267–1276.

12. Macaskill MR, Graham CF, Pitcher TL, et al. The influence of motor and cognitive impairment upon visually guided saccades in Parkinson's disease. Neuropsychologia 2012; **50**(14): 3338–3347.

13. Terao Y, Fukuda H, Yugeta A, et al. Initiation and inhibitory control of saccades with the progression of Parkinson's disease – changes in three major drives converging on the superior colliculus. Neuropsychologia 2011; **49**(7): 1794–1806.

14. Anderson TJ, MacAskill MR. Eye movements in patients with neurodegenerative disorders. Nat Rev Neurol 2013; **9**(2): 74–85.

15. Stuart S, Lawson RA, Yarnall AJ, et al. Pro-saccades predict cognitive decline in Parkinson's disease: ICICLE-PD. Mov Disord 2019; **34**(11): 1690–1698.

16. Chan F, Armstrong IT, Pari G, et al. Deficits in saccadic eye-movement control in Parkinson's disease. Neuropsychologia 2005; **43**(5): 784–796.

17. Pinkhardt EH, Jurgens R, Becker W, et al. Differential diagnostic value of eye movement recording in PSP-parkinsonism, Richardson's syndrome, and idiopathic Parkinson's disease. J Neurol 2008; **255**(12): 1916–1925.

18. Pinkhardt EH, Kassubek J. Ocular motor abnormalities in Parkinsonian syndromes. Parkinsonism Relat Disord 2011; **17**(4): 223–230.

19. Nakashima H, Terada S, Ishizu H, et al. An autopsied case of dementia with Lewy bodies with supranuclear gaze palsy. Neurol Res 2003; **25**(5): 533–537.

20. Grotzsch H, Sztajzel R, Burkhard PR. Levodopa-induced ocular dyskinesia in Parkinson's disease. Eur J Neurol 2007; **14**(10): 1124–1128.

21. Racette BA, Gokden MS, Tychsen LS, Perlmutter JS. Convergence insufficiency in idiopathic Parkinson's disease responsive to levodopa. Strabismus 1999; **7**(3): 169–174.

22. Sharpe JA, Fletcher WA, Lang AE, Zackon DH. Smooth pursuit during dose-related on-off fluctuations in Parkinson's disease. Neurology 1987; **37**(8): 1389–1392.

23. Gilman S, Wenning GK, Low PA, et al. Second consensus statement on the diagnosis of multiple system atrophy. Neurology 2008; **71**(9): 670–676.

24. Anderson T, Luxon L, Quinn N, et al. Oculomotor function in multiple system atrophy: clinical and laboratory features in 30 patients. Mov Disord 2008; **23**(7): 977–984.

25. Lee JY, Lee WW, Kim JS, et al. Perverted head-shaking and positional downbeat nystagmus in patients with multiple system atrophy. Mov Disord 2009; **24**(9): 1290–1295.

26. Chen AL, Riley DE, King SA, et al. The disturbance of gaze in progressive supranuclear palsy:

implications for pathogenesis. Front Neurol 2010; **1**: 147.

27. Litvan I, Agid Y, Calne D, et al. Clinical research criteria for the diagnosis of progressive supranuclear palsy (Steele-Richardson-Olszewski syndrome): report of the NINDS-SPSP international workshop. Neurology 1996; **47**(1): 1–9.

28. Troost BT, Daroff RB. The ocular motor defects in progressive supranuclear palsy. Ann Neurol 1977; **2**(5): 397–403.

29. Altiparmak UE, Eggenberger E, Coleman A, Condon K. The ratio of square wave jerk rates to blink rates distinguishes progressive supranuclear palsy from Parkinson disease. J Neuroophthalmol 2006; **26**(4): 257–259.

30. Williams DR, de Silva R, Paviour DC, et al. Characteristics of two distinct clinical phenotypes in pathologically proven progressive supranuclear palsy: Richardson's syndrome and PSP-parkinsonism. Brain 2005; **128**(Pt 6): 1247–1258.

31. Williams DR, Holton JL, Strand K, Revesz T, Lees AJ. Pure akinesia with gait freezing: a third clinical phenotype of progressive supranuclear palsy. Mov Disord 2007; **22**(15): 2235–2241.

32. Stell R, Bronstein AM. Eye movement abnormalities in extra pyramidal disease. In: Marsden CD, Fahn S (eds.). *Movement Disorders 3.* Butterworth-Heinemann Ltd; 1994, 88–113.

33. Vidailhet M, Rivaud-Pechoux S. Eye movement disorders in corticobasal degeneration. Adv Neurol 2000; **82**: 161–167.

34. Boxer AL, Garbutt S, Seeley WW, et al. Saccade abnormalities in autopsy-confirmed frontotemporal lobar degeneration and Alzheimer disease. Arch Neurol 2012; **69**(4): 509–517.

35. Bejjani BP, Arnulf I, Houeto JL, et al. Concurrent excitatory and inhibitory effects of high frequency stimulation: an oculomotor study. J Neurol Neurosurg Psychiatry 2002; **72**(4): 517–522.

36. Shaikh AG, Antoniades C, Fitzgerald J, Ghasia FF. Effects of deep brain stimulation on eye movements and vestibular function. Front Neurol 2018; **9**: 444.

37. Khan AN, Bronstein A, Bain P, Pavese N, Nandi D. Pedunculopontine and subthalamic nucleus stimulation effect on saccades in Parkinson disease. World Neurosurg 2019; **126**: e219–e31.

38. Fasano A, Aquino CC, Krauss JK, Honey CR, Bloem BR. Axial disability and deep brain stimulation in patients with Parkinson disease. Nat Rev Neurol 2015; **11**(2): 98–110.

39. Krack P, Batir A, Van Blercom N, et al. Five-year follow-up of bilateral stimulation of the subthalamic nucleus in advanced Parkinson's disease. N Engl J Med. 2003; **349**(20): 1925–1934.

40. Bostan AC, Strick PL. The cerebellum and basal ganglia are interconnected. Neuropsychol Rev 2010; **20**(3): 261–270.

41. Shaikh AG, Straumann D, Palla A. Motion illusion-evidence towards human vestibulo-thalamic projections. Cerebellum 2017; **16**(3): 656–663.

42. Stuart S, Alcock L, Galna B, Lord S, Rochester L. The measurement of visual sampling during real-world activity in Parkinson's disease and healthy controls: a structured literature review. J Neurosci Methods 2014; **222**: 175–188.

43. Anastasopoulos D, Ziavra N, Savvidou E, Bain P, Bronstein AM. Altered eye-to-foot coordination in standing parkinsonian patients during large gaze and whole-body reorientations. Mov Disord 2011; **26**(12): 2201–2211.

44. Glickstein M, Stein J. Paradoxical movement in Parkinson's disease. Trends Neurosci 1991; **14** (11): 480–482.

45. Vitorio R, Lirani-Silva E, Pieruccini-Faria F, et al. Visual cues and gait improvement in Parkinson's disease: which piece of information is really important? Neuroscience 2014; **277**: 273–280.

46. Lohnes CA, Earhart GM. Saccadic eye movements are related to turning performance in Parkinson disease. J Parkinsons Dis 2011; **1**(1): 109–118.

47. Matsumoto H, Terao Y, Furubayashi T, et al. Small saccades restrict visual scanning area in Parkinson's disease. Mov Disord 2011; **26**(9): 1619–1626.

48. Archibald NK, Hutton SB, Clarke MP, Mosimann UP, Burn DJ. Visual exploration in Parkinson's disease and Parkinson's disease dementia. Brain 2013; **136**(Pt 3): 739–750.

49. Jehangir N, Yu CY, Song J, et al. Slower saccadic reading in Parkinson's disease. PLoS One 2018; **13** (1): e0191005.

50. Moes E, Lombardi KM. The relationship between contrast sensitivity, gait, and reading speed in Parkinson's disease. Neuropsychol Dev Cogn B Aging Neuropsychol Cogn 2009; **16**(2): 121–132.

51. Pascoe M, Alamri Y, Dalrymple-Alford J, Anderson T, MacAskill M. The symbol-digit modalities test in mild cognitive impairment: evidence from Parkinson's disease patients. Eur Neurol 2018; **79**(3–4): 206–210.

52. Cano Porras D, Siemonsma P, Inzelberg R, Zeilig G, Plotnik M. Advantages of virtual reality in the rehabilitation of balance and gait: systematic review. Neurology 2018; **90**(22): 1017–1025.

53. Marazzi S, Kiper P, Palmer K, Agostini M, Turolla A. Effects of vibratory stimulation on balance and gait in Parkinson's disease: a systematic review and meta-analysis. Eur J Phys Rehabil Med 2020; DOI: 10.23736/S1973-9087.20.06099-2

54. Olson M, Lockhart TE, Lieberman A. Motor learning deficits in Parkinson's disease (PD) and their effect on training response in gait and balance: a narrative review. Front Neurol 2019; 10: 62.

55. Reichert WH, Doolittle J, McDowell FH. Vestibular dysfunction in Parkinson disease. Neurology 1982; 32(10): 1133–1138.

56. Cipparrone L, Ginanneschi A, Degl'Innocenti F, et al. Electro-oculographic routine examination in Parkinson's disease. Acta Neurol Scand 1988; 77 (1): 6–11.

57. Venhovens J, Meulstee J, Bloem BR, Verhagen WI. Neurovestibular analysis and falls in Parkinson's disease and atypical parkinsonism. Eur J Neurosci 2016; 43(12): 1636–1646.

58. Scocco DH, Wagner JN, Racosta J, Chade A, Gershanik OS. Subjective visual vertical in Pisa syndrome. Parkinsonism Relat Disord 2014; 20(8): 878–883.

59. Vitale C, Marcelli V, Furia T, et al. Vestibular impairment and adaptive postural imbalance in parkinsonian patients with lateral trunk flexion. Mov Disord 2011; 26(8): 1458–1463.

60. Bronstein AM, Yardley L, Moore AP, Cleeves L. Visually and posturally mediated tilt illusion in Parkinson's disease and in labyrinthine defective subjects. Neurology 1996; 47(3): 651–656.

61. White OB, Saintcyr JA, Tomlinson RD, Sharpe JA. Ocular motor deficits in Parkinson's disease. 3. Coordination of eye and head movements. Brain 1988; 111: 115–129.

62. Lv W, Guan Q, Hu X, et al. Vestibulo-ocular reflex abnormality in Parkinson's disease detected by video head impulse test. Neurosci Lett 2017; 657: 211–214.

63. Bronstein AM, Kennard C. Predictive ocular motor control in Parkinson's disease. Brain 1985; 108: 925–940.

64. Waterston JA, Barnes GR, Grealy MA, Collins S. Abnormalities of smooth eye and head movement control in Parkinson's disease. Ann Neurol 1996; 39(6): 749–760.

65. Cronin T, Arshad Q, Seemungal BM. Vestibular deficits in neurodegenerative disorders: balance, dizziness, and spatial disorientation. Front Neurol 2017; 8: 538.

66. Bisdorff AR, Bronstein AM, Wolsley C, et al. EMG responses to free fall in elderly subjects and akinetic rigid patients. J Neurol Neurosurg Psychiatry 1999; 66(4): 447–455.

67. Shalash AS, Hassan DM, Elrassas HH, et al. Auditory- and vestibular-evoked potentials correlate with motor and non-motor features of Parkinson's disease. Front Neurol 2017; 8: 55.

68. Cicekli E, Titiz AP, Titiz A, Oztekin N, Mujdeci B. Vestibular evoked myogenic potential responses in Parkinson's disease. Ideggyogyaszati szemle 2019; 72(11–12): 419–425.

69. de Natale ER, Ginatempo F, Paulus KS, et al. Paired neurophysiological and clinical study of the brainstem at different stages of Parkinson's disease. Clin Neurophysiol 2015; 126(10): 1871–1878.

70. de Natale ER, Ginatempo F, Paulus KS, et al. Abnormalities of vestibular-evoked myogenic potentials in idiopathic Parkinson's disease are associated with clinical evidence of brainstem involvement. Neurol Sci 2015; 36(6): 995–1001.

71. Pollak L, Prohorov T, Kushnir M, Rabey M. Vestibulocervical reflexes in idiopathic Parkinson disease. Clin Neurophysiol 2009; 39(4–5): 235–240.

72. Potter-Nerger M, Govender S, Deuschl G, Volkmann J, Colebatch JG. Selective changes of ocular vestibular myogenic potentials in Parkinson's disease. Mov Disord 2015; 30(4): 584–589.

73. Potter-Nerger M, Reich MM, Colebatch JG, Deuschl G, Volkmann J. Differential effect of dopa and subthalamic stimulation on vestibular activity in Parkinson's disease. Mov Disord 2012; 27(10): 1268–1275.

74. Bronstein AM, Hood JD, Gresty MA, Panagi C. Visual control of balance in cerebellar and parkinsonian syndromes. Brain 1990; 113(Pt 3): 767–779.

75. Cooke JD, Brown JD, Brooks VB. Increased dependence on visual information for movement control in patients with Parkinson's disease. Can J Neurol Sci 1978; 5(4): 413–415.

76. Martin JP. The Basal Ganglia and Posture. Lippincott; 1967.

77. Nakamura T, Bronstein AM. The perception of head rotation in Parkinson's disease. Acta Otolaryngol Suppl 1995; 520(Pt 2): 387–391.

78. Nakamura T, Bronstein AM, Lueck C, Marsden CD, Rudge P. Vestibular, cervical and visual remembered saccades in Parkinson's disease. Brain 1994; 117(Pt 6): 1423–1432.

79. Pastor MA, Day BL, Marsden CD. Vestibular induced postural responses in Parkinson's disease. Brain 1993; 116(Pt 5): 1177–1190.

80. Rothwell JC, Obeso JA, Traub MM, Marsden CD. The behaviour of the long-latency stretch reflex in patients with Parkinson's disease. J Neurol Neurosurg Psychiatry 1983; **46**(1): 35–44.

81. Berardelli A, Rothwell JC, Thompson PD, Hallett M. Pathophysiology of bradykinesia in Parkinson's disease. Brain 2001; **124**(Pt 11): 2131–2146.

82. Delval A, Tard C, Defebvre L. Why we should study gait initiation in Parkinson's disease. Clin Neurophysiol 2014; **44**(1): 69–76.

83. Beylergil SB, Ozinga S, Walker MF, McIntyre CC, Shaikh AG. Vestibular heading perception in Parkinson's disease. Prog Brain Res 2019; **249**: 307–319.

84. Yakubovich S, Israeli-Korn S, Halperin O, et al. Visual self-motion cues are impaired yet over-weighted during visual-vestibular integration in Parkinson's disease. Brain Commun 2020; **2**(1): 1–15.

85. Bertolini G, Wicki A, Baumann CR, Straumann D, Palla A. Impaired tilt perception in Parkinson's disease: a central vestibular integration failure. PLoS One 2015; **10**(4): e0124253.

86. Putcha D, Ross RS, Rosen ML, et al. Functional correlates of optic flow motion processing in Parkinson's disease. Front Integr Neurosci 2014; **8**: 57.

87. Amick MM, Schendan HE, Ganis G, Cronin-Golomb A. Frontostriatal circuits are necessary for visuomotor transformation: mental rotation in Parkinson's disease. Neuropsychologia 2006; **44** (3): 339–349.

88. Gitchel GT, Wetzel PA, Baron MS. Pervasive ocular tremor in patients with Parkinson disease. Arch Neurol 2012; **69**(8): 1011–1017.

89. Kaski D, Saifee TA, Buckwell D, Bronstein AM. Ocular tremor in Parkinson's disease is due to head oscillation. Mov Disord 2013; **28**(4): 534–537.

90. Leigh RJ, Martinez-Conde S. Tremor of the eyes, or of the head, in Parkinson's disease? Mov Disord 2013; **28**(6): 691–693.

91. Kaski D, Bronstein AM. Ocular tremor in Parkinson's disease: discussion, debate, and controversy. Front Neurol 2017; **8**: 134.

92. MacAskill M, Myall D. "Pervasive ocular tremor of Parkinson's" is not pervasive, ocular, or uniquely parkinsonian. 2020. Doi: 10.31219/osf. io/s8rwt

93. Roze E, Coelho-Braga MC, Gayraud D, et al. Head tremor in Parkinson's disease. Mov Disord 2006; **21**(8): 1245–1248.

94. Coe BC, Trappenberg T, Munoz DP. Modeling saccadic action selection: cortical and basal ganglia signals coalesce in the superior colliculus. Front Syst Neurosci 2019; **13**: 3.

95. Bronstein AM, Gresty MA, Rudge P. Neuro-otological assessment in the patient with balance and gait disorder. In: Bronstein AM, Brandt T, Woollacott M, (eds.). *Clinical Disorders of Balance, Posture and Gait*. Hodder Arnold; 1996.

Chapter 12

Autonomic Dysfunction and Failure in Parkinson's Disease

Thomas Foki, Birgit Riemer, Bianca Brim, Walter Struhal

Introduction

Autonomic complications in Parkinsonian syndromes present a considerable cause of reduced quality of life, morbidity, and mortality [1]. Recognition, evaluation, and management are of utmost importance.

The autonomic nervous system is still a field that to many clinicians is obscure or at least its involvement in the clinical course is hard to grasp. This may be based on the considerable widespread knowledge gap and lack of access in electrophysiology evaluation of the autonomic nervous system [2]. However, autonomic syndromes in several autonomic domains are easily evaluable at the bedside, with electrophysiologic autonomic evaluation only necessary in a minority of patients [3]. This chapter will provide a clinical focus on the autonomic cardiovascular, thermoregulatory, urogenital, and gastrointestinal systems.

Cardiovascular Dysfunction

Among the non-motor Parkinson features, dysfunction of the cardiovascular autonomic nervous system shows different degrees of severity – not always corresponding to the disease progression.

In evaluation of autonomic signs, a focused history is mandatory and usually guides the questioner to the succeeding examinations. This history should cover the following fields:

Cardiovascular Symptoms

Cardiovascular symptoms are the result of temporary cerebral or retinal hypoperfusion. Affected people might report symptoms such as "brain fog", blurred, obscured, or reduced color vision, "coat hanger pain" (temporary pain in neck area or between the shoulders),

lumbar pain, orthostatic weakness, impaired cognitive performance, or mock angina pectoris. Syncope is not obligatory in cardiovascular autonomic dysfunction but may be present. A main feature of autonomic malfunction is intolerance of upright posture whereas the lying posture is associated with normal well-being. Aggravation of symptoms is typical in hot weather, fever, after heavy meals, prolonged standing, humid crowded rooms, and during the early morning after bed rest.

Assessing the function of the cardiovascular autonomic nervous system during orthostatic changes is easily achievable (Figure 12.1). The first step is imperative and consists of a good and complete **disease history** including the carer's observations. Next step in orthostatic hypotension (OH) screening should be the **standing test**. The use of a sphygmomanometer is highly recommended, because by using an automatic hand-cuff device one might miss a rapid change in blood pressure value in orthostatic hypotension. Gold standard for evaluation of rapid changes in blood pressure is continuous non-invasive beat-to-beat blood pressure measurement. This method also allows the detection of initial orthostatic hypotension within the first 15 seconds of standing. Very helpful in assessment is a **24-hour ambulatory blood pressure monitoring** with personal notes of the patient indicating the times of symptoms and drug intake. An optional step of evaluation in suspected OH is the **tilt table assessment**. The tilt table should be considered if a Parkinson patient's symptoms point towards OH, but preceding tests were not indicative. Due to tilt duration which can be prolonged to 30 minutes of tilt time, it is possible to detect delayed OH [4], which occurs after more than 10 minutes of tilt.

Stepwise assessment of autonomic function in Parkinson's disease

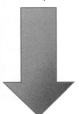

- Patient's history ——————— general history
  medication
  carer's observation

- Standing test
- 24-hour ambulatory blood pressure monitoring
- Tilt table assessment

Figure 12.1

More than 60% of Parkinson patients fulfil the criteria of OH during the course of the disease. Symptom severity correlates with stage of the disease and predicts disease course. Some patients struggle with mild symptoms like short-lasting dizziness when rising from bed in the morning, but OH can also lead to severe symptoms like syncope and falls with fractures. The prevalence of symptomatic OH is calculated as high as 20% in PD patients [5].

In Parkinson patients, OH is often due to impaired autonomic neurotransmission. This is **neurogenic OH (nOH)**. Hallmarks are impaired autonomic postural responses with focus on malfunctioning systemic vasoconstriction and lack of compensatory increasing heart rate to maintain a sufficient blood pressure because of insufficient norepinephrine release from sympathetic nerves [6]. The pathophysiology of nOH is not clearly understood, but Lewy pathology involvement in peripheral and to a lesser extent involvement in central autonomic structures seems to play a key role.

Neurogenic orthostatic hypotension is diagnosed if an individual meets the criteria of OH and simultaneously does not augment heart rate adequately. A blunted rise in HR of <0.49 beats/minute per mmHg of systolic BP fall is an easy bedside marker to differentiate between structural baroreflex arch (nOH) lesion from dehydration or polypharmacy (OH) [7].

According to the time of manifestation of blood pressure fall during standing test or tilt maneuver we can differentiate the following **sub classes of OH: initial OH, classical OH, and delayed OH**.

Initial OH may be found in the first 15 seconds of active standing and is characterized by systolic blood pressure decrease of >40 mmHg on standing and/or diastolic blood pressure decrease of > 20 mmHg. After these initial seconds blood

pressure rapidly returns to normal. Therefore, it is impossible to catch initial OH with a commonly used sphygmomanometer or automatic arm-cuff device. Only systems working with continuous beat-to-beat blood pressure measurement will detect it. However, initial OH is prominent in young individuals.

According to recent ESC guidelines [8], **classical OH** is defined as a drop in systolic blood pressure minus >20 mmHg and/or drop in diastolic blood pressure minus >10 mmHg or measures of blood pressure below 90 mmHg in an upright posture on tilt table test with a tilt angle between 60 and 70 degrees or standing test. The fall in blood pressure correlates with an insufficiency of the autonomic nervous system in Parkinson patients in maintaining a sufficient cerebral perfusion pressure during orthostatic movement. Vasoconstriction in these patients does not work promptly. Therefore, gravitationally mediated considerable blood volume (estimated 500–1,000 ml) sinks in splanchnic vessels and vessels of lower limbs. This leads to a temporary decrease in venous return and cardiac output. The compensatory reflex response is mainly induced by the baroreceptors which are mechanical arterial receptors located at the sinus caroticum in the vessel wall of the carotid arteries. Activation of the baroreceptors leads to an increase of peripheral resistance and improvement of venous return and therefore improved cardiac output. In neurogenic OH patients impaired baroreceptor function is obvious. Disability of the autonomic nervous system in PD patients not only results from impaired baroreceptor reflex, but also from cardiac noradrenergic sympathetic denervation and central and peripheral noradrenaline deficiency. This leads to impaired regulation of cardiac output and vasoconstriction.

In **delayed OH** significant blood pressure fall – as mentioned above at "classical OH" – does not

131

occur promptly after being tilted but takes more than 3 minutes of upright posture. According to Gibbons and Freeman [9], the examiner can expect 46% of OH cases within 3 minutes of head up tilt; 15% of the patients showed OH between 3 and 10 minutes and 39% had OH only after 10 minutes of tilt table testing.

Orthostatic hypotension may be differentiated into **symptomatic and asymptomatic form**. Symptomatic and asymptomatic OH are both equally associated with increased prevalence of falls and healthcare utilization. In symptomatic form patients might report feelings like dizziness or light-headedness along with blood pressure fall, but seemingly 6% of patients do not report any symptoms when they have a significant blood pressure drop. These patients are at high risk of a negative outcome.

In progressive Parkinson's disease, **supine hypertension** (SH) may occur and show correlation to negative prognosis in survival, cardiovascular and cerebrovascular outcomes, and cognitive decline [10]. Supine hypertension is defined as systolic blood pressure of 140 mmHg, diastolic blood pressure of 90 mmHg or more while in recumbent position [11]. Severity is graded as follows [11]:

Mild nSH: systolic BP 140–159 mmHg or diastolic BP values of 90–99 mmHg

Moderate nSH: systolic BP 160–179 mmHg or diastolic BP 100–109 mmHg

Severe nSH: systolic BP values of ≥ 180 mmHg or diastolic BP values of ≥ 110 mmHg

Supine hypertension during bed rest at night causes forced nocturnal diuresis. This leads to forced urine production. Consequently, patients have a relative lack of blood volume in the morning and are more likely to have OH symptoms. On the other hand, patients with chronic SH may be prone for end-organ damage. In non-pharmacological as well as pharmacological management of nOH, it is of the utmost importance to screen for SH. Twenty-four-hour ambulatory BP measurements are helpful. Espay et al. [12] presented positive arguments for prioritization of nOH over SH when coexisting in a PD patient. These are mainly based on a small modified cardiovascular risk in PD patients, since smoking and atherosclerosis are not the predominant causes of hypertension, but a failure in autonomic nervous function.

Non-pharmacological measures of autonomic symptoms are the cornerstone in managing OH and SH. There are various non-pharmacological methods to treat orthostatic symptoms which should be explained to the patient and used initially as first-line of treatment. These comprise drinking a glass of water in the morning before getting up, sitting at bedside and activating the muscle pump of the legs, avoiding heavy meals, alcohol, and high surrounding temperature.

The following table gives an overview of the most important conservative lifestyle approaches in treating OH and SH [13] (Table 12.1).

Table 12.1 Lifestyle Approaches in (Neurogenic) Orthostatic Hypotension and Supine Hypertension

Neurogenic orthostatic hypotension:
- Avoid heavy meals
- Avoid alcohol
- Avoid hot surroundings
- Stand up slowly and activate your muscle pumps in the legs before standing up
- Increase water and salt intake
- Perform rescue movements like squatting, sitting down, squeezing the buttocks when feeling hypotensive symptoms
- Consider wearing thigh-high compression stockings or abdominal binder
- Sleep with the head of the bed elevated at 30 degrees

Supine hypertension:
- Eat a small meal before going to bed (this will induce postprandial hypotension)
- Avoid the supine position during the day
- Sleep with the head of the bed elevated at 30 degrees

Thorough evaluation of prevailing medication of the patient is necessary since there are many interfering and negatively influencing substances with the autonomic nervous system. Often adjusting or changing drug classes or agents can lead to elimination or alleviation of orthostatic dysfunction symptoms. These drugs or agents are known to boost orthostatic hypotension: alpha blockers, antipsychotics, beta blockers (might also alleviate OH), nitrates, hypnotics, ACE inhibitors, anesthetics, AT2 inhibitors, barbiturates, calcium antagonists, clonidine, diuretics, levodopa, dopamine agonists, methyldopa, phenothiazines, sildenafil, tricyclic antidepressants, and MAO inhibitors [13]. Treatment adjustments can often lead to amelioration of the blood pressure profile with avoidance of a) early morning low blood pressure levels and b) high supine blood pressure during sleep.

Pharmacological management is based on the skillful use of a number of drugs. In pharmacological OH management, the first important clinical question is whether SH is present. In SH, only short-acting drugs such as droxidopa or midodrine are used if needed.

Dysfunction of Thermoregulation

Abnormal sweating and temperature sensation have long been recognized in PD. These disorders of thermoregulation affect approximately two-thirds of patients, and they have significant impact on well-being and the quality of life of patients and their caregivers. Symptoms tend to correlate with disease severity. They are disturbing both at night as well as daytime, which may lead to disturbed sleep and social embarrassment, respectively. Patients with hyperhidrosis tend to present higher dyskinesia symptoms and increased levels of anxiety and depression [14].

Episodic excessive sweating is the most frequently reported and disturbing symptom of thermoregulatory dysfunction. In addition, heat or cold intolerance, night sweats, but also hypohidrosis and the sense of cold limbs are observed.

Hyperhidrosis is present in up to 30% of PD patients. It is often regarded as a compensatory phenomenon in response to areas of lower-body hypohidrosis. Hyperhidrosis has been found at rest as well as a response to a heat stimulus. Trunk and head are most often affected by excessive sweating, although generalized patterns and asymmetric hyperhidrosis with involvement of the side with pronounced motor deficit are also observed. Importantly, hyperhidrosis may also interfere with transdermally applied therapies. Sialorrhea and constipation are correlated with hyperhidrosis. In patients with symptomatic orthostatic hypotension, sweating episodes are likely to occur after meals or at night.

Although less bothersome, hypohidrosis is reported more often in PD patients than in controls [15]. Distal parts of the extremities are most

often implicated. The feeling of heat intolerance also represents a correlate of reduced sweating. It may be the only manifestation of hypohidrosis or anhidrosis.

ON and OFF states likely play a major role in symptoms of thermoregulatory dysfunction in PD. Typically, sweating is increased in OFF periods. Nevertheless, severe dyskinesias may also give rise to excessive sweating.

Regarding the feeling of coldness of the distal limbs, prolonged vasoconstriction represents the main pathophysiological source in affected individuals.

Particular medications have the potential to interfere with thermoregulatory function in PD, such as SNRIs causing hyperhidrosis and cholinergics giving rise to heat intolerance due to decreased sweating.

Sweating is controlled by sympathetic signals originating in the hypothalamic preoptic sweat center, synapsing with neurons in the intermediolateral cell columns projecting to unmyelinated post-ganglionic class C fibers in the paravertebral ganglia that form peripheral nerves to reach the sweat glands [16]. Cholinergic, noradrenergic, and adrenergic pathways are involved.

When it comes to the underlying pathophysiological processes of thermoregulatory deficits in PD, the autonomic nervous system is affected both at the peripheral and central level.

Regarding *central* changes, degenerative processes with Lewy body formation in hypothalamus and sympathetic cell groups of the brainstem play major roles for thermoregulatory dysfunction in PD. Preganglionic neurons in the intermediolateral cell column of the spinal cord are also affected by α-synuclein pathology.

Physiologically, *peripheral* thermoregulatory processes are largely influenced by sympathetic outflow using cholinergic input to sweat glands (sudomotor) and noradrenergic vasoconstriction [17]. Skin biopsies have demonstrated lower cutaneous autonomic innervation in blood vessels, sweat glands, and erector pili muscles in PD. Eccrine, cholinergic sweat glands are distributed over nearly the entire body with greatest density in the forehead followed by the upper limbs, trunk, and lower limbs. Peripheral thermoregulatory function is largely mediated by small-fiber axons, which are affected by neuropathic changes in PD. Those changes become more prominent late in disease. Quantitative sudomotor axon

133

reflex testing (QSART) provides information on the postganglionic sympathetic sudomotor axon. In PD, QSART abnormalities tend to be in a distal or length-dependent pattern. Decreased sweat volumes with a distal predominance of the lower extremities are the respective correlates [18]. Indeed, the most common pattern of anhidrosis on thermoregulatory sweat test in PD is distal or length-dependent sweat loss with a low percentage of total body anhidrosis [17]. This is in contrast to MSA patients, whose anhidrotic pattern is predominantly caused by preganglionic sympathetic dysfunction with acral sparing. In addition to the neuropathic mechanisms mentioned above, a reduction of intraepidermal nerve fiber density and an increase in skin α-synuclein deposition may also be involved. Cutaneous autonomic pilomotor testing, in which iontophoresis of phenylephrine induces a local neurogenic pilomotor erection ("goose bumps") as a measure of functional integrity of autonomic skin nerve fibers, is an approach to capture the progression of autonomic nerve dysfunction and α-synuclein deposition [19].

A careful history of thermoregulatory symptoms and review of medications represent a fundamental part of any therapeutic approach for thermoregulatory dysfunction in PD. Any association with dopaminergic medication should be noticed, and the dopaminergic regimen should be adapted accordingly. Episodes of enhanced sweating may be the first sign of wearing-off, preceding classical motor signs of wearing-off. As a rule of thumb, sweating during the day is more frequently associated with dopaminergic therapy and fluctuations, whereas non-dopaminergic mechanisms rather underly excessive sweating at night.

If adaptation of dopaminergic therapy does not control hyperhidrosis, anticholinergic treatment represents a pharmacological alternative. Here, anticholinergic side effects, especially cognitive deterioration and risk of delirium, should be taken into account. Moreover, patients should also be counseled regarding heat intolerance and the risk of heat stroke when put on anticholinergic medication. Glycopyrrolate (1–3 mg/day) or pirenzepine (25–100 mg/day) may be used.

In case of sweating attacks in association with emotional arousal, propranolol may be administered. Focal hyperhidrosis, though rare in PD, responds well to 15–25% aluminium chloride. If

ineffective, steady current iontopheresis and the application of botulinum toxin A may be used for local hyperhidrosis.

Deep brain stimulation (DBS) of the subthalamic nucleus may improve drenching sweats [20]. This holds especially true for OFF-associated sweating. Other factors, including reduced dopaminergic medication, excessive movement from dyskinesias, and direct effect of DBS on central autonomic control may also contribute to a reduction in sweating. Nevertheless, thermoregulatory problems per se do not represent an indication for DBS surgery [21], and DBS of other targets such as the thalamus may give rise to hyperhidrosis.

It is important to mention that excessive sweating, according to some experts, may be a seasonal symptom occurring more frequently in spring and fall. A self-limitation of symptoms is hence possible.

Pupillo-Motor and Tear Regulation

Parkinson's disease patients suffer from impairment of the pupillary light reflex. Moreover, pupillary responses to dark or light adaptation and near vision reaction are affected. In addition, pupils are hypersensitive to sympathetic drugs. Impaired tear function is another manifestation of autonomic dysfunction concerning the ocular region.

Pupillo-motor abnormalities are associated with blurred vision, hypersensitivity to light, and involuntary blink reflex. If impaired tear function becomes clinically manifest, xeropthalmic changes can be assessed.

Only a limited number of studies have focused on pupillo-motor and tear abnormalities and their sources in PD [16]. In accordance with the aforementioned symptoms, the Edinger-Westphal nucleus has been shown to suffer from Lewy body pathology. Reports of the light reflex in PD have observed reduced constriction velocity compared to controls, considered to reflect a parasympathetic deficit. Comparisons of PD patients with and without dementia reveal lower constriction velocities in PD with dementia, confirming that the parasympathetic system is critically implicated and that autonomic dysfunction in general correlates with overall disease severity.

Although the burden of this symptom complex has not been systematically assessed, from a clinical point of view several simple therapeutic measures such as wearing sunglasses and the replacement of tear fluids have proven effective according to personal experiences.

The education of ophthalmologists about possible ocular symptoms due to PD is another critical issue.

The Enteric Nervous System

The occurrence of gastrointestinal symptoms is widespread in patients with PD. A large variety of symptoms can cause a significant reduction in quality of life for patients and a challenge for their caregivers. As we know, digestive symptoms often appear in the premotor phase. In many cases the symptoms are mild, so they may remain unrecognized for a long period. However, it has been reported that 88.9% of PD patients develop gastrointestinal symptoms before the onset of motor symptoms [22]. Basically, the symptoms can occur in every stage of the disease.

Concerning the pathophysiological foundations, degeneration of serotonergic and dopaminergic neurons plays a major role in the dysregulation of the autonomic nervous system (ANS) as well as in the enteric nervous system (ENS). The central autonomic control centers and the peripheral autonomic nervous system are damaged by neuronal destruction and accumulation of α-synuclein [23]. Since almost every PD patient shows signs of Lewy body pathology, it is suspected that these lesions are already developed in enteric neurons before the substantia nigra shows signs of destruction [24, 25]. Furthermore, it is remarkable that the upper gastrointestinal plexuses are characterized by a presence of 15–20% of dopaminergic neurons of the total number of enteric neurons. In comparison the large intestine expresses 2–4% dopaminergic neurons [24].

Dysregulations in the brain-gut-microbiota-axis are influenced by neuroendocrine, immunological, and direct neural mechanisms. It has also been discussed whether dysregulations in the brain-gut-axis play a role in the pathogenesis of PD itself [23].

Nevertheless, gastrointestinal function can be impaired at all levels of the digestive tract, from ingestion to defecation.

Weight Loss

Over 50% of PD patients experience weight loss at the onset of the disease [24]. The pathophysiological processes are still not well understood. Several factors can interact here. Disturbance of the energy balance can be caused by reduced ingestion on one hand, but on the other hand by increased energy consumption. The following factors play an important role: dysphagia, olfactory impairment, reduced sense of taste, rigidity, tremor, and nausea. Moreover, weight loss can also be associated with Parkinson medication, especially levodopa [22, 24].

Oropharyngeal Dysfunction

People with PD may have problems with chewing, swallowing, and controlling their saliva. Drooling, inability to clear food from the mouth, and swallowing problems can lead to an enormous loss of quality of life, including social stigma, embarrassment, and social isolation. In addition patients may suffer from malnutrition, dehydration, a higher risk for gastroesophageal reflux disease (GERD), and aspiration pneumonia [22, 26].

Hypersalivation, with or without drooling, occurs in over 70% during the course of the disease [24]. Sialorrhea is more likely caused by impaired automatic swallowing as a result of dysphagia rather than increased salivary secretion [27]. Saliva production is often reduced in Parkinson's disease and many patients suffer from mouth dryness before the onset of motor symptoms.

Hypersalivation can be objectivized with saliva collecting and analysis. It has also been reported that scintigraphy of the salivary glands found a higher speed of parotic excretion in PD patients than in healthy persons [22].

Common treatments for hypersalivation are anticholinergic agents, but several side effects such as constipation, urinary retention, blurred vision, or cognitive impairment are notable. There are positive experiences with botulinum toxin injections, oral glycopyrrolate or clonidin, local administration of ipratropium bromide, scopolamine, and tropicamide. In the future radiotherapy on the salivary glands could also be a promising method [22, 26].

Dysphagia, which is experienced by over 50% of PD patients [24], correlates with α-synuclein aggregates in the glossopharyngeal and the vagus nerve [22, 28]. Every stage of swallowing can be affected to different degrees. Usually dysphagia occurs in later stages of the disease but in some cases it may also occur as an early symptom. In fact, dysphagia is a predictor of poorer outcome [22]. Dysphagia may also be a side effect of levodopa medication.

Swallowing ability can be assessed with bedside swallowing screening tests, such as the Gugging swallowing screen (GUSS) [29]. Pharyngo-esophageal motility and laryngeal functions can be tested with fiberoptic endoscopic evaluation of swallowing (FEES), which is also helpful to study the pathophysiology of dysphagia and to control the success of dysphagia therapy. In some cases, high resolution manometry (HRM) may also be useful to evaluate swallowing and esophageal motility [22].

Patients with dysphagia benefit from logopedic and behavioral therapy (e.g. minimize meal volumes, modified meal consistency, liquid thickeners). Expiratory muscle strength training and video-assisted swallowing therapy improve swallowing and cough functions. Sometimes vocal fold augmentation with injection laryngoplasty or the usage of botulinum toxin injections in the distal esophagus may also improve dysphagia [22]. The effect of dopaminergic medication and DBS is controversial [28].

Gastric Dysfunction

Gastroparesis may be accompanied by nausea, postprandial bloating, acid indigestion, lack of appetite, early satiety, vomiting, and weight loss. In addition impaired gastric emptying can also lead to reduced levodopa absorption.

The prevalence of gastric emptying delay is not known exactly; it is suspected to range between 70% and 100% [22]. Dopaminergic, cholinergic muscarinic, cholinergic nicotinic, and serotinergic receptors are involved in the complex modulation of gastric motility [28]. α-synuclein pathology is assumed to interrupt the pathophysiological processes in the submucosal Meissner's plexus, in the gastric mucosa as well as in the fundus glands [24].

The gold standard to test gastric emptying time (GET) is gastric scintigraphy. Furthermore the (13)C-octanoate breath test can also be used to measure gastric emptying time. Functional magnetic resonance imaging can find smaller amplitudes of peristaltic contractions in PD patients with gastroparesis [22].

With mild symptoms patients could benefit from behavioral methods, such as taking small frequent meals, avoiding high-fat foods, and taking walks after meals. Regarding the pharmacological treatments of gastroparesis, caution is required because of possible side effects. D2 receptor blockers, especially Domperidone can improve gastric motility as well as levodopa adsorption but the potential cardiotoxicity has to be observed [22, 24]. Motility receptor agonists, such as Erythromycine and Azithromycine, may also have adverse effects including antibiotic resistance, gastrointestinal toxicity, ototoxicity, and cardiac arrhythmias, especially QT prolongation [28].

Small Intestinal Bacterial Overgrowth Syndrome

It is thought that impaired intestinal sluggishness favors the occurrence of small intestinal bacterial overgrowth syndrome (SIBO). Between 20% and 60% of individuals with PD suffer from the consequences of bacterial overgrowth in the small intestine, which exacerbates gastrointestinal symptoms and may also worsen motor functions [22]. SIBO has been reported to cause a secondary inflammatory response of the mucosa and worsen levodopa absorption in some cases [24]. Studies show that antibiotic eradication therapy with rifaximin improves motor fluctuations [30]. In addition, probiotics can also be helpful.

Constipation and Defecatory Dysfunction

Constipation, which is defined as a dysfunction of the colon, often occurs in the premotor stage and is reported to affect over 50% of PD patients [24]. Related to this, anorectal dysfunction occurs in over 70% of patients with PD [22].

Patients complain about lower abdominal discomfort and incomplete defecation with increased effort and pain, rectal sensation diminishment, or even fecal incontinence as a result of a failure of the rectoanal inhibitory reflex. Feared complications of constipation are ileus, intestinal perforation, volvulus, or megacolon.

Lewy body pathology is suspected to be causally responsible for the damage of enteric neurons. Investigations have shown prolonged colon transit time, dysfunction of rectal phasic contractions, paradoxical ineffective sequence of sphincter contraction and relaxation during defecation, as well as abdominal muscle weakness [26]. In addition, they also show decreased anal tone and impaired voluntary sphincter squeeze in anorectal manometry studies [22]. It should also be mentioned that obstipation may be aggravated by several consequences of the disease, such as dehydration, lack of movement, or side effects of anticholinergic medications.

Intestinal motility and the resulting gastrointestinal transit time can be measured with the radio-opaque marker (ROM)-technique. Furthermore, CT or MRI can be used to evaluate colonic functions [22]. It was found that PD patients often have increased colonic volumes, particularly in distal colonic segments [22]. A further possibility for the assessment of intestinal passage time is intestinal scintigraphy. Anorectal functions are evaluated by anorectal manometry, electromyography (EMG), and defecography [22].

Treatment options for constipation include primarily non-pharmacological methods. The adherence to a diet is recommended (especially fiber supplements and increased fluid intake); physical exercise is given high priority as well [24]. A restrained use of medications which are known to worsen constipation (opioids for example) is necessary. If the methods above are not sufficient, various laxatives are available. Prokinetic agents, such as serotonin agonists, muscarinic agonists, or acetylcholinesterase inhibitors can be used with caution for side effects. Levodopa could also help improve constipation symptoms [22, 26, 28]. Functional magnetic stimulation also improves colonic motility in some cases [22].

Disorders of anorectal function are reported to respond well to levodopa [26] or subcutaneous injection of apomorphine [24]. In PD patients, defecation is known to be interrupted by an incomplete or missing relaxation in the external anal sphincter and the puborectal muscle. Local injection of botulinum toxin into these muscles is another therapy option, which may lead to improvement for several months [24, 26]. Sometimes enemas and manual disimpactions will be needed too.

Urogenital Autonomic Innervation

Urinary Dysfunction

The bladder is primarily *activated* by the parasympathetic pelvic nerve (muscarinic) and the urethra/sphincter by the sympathetic hypogastric nerve (adrenergic) and the somatic pudendal (nicotinic-cholinergic) nerve. Both bladder and urethra/sphincter have their sympathetic and parasympathetic antagonists, respectively, that mediate *relaxation*. Voiding is associated with activation of the detrusor muscle of the bladder and relaxation of urethra/sphincter. All above receive descending projections from the pontine micturition center. The latter is controlled by cortical and subcortical structures, with a particular implication of D1-mediated basal ganglia projections.

Previous studies consistently identified frequent and less controllable detrusor muscle activity as the main pathophysiological source of urgency and frequency. It is assumed that basal ganglia dysfunction due to an impaired frontal-basal ganglia dopaminergic D1 circuit causes disinhibition of the pontine micturition center, resulting in frequency and urgency.

Also due to the dysfunction at spinal and peripheral level as mentioned below, smaller bladder volumes (100–250 ml) than usual (400–500 ml) can initiate detrusor activation. At the spinal and peripheral level, the autonomic nervous system is severely affected by Lewy pathology throughout the sympathetic ganglia and parasympathetic nuclei [31]. Their definite role in urological dysfunction in PD is not as clear as with subcortical and pontine dysfunction, but they are co-responsible for the symptoms of urinary dysfunction in PD. Correspondingly, a recent study showed that detrusor overactivity is almost universal in all patients with PD complaining of overactive bladder symptoms (97.1%), but a significant percentage of patients also had bladder outlet obstruction (36.8%), voiding detrusor underactivity (47%), and increased post void residual volume (16.7%) indicating that detrusor overactivity may not be the only cause of bladder dysfunction in PD [32].

However, despite the voiding symptoms, PD patients have low post void residuals. Therefore, it seems reasonable to regard overactive bladder (urgency/frequency syndrome) as the most typical feature of bladder dysfunction in PD [33].

At least 50% of PD patients suffer from urological symptoms due to their neurological disease. The associated reduction of quality of life is comparable to other symptoms caused by autonomic dysfunction. Although urological symptoms are usually part of the advanced disease stages, they may be present at the beginning or even before the classical motor symptoms in PD. The extent of symptoms directly correlates with age and disease stage according to Hoehn and Yahr [34]. Patients with PD dementia are at higher risk to suffer from urological dysfunction.

In a simplified manner, urological dysfunction can be dichotomized into storage dysfunction and voiding dysfunction. The storage dysfunction, which predominates in PD, is associated with incontinence and reduced quality of life. The voiding dysfunction is associated with retention, leading to reduced life expectancy. Clinical correlates of the storage dysfunction are urinary urgency (sudden need to void that is difficult to defer), increased daytime frequency (voiding more than eight times during the day), and nocturia. Voiding deficits are typically associated with the feeling of retention, hesitancy, and poor urinary stream. Nevertheless, micturition depends on the thorough interplay between these two key mechanisms.

Patients typically report frequent urge to urinate with increased risk of incontinence and/or low volumes during frequent micturition.

Nocturia represents the most frequent symptom of bladder dysfunction in PD. It is associated with poor sleep quality, falls, and institutionalization. Two or more voids per night are perceived as troublesome [35]. The two main sources of nocturia are reduced functional bladder capacity and/or nocturnal polyuria (defined as the proportion of 24-hour urine voided between midnight and 8 AM being more than 33%). Nocturnal polyuria represents a compensatory mechanism of cardiovascular diseases (e.g. congestive heart disease) or PD-associated cardiovascular dysfunction during daytime; redistributing blood volume enhances brain natriuretic peptide (BNP) excretion and hence pressure natriuresis. Importantly, nocturia is a multifactorial disorder, since disorders of circadian rhythm regulation also impact sleep and nighttime voiding in PD.

A smaller fraction of PD patients (about 25% according to [36]) suffer from insufficient bladder emptying with increased risk of recurrent lower urinary tract infections.

Particular characteristics of urogenital symptoms provide the possibility to differentiate between PD and MSA. In MSA, symptoms usually develop earlier, and they are on average more severe and more frequent than in PD. Moreover, MSA patients often suffer from erectile dysfunction before the onset of motor symptoms, and significant post voiding bladder volumes (> 100 ml) occur more frequently, especially as a complication of anticholinergic treatment. As a rule of thumb, micturition problems precede sexual dysfunction in PD, whereas the opposite timing is described for MSA. Sphincter EMG provides another means to differentiate these disorders, with neurogenic changes of sphincter potentials typical of MSA.

As PD predominantly affects the elderly population, particular physiological changes predispose these patients to urological dysfunction: bladder capacity and detrusor muscle strength decrease during physiological aging. Further, endocrinological changes in the elderly lead to one or two additional micturitions at nighttime. In men, prostatic changes have the potential to aggravate neurologically determined urological dysfunction. Likewise, pelvic floor symptoms can enhance stress incontinence and urge in women. Side effects of medications do affect women as well as men. Actually, urological diseases increase with age and disease severity: 90% of PD patients with Hoehn and Yahr stage 4 or 5 suffer from incontinence for any reason.

The diagnostic work-up of urological symptoms in PD has to be performed systematically. A urological consultation is mandatory whenever urological symptoms in a PD patient arise. This includes work-up of possible urinary tract infections, especially if new novel urological signs arise. Since women can suffer from gender-specific sources of urinary dysfunction as mentioned above, it is important not to miss those diseases. Consequently, female PD patients should also be referred to gynecologists. Further, careful screening of medications with potential influence on bladder and voiding function is mandatory.

As non-motor symptoms including autonomic dysfunction may fluctuate with dopaminergic medication and are reported more frequently in OFF-episodes, a critical part of the neuro-urological history is the assessment of any association with time points of dopaminergic medication.

Following a careful history of urological problems including sexual problems, the most important instrument to assess bladder function is the generation of a micturition diary. Patients take notes of time and volume of all micturition episodes, along with the assessment of orally administered liquids and episodes of incontinence. Medications are noted as well. Moreover, night-time symptoms such as cramping, pain, and nightmares should also be noted since they may be co-responsible for nocturia as well.

In addition, ultrasonographic assessment of post void residual bladder volume is mandatory. Compared to MSA, significant post void volumes in PD are rare.

Further examinations are usually performed by neuro-urologists, such as urodynamic testing. It should be performed in patients with suspected additional urological diseases, patients not responding to standard treatments, patients with raised post void volumes, or before prostate surgery [37]. The latter indication is a crucial diagnostic step to confirm a urodynamic profile as typical for PD, since MSA patients misdiagnosed as PD typically suffer from a deterioration of urological problems after prostate surgery. A urodynamic work-up may be the only method to differentiate whether raised post void volume is caused by poor detrusor contractility or by obstruction. Urodynamic abnormalities in PD include reduced bladder capacity, detrusor over-activity, external sphincter relaxation, detrusor weakness, and mild urethral obstruction. As mentioned, the most frequent finding is detrusor hyperreflexia, which can be combined with impaired contractile function during voiding or, even rarer in PD, detrusor-sphincter dyssynergia in a minority of patients [38]. The two latter findings put patients at particular risk of raised post void volume in addition to the classical symptoms of storage dysfunction.

In order to assess the extent of symptoms and their impact on quality of life, several scales are in use. Urological symptoms are embedded in scales for the assessment of all autonomic dysfunctions in PD. Several scales are specifically dedicated to urologic problems, but they are not well-validated in PD populations [39].

As soon as symptoms are irritative and/or associated with decreased quality of life, specific treatments are necessary. Kidney protection and avoidance of lower urinary tract infections with potential risk of urosepsis and death represent indications of treatment, too. General goals of any therapeutic measure are well-controlled and complete micturition and the avoidance of incontinence. Any therapeutic intervention has to be preceded by careful diagnostic evaluation.

The discontinuation of related aggravating drugs such as diuretics, psychopharmacological substances, benzodiazepines, and treatment of other relevant diseases should be considered first.

Numerous non-pharmacological measures are helpful to treat urological symptoms in PD. They are side-effect free and should represent the initial management strategy. As soon as a micturition diary is available, the time points of voiding episodes can be pre-scheduled, for example, every two hours. This avoids unpredictable urge with potential incontinence and embarrassing situations. Further, the amount of orally administered fluids can be limited or kept within a particular range. Large evening drinks should be avoided.

Physiotherapeutic practice focusing on pelvic floor muscle exercises has the potential to strengthen pelvic muscles aiming to support sphincter function. Biofeedback training may be successfully applied as well [40]. To specifically treat nocturia, reducing fluid intake, caffeine, and alcohol a few hours before going to bed may be effective. Patients are encouraged to empty the bladder before going to bed. To avoid absorption of dependent edema fluid at night that may cause nocturia, lower limb elevation above the heart level in the afternoon and the use of compression stockings are advised.

In cases of fluctuating urological symptoms that correlate with dopaminergic treatment, improvement of dopaminergic therapy aiming to reduce OFF-time is warranted. Off-associated urgency and frequency may benefit best. Nevertheless, reports on changes of urinary dysfunction due to dopaminergic agents are contradictory. In line with this observation, dopaminergic therapy in PD has been shown to have an unpredictable effect on urodynamic parameters [41].

If these dopaminergic measures do not show significant benefit or even deterioration of symptoms, different pharmacological strategies are available (see Table 12.2). Generally, the number of RCTs examining pharmacologic treatment of urological symptoms in PD is scarce.

Antimuscarinic medications (anticholinergics) are the first-line treatment for bladder storage symptoms and detrusor overactivity. Those agents antagonize muscarinic M2- and M3-receptors, so they prevent detrusor contraction and lower intravesical storage pressure. The storage capacity of urine volume is hence increased. They are most frequently used in a gradually increasing manner. Here, substances with low or absent CNS-penetrance should be preferred, in order to avoid classic anticholinergic side effects such as cognitive dysfunction/delirium. In addition, dry mouth, blurred vision, constipation, arrhythmias, and falls are well-known side effects. Target symptoms of anticholinergics are the reduction of frequency and urgency both at daytime and nighttime. Due to their pharmacodynamic effect, anticholinergics increase the likelihood of raised post void volume, which has to be monitored. Trospium chloride, oxybutinin, tolterodine, and darifenacin are the most frequently used substances. Trospium chloride is least associated with cognitive side effects. Recently, solifenacin, a selective blocker of cholinergic M3-receptors, was rated possibly effective to treat overactive bladder by a MDS-commissioned review on non-motor symptoms in PD [42].

Beta 3-adrenergic agonists can also reduce detrusor overactivity in PD. They are not associated with cognitive side effects. Mirabegron is the only β 3-adrenergic agonist examined in PD with proven effect on the improvement of urgency symptoms. It mediates its effect via the sympathetic hypogastric nerve, improving bladder

Table 12.2 Pharmacological treatment of urogenital dysfunction in Parkinson's disease

Overactive bladder Antimuscarinic	Dose	Regimen	CNS penetrance
Trospium chloride	15–45 mg/day	bid/tid	low
Tolterodine	1–2 mg/day	bid/tid	moderate
Solifenacin	5–10 mg/day	oid	moderate
Fesoterodine	4–8 mg/day	oid	moderate
Darifenacin	7.5–15 mg/day	oid	low
Oxybutinin	5 mg/day	bid/tid	moderate
β3-adrenergic agonists			
Mirabegron	25–50 mg/day	oid	low
Arginin-vasopressin analog			
Desmopressin nasal spray	10–40 microgram	bed-time	
Botulinum toxin (detrusor)	200–300 units	3–6 months	
Incomplete bladder emptying			
Prazosin	1 mg	tid	
Alfuzosin	5 mg	bid	
Terazosin	2–10 mg	oid	
Doxazosin	2–4 mg	oid	
Tamsulosin	0.4 mg	oid	
Sexual dysfunction			
Phosphodiesterase 5 – Inhibitors		**Before sexual intercourse**	
Sildenafil	50–100 mg	30–60 minutes	
Tadalafil	10 mg	30 minutes	
Vardenafil	10 mg	30–60 minutes	
Apomorphine sublingual/subcutaneous	2–5 mg	10–25 minutes	
Alprostadil intracavernous injection	10–20 micrograms	5–10 minutes	

capacity. Caution is required in patients with uncontrolled hypertension or arrhythmias. On the other hand, elevating blood pressure may be a synergistic and desired side effect in patients with orthostatic hypotension. Vibegron, another beta 3-adrenergic receptor agonist, has proven effective for overactive bladder symptoms and has just recently been approved in Japan [43].

If orally administered substances are ineffective for storage symptoms, the injection of botulinum toxin A into the muscular layers of the bladder is another interesting, safe, and effective approach. It is associated with positive effects on quality of life documented up to nine months. Periodical monitoring of raised post void volume is mandatory, since its likelihood is increased.

Regarding DBS therapy, which partially restores basal ganglia dysfunction, most studies report improvement of urgency, mediated by the improvement of bladder storage function. This conclusion was mainly drawn by studies targeting the subthalamic nucleus (STN) [44]. The observation is in line with the crucial implication of basal ganglia function for correct detrusor function.

Sacral and/or pudendal nerve modulation and percutaneous tibial nerve stimulation are other neuromodulatory options that can be tried in refractory cases of storage symptoms. Its definite mechanisms of action still need to be clarified.

Symptoms due to incomplete bladder emptying, which are less common in PD, can be alleviated by adrenoceptor antagonists (tamsulosin, alfuzosin, doxazosin, prazosin). Nevertheless, one needs to be aware of the risk of postural hypotension in PD patients using these substances.

If pharmacological approaches do not improve emptying deficits significantly, intermittent self-catheterization has to be applied. Persistent elevation of post void residual volume above 200 ml requires intermittent self-catheterization. Due to continuous irritation of the lower urinary tract with risks of mechanical injuries and infections, a permanent suprapubic catheter may be a rational solution in selected patients.

Since nocturia may also be due to increased brain natriuretic peptide (BNP) release during supine position, desmopressin, a potent analogue of arginin-vasopressin, can counter act nocturnal diuresis. Using this pharmacological approach, nocturia mainly due to nocturnal polyuria can be improved, as well as early morning symptoms of orthostatic hypotension. Due to the risk of hyponatremia, caution is required regarding its use.

Interestingly, melatonin has been used successfully to treat nocturia in one study, targeting the regularity of the circadian cycle [35].

Sexual Dysfunction

Sexual dysfunction in PD is associated with reduced quality of life and psychological strain. It means frustration to both the patient and the partner, and it occurs more frequently than in age-matched controls.

Regarding the whole span of the disease, up to 80% of male PD patients suffer from decreased libido, which is accompanied by erectile dysfunction in eight out of ten patients. Erectile dysfunction is defined as the incapacity to achieve or maintain a penile erection long enough to allow a sexual relation.

At least two-thirds of female PD patients lose a significant amount of sexual drive and arousal [45].

There is a bi-directional association between sexual dysfunction and depression/apathy, and a multidimensional nature is assumed. Here, extent of motor symptoms (especially the akinetic-rigid type of parkinsonism), age, pain, and other factors contribute to the disorder [46].

Although very early sexual dysfunction, particularly erectile dysfunction, is pathognomonic for MSA, up to 50% of PD patients are also affected at early disease stages or even before motor symptoms [47]. Interestingly, bladder dysfunction and erectile dysfunction are not correlated in PD. Moreover, erectile dysfunction confers a significant risk of PD, even in younger men [48].

Difficulties achieving orgasm are common to both men and women with PD [40]. When it comes to gender-specific symptoms, erectile dysfunction and ejaculation abnormality occur specifically in men, while female patients typically report loss of lubrication and involuntary urination during sexual intercourse. Older age and pronounced depressive symptoms are the most relevant factors for sexual dysfunction in women. Nevertheless, female sexual dysfunction has been less studied in PD.

Of course, impulse control disorders are implicated in sexual behavior. Since dopamine replacement induced or aggravated hypersexuality and aberrant sexual behavior are not due to dysautonomia itself, they are discussed elsewhere in this book. Although the genital organ primarily shares lumbosacral innervation with the lower urinary tract, regular erection is a vascular event occurring secondarily after (cholinergically mediated) dilation of the cavernous helical artery and compression of the cavernous vein to the tunica albuginea. Ejaculation is brought about by contraction of the vas deferens and the bladder neck, in order to prevent retrograde ejaculation (by activation of adrenergic nerves). In men, sexual intercourse is divided into desire, erection/excitement, and orgasm/ejaculation.

Concerning the underlying pathophysiological processes, a dysfunction due to central and peripheral (parasympathetic and sympathetic) degenerative processes is discussed to be implicated in the changes of all aspects of sexual intercourse in PD. The dopaminergic deficit definitely has a detrimental role on libido and arousal-related vasodilatation of structures associated with penile erection.

Regarding further central mechanisms, hypothalamic dysfunction seems to be involved in decreased libido and erection, via altered dopamine-oxytocin pathways [33]. Interestingly, reduced testosterone levels have been linked to non-motor symptoms in men with PD, but the association is not clear, and testosterone substitution is not clearly effective to treat sexual dysfunction.

Taken together, the pathophysiological background of autonomic sexual dysfunction is still under investigation.

Taking a detailed history together with the partner, if available, represents the most important diagnostic step. Further tests including penile plethysmography, Doppler ultrasound, penile arteriography, and nocturnal penile tumescence are usually not necessary, but they are used for research purposes.

Any treatment goal for sexual dysfunction in PD is the improvement of sexual satisfaction and hence quality of life.

First, comorbid conditions and current medications need to be assessed, since they may represent the primary source of sexual dysfunction. Here, it is paramount to consider illnesses like cardiovascular disease, diabetes mellitus,

hypertension, pre-existing genitourinary disorders and radiation therapy, depression, anxiety as well as personal habits such as smoking, consumption of tea or coffee, alcohol or any substance abuse [49]. Regarding medications with negative effect on sexual function, beta-blockers, hydrochlorothiazides, and SSRIs are of particular importance.

Effectiveness and safety of the cGMP-specific phosphodiesterase type 5 inhibitor, sildenafil, has been documented in men with PD. It augments the nitric oxide mediated relaxation pathway in the corpora cavernosum and spongiosum. Thus, it does not increase the arousal, it only helps to maintain the erection. It is usually taken 30 to 60 minutes before intercourse. Improvement was reported with regard to erectile function, the ability to reach orgasm, and overall sexual satisfaction [50]. Notably, the class of phosphodiesterase inhibitors can produce symptomatic orthostatic hypotension, especially in patients with (subclinical) cardiovascular autonomic dysfunction. Nevertheless, it is the most frequently used substance class to treat erectile dysfunction in men with PD, and sildenafil is the only substance recommended by the American Academy of Neurology for urogenital dysfunction in PD, with approval by the Food and Drug Administration.

Though not formally tested in PD, tadalafil (with a longer duration of action than sildenafil) or vardenafil are equally effective. Nevertheless, it is important to notify patients that these drugs may not work every time.

There are reports on a beneficial effect of sublingual apomorphine on sexual dysfunction in PD, which is probably centrally mediated via D2-related stimulation of oxytocinergic neurons. Pharmacological treatment strategies are listed in Table 12.2.

If the above-mentioned approaches lack success or are contraindicated, intracavernosal injections of alprostadil and moxisylyte are effective (although not formally assessed by appropriate studies in PD), but the injection is very painful and can result in noduli formation. Vacuum devices in combination with constrictor bands, intraurethral prostaglandin suppositories, and implantable inflatable prostheses are additional treatment possibilities, but not straightforward to handle. Any therapeutic approach needs to be discussed with the partner.

Therapeutics for sexual dysfunction in female patients are limited, but the use of vaginal lubrication and hormonal therapy can be recommended. Phosphodiesterase 5 inhibitors have been used with some success.

Psychotherapy and counseling may be effective for some patients and their partners.

References

1. Freeman R, Abuzinadah AR, Gibbons C, et al. Orthostatic hypotension. J Am Coll Cardiol 2018; **72**(11): 1294–1309.

2. Novak P. Quantitative autonomic testing. J Vis Exp 2011; **53**: 2502.

3. Struhal W, Lahrmann H, Fanciulli A, Wenning GK (eds.). *Bedside Approach to Autonomic Disorders: A Clinical Tutor.* Springer; 2017.

4. Gibbons CH, Freeman R. Delayed orthostatic hypotension – a frequent cause of orthostatic intolerance. Neurology 2006; **67**(1): 28–32.

5. Senard JM, Rai S, Lapeyre-Mestre M, et al. Prevalence of orthostatic hypotension in Parkinson's disease. J Neurol Neurosurg Psychiatry 1997; **63**: 584–589.

6. Metzler M, Duerr S, Granata R, et al. Neurogenic orthostatic hypotension: pathophysiology, evaluation, and management. J Neurol 2013; **260** (9): 2212–2219.

7. Norcliffe-Kaufmann L, Kaufmann H, Palma JA, et al. Orthostatic heart rate changes in patients with autonomic failure caused by neurodegenerative synucleinopathies. Ann Neurol 2018; **83**(3): 522–531.

8. Michele B, Moya A, de Lange FJ, et al. 2018 ESC Guidelines for the diagnosis and management of syncope. Eur Heart J 2018; **39** (21): 1883–1948.

9. Gibbons CH, Freeman R. Delayed orthostatic hypotension – a frequent cause of orthostatic intolerance. Neurology 2006; **67**(1): 28–32.

10. Fanciulli A, Strano S, Ndayisaba JP, et al. Detecting nocturnal hypertension in Parkinson's disease and multiple system atrophy: proposal of a decision-support algorithm. J Neurol 2014; **261**(7): 1291–1299.

11. Fanciulli A, Jordan J, Biaggioni I, et al. Consensus statement on the definition of neurogenic supine hypertension in cardiovascular autonomic failure by the American Autonomic Society (AAS) and the European Federation of Autonomic Societies (EFAS). Clin Auton Res 2018; **28**: 355–362.

12. Espay AJ, Lewitt PA, Hauser RA, et al. Neurogenic orthostatic hypotension and supine hypertension in Parkinson's disease and related synucleinopathies: prioritisation of treatment targets. Lancet Neurol 2016; **15**(9): 954–966.

13. Maule S, Papotti G, Naso D, et al. Orthostatic hypotension: evaluation and treatment. Cardiovasc Hematol Disord Drug Targets 2007; **7**(1): 63–70.

14. van Wamelen DJ, Leta V, Podlewska AM, et al. Exploring hyperhidrosis and related thermoregulatory symptoms as a possible clinical identifier for the dysautonomic subtype of Parkinson's disease. J Neurol 2019; **266**: 1736–1742.

15. Swinn L, Schrag A, Viswanathan R, et al. Sweating dysfunction in Parkinson's disease. Mov Disord 2003; **18**: 1459–1463.

16. Jain S. Multi-organ autonomic dysfunction in Parkinson disease. Parkinsonism Relat Disord 2011; **17**: 77–83.

17. Coon EA, Low PA. Thermoregulation in Parkinson disease. Handb Clin Neurol 2018; **157**: 715–725.

18. Kim JB, Kim BJ, Koh SB, et al. Autonomic dysfunction according to disease progression in Parkinson's disease. Parkinsonism Relat Disord 2014; **20**: 303–307.

19. Mendoza-Velásquez JJ, Flores-Vázquez JF, Barrón-Velázquez E, et al. Autonomic dysfunction in α-synucleinopathies. Front Neurol 2019; **10**: 363.

20. Sanghera MK, Ward C, Stewart RM, et al. Alleviation of drenching sweats following subthalamic deep brain stimulation in a patient with Parkinson's disease–a case report. J Neurol Sci 2009; **285**: 246–249.

21. Bellini G, Best LA, Brechany U, et al. Clinical impact of deep brain stimulation on the autonomic system in patients with Parkinson's disease. Mov Disord Clin Pract 2020; **7**: 373–382.

22. Chen Z, Li G, Liu J. Autonomic dysfunction in Parkinson's disease: implications for pathophysiology, diagnosis, and treatment. Neurobiol Dis 2020; **134**: 104700.

23. Mulak A, Bonaz B. Brain-gut-microbiota axis in Parkinson's disease. World J Gastroenterol 2015; **21**(37): 1060920.

24. Kim JS, Sung HY. Gastrointestinal autonomic dysfunction in patients with Parkinson's disease. J Mov Disord 2015; **8**(2): 76–82.

25. Palma JA, Kaufmann H. Autonomic disorders predicting Parkinson's disease. Parkinsonism Relat Disord 2014; **20**(S1): S94–S98.

26. Csoti I, Jost WH, Reichmann H. Parkinson's disease between internal medicine and neurology. J Neural Transm 2016; 123(1): 3–17.

27. Ziemssen T, Schmidt C, Herting B, Reichmann H. *Autonome Dysfunktion beim idiopathischen Parkinson-Syndrom und der Multisystematrophie* [Autonomic Dysfunction in Parkinson's Disease and Multiple System Atrophy]. Georg Thieme Verlag; 2006.

28. Palma JA, Kaufmann H. Treatment of autonomic dysfunction in Parkinson disease and other synucleinopathies. Mov Disord 2018; 33(3): 372–390.

29. Trapl M, Enderle P, Nowotny M, et al. The Gugging Swallowing Screen. Stroke 2007; 38: 2948.

30. Fasano A, Bove F, Gabrielli M, et al. The role of small intestinal bacterial overgrowth in Parkinson's disease. Mov Disord 2013; 28(9): 1241–1249.

31. Wakabayashi K, Takahashi H. Neuropathology of autonomic nervous system in Parkinson's disease. Eur Neurol 1997; 38(Suppl 2): 2–7.

32. Vurture G, Peyronnet B, Palma JA, et al. Urodynamic mechanisms underlying overactive bladder symptoms in patients with Parkinson disease. Int Neurourol J 2019; 23: 211–218.

33. Sakakibara R, Uchiyama T, Yamanishi T, et al. Genitourinary dysfunction in Parkinson's disease. Mov Disord 2010; 25: 2–12.

34. Barone P, Antonini A, Colosimo C, et al. The PRIAMO study: a multicenter assessment of nonmotor symptoms and their impact on quality of life in Parkinson's disease. Mov Disord 2009; 24: 1641–1649.

35. Batla A, Phé V, De Min L, et al. Nocturia in Parkinson's Disease: why does it occur and how to manage? Mov Disord Clin Pract 2016; 3: 443–451.

36. Campos-Sousa RN, Quagliato E, da Silva BB, et al. Urinary symptoms in Parkinson's disease: prevalence and associated factors. Arq Neuropsiquiatr 2003; 61(2B): 359–363.

37. Kapoor S, Bourdoumis A, Mambu L, et al. Effective management of lower urinary tract dysfunction in idiopathic Parkinson's disease. Int J Urol 2013; 20: 79–84.

38. Chen Z, Li G, Liu J. Autonomic dysfunction in Parkinson's disease: implications for pathophysiology, diagnosis, and treatment. Neurobiol Dis 2020; 134: 104700.

39. Pavy-Le Traon A, Cotterill N, Amarenco G, et al. Clinical rating scales for urinary symptoms in Parkinson disease: critique and recommendations. Mov Disord Clin Pract 2018; 5 :479–491.

40. Palma JA, Kaufmann H. Treatment of autonomic dysfunction in Parkinson disease and other synucleinopathies. Mov Disord 2018; 33: 372–390.

41. Winge K, Werdelin LM, Nielsen KK, et al. Effects of dopaminergic treatment on bladder function in Parkinson's disease. Neurourol Urodyn 2004; 23: 689–696.

42. Seppi K, Chaudhuri KR, Coelho M, et al. Update on treatments for nonmotor symptoms of Parkinson's disease: an evidence-based medicine review. Mov Disord 2019; 34: 180–198.

43. Keam SJ. Vibegron: first global approval. Drugs 2018; 78: 1835–1839.

44. Basiago A, Binder DK. Effects of deep brain stimulation on autonomic function. Brain Sci 2016; 6: 33.

45. Bronner G, Royter V, Korczyn AD, et al. Sexual dysfunction in Parkinson's disease. J Sex Marital Ther 2004; 30: 95–105.

46. Pfeiffer RF. Management of autonomic dysfunction in Parkinson's disease. Semin Neurol 2017; 37: 176–185.

47. Malek N, Lawton MA, Grosset KA, et al. Autonomic dysfunction in early Parkinson's disease: results from the United Kingdom Tracking Parkinson's Study. Mov Disord Clin Pract 2016; 4: 509–516.

48. Gao X, Chen H, Schwarzschild MA, et al. Erectile function and risk of Parkinson's disease. Am J Epidemiol 2007; 166: 1446–1450.

49. Bhattacharyya KB, Rosa-Grilo M. Sexual dysfunctions in Parkinson's disease: an underrated problem in a much discussed disorder. Int Rev Neurobiol 2017; 134: 859–876.

50. Hussain IF, Brady CM, Swinn MJ, et al. Treatment of erectile dysfunction with sildenafil citrate (Viagra) in parkinsonism due to Parkinson's disease or multiple system atrophy with observations on orthostatic hypotension. J Neurol Neurosurg Psychiatry 2001; 71: 371–374.

Chapter 13

Gastrointestinal Disturbances in Parkinson's Disease Including the Management of Sialorrhea

Wolfgang H. Jost and Lisa Klingelhoefer

Introduction

Gastrointestinal complaints are the most frequent autonomic symptoms in Parkinson's disease (PD) and affect almost all patients over the course of time [1, 2, 3]. The causes are not clear. It is likely to be a multifactorial event in which both central and peripheral degenerative processes play a role [4, 5]. In addition, influences from the medication have to be considered, which are certainly not predominant. The central degenerative process involving the dorsal vagal nucleus is certainly significant, but it does not explain the range of symptoms. Involvement of the enteric nervous system is likely to be more crucial, with PD typical changes involving the presence of Lewy bodies extending from the upper esophagus down to the rectum in the Plexus myentericus Auerbach and the Plexus submucosus Meissner [4, 6, 7, 8, 9, 10]. The functional disturbance can therefore affect the entire gastrointestinal tract [5]. Thus dysphagia can occur in addition to delayed gastric emptying and extended intestinal transit. Very common is sialorrhea due to impaired and less frequent swallowing. Constipation and dysphagia are described by patients as particularly afflicting [5].

Sialorrhea in Parkinson's Disease

Extensive sialorrhea is a common complaint in PD and presents in 50% to 75% of cases [9, 11, 12], but it is frequently and erroneously viewed as an increased salivary production. This is an inference based on the clinical observation of saliva exuding from the corner of the mouth when only slightly open. Numerous studies have however demonstrated that sialorrhea results from dysphagia and not from an increase in salivary production [5, 9]. Rather it has been conclusively shown that in PD patients absolute saliva amounts are reduced both under resting conditions and under provocation when compared with a normal juvenile population and that in fact no differences could be found in salivary production between patients with and without sialorrhea. Dysphagia is a major problem for the patients, complicated when (1) forward-leaning posture positions the head farther forward as well as (2) when the mouth remains slightly opened which is common due to hypomimia. A further complication arises when the M. orbicularis oris presents with reduced muscle tonus. Recent probes have also demonstrated neuropathological changes in the salivary gland itself [9].

Given a tentative diagnosis, sialorrhea patients should undergo a timely screening for their swallowing ability and an examination by the swallowing therapist, for example, speech therapists. Recommended is a fiberoptic endoscopic evaluation of swallowing (FEES, see Figure 13.1), which today constitutes an indispensable standard examination [13].

A basic intervention involves therapeutic measures for swallowing, in particular, functional dysphagia therapy (FDT) [13]. The medical treatment of sialorrhea recommended for the patient usually involves anticholinergics, for example, scopolamine, which do reduce the salivation and this should become apparent after only a few weeks; but these medications unfortunately induce considerable adverse reactions [5]. After discontinuing the anticholinergics salivation is reported to return to pre-medication levels. The parasympatholyticum glycopyrrolate can be recommended, because of fewer central nervous side effects [14]. But it would be medically more sensible to directly treat the primary dysphagic factor and to be more restrictive in administering anticholinergics [5].

A significant therapeutic option can be found in injections of botulinumtoxin, involving

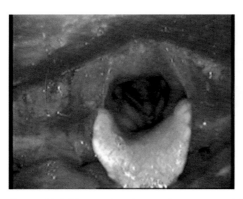

Figure 13.1 Fiber optic endoscopy in a patient with PD. (For the color version, please refer to the plate section.)

particularly Gl. submandibularis and also Gl. parotis [15, 16, 17]. Injections are generally done transcutaneously directly into the salivary glands.

In July 2018 incobotulinumtoxinA was approved for the treatment of chronic sialorrhea in adults without restrictions, independent of the underlying disease. The recommended treatment dose is 100 units, with 30 units given to each of the two parotid glands and 20 units to the two submandibular glands; a possible repetition can be undertaken after 16 weeks [16, 17]. In August 2019 the FDA (US Food and Drug Administration) approved rimabotulinumtoxinB for chronic sialorrhea in adults [15]. The recommended dose is 500–1,500 units per parotid gland and 250 units per submandibular gland (total dose of 1,500–3,500 units). Transient dry mouth and dysphagia have been described as frequent side effects of botulinumtoxin injections. It is recommended to inject with ultrasound control if possible [13].

Dysphagia in Parkinson's Disease

Parkinson already described such pronounced problems in swallowing in his patients that assimilating foods was limited to only fluids [5]. Dysphagia has been found in 50% to 75% of Parkinson patients [5, 9]. These dysphagic symptoms can only be partially explained by the dopaminergic deficit. It is important to note that a good number of PD medications themselves can reinforce dysphagia, especially anticholinergics [5].

The overall process of swallowing is deficient [18]. Swallowing is made difficult by insufficient mastication which is itself a result of weakened

musculature or "rigid" chewing muscles [5]. Foodstuffs are insufficiently transmitted to the throat when swallowing, and transport through the esophagus is retarded. This is typically explained by a reduced peristalsis [5], or otherwise by inadequate coordination due to insufficient muscle relaxation in the esophageal sphincter [5, 9]. In a large number of PD patients dysphagia, though present, remains asymptomatic, but it is possible even in these cases to observe the functional disturbance [5]. A relationship to achalasia has been posited [5]. Furthermore, there are observations of increased numbers of hiatus hernias, gastroesophageal reflux, segmental spasms in the esophagus, and an increase in passage duration in the esophagus [5]. The most frequent complications include chronic laryngitis, acute and chronic tracheobronchitis, and aspiration pneumonia. Severe cases of pneumonia, abscesses, and bronchiectasis are rather seldom [5]. There are, however, reports of pronounced forms, even including medically necessary esophagus dilatation and gastrostomy [5]. One explanation for this case involves the reduced muscle tone in the esophagus or otherwise insufficient muscle relaxation and coordination of the lower esophagus sphincter [5].

For screening, both by a trained physician or by a speech therapist, a standardized swallowing assessment in the form of the three-ounce water swallow test [19, 20] and the swallowing of pasty and crumbly food can be performed [21]. As an indication for dysphagia, the behavior of the patients should be observed during the swallowing test with special focus on whether any coughing, harrumphing, throaty voice, or compensation mechanisms such as chin tuck, head turn, effortful swallow, supraglottic and super-supraglottic swallowing, and Mendelsohn Maneuver appear. As the gold standard for objective assessment of dysphagia, a fiberoptic endoscopic evaluation of swallowing (FEES) can be performed which provides a detailed analysis about the late oral and pharyngeal phases of swallowing of liquid and different food consistencies. Alternatively, videofluoroscopy swallowing studies (VFSS) may be performed to indirectly visualize the structures involved in swallowing and analyze the bolus flow and kinematic events of the oropharyngeal swallowing phases via real-time diagnostic X-ray during actual swallowing of the radiopaque fluid and food [22, 23].

To date, treating dysphagia is still unsatisfactory [18]. Present-day emphasis is placed on optimizing dopaminergic therapy and speech therapy measures for swallowing. Patients can be given specific dysphagic diets or pureed foods or should be recommended to avoid swallowing larger pieces of food. This, however, seldom achieves any substantial improvement [5, 18]. Medically, administering prokinetic agents can be useful. In the case of insufficient relaxation of the esophagus sphincter, the sphincter can be extended by dilatation or a posterior cricopharyngeal sphincterotomy (though extremely rare) can be performed [5, 13]. Alternatively, injecting botulinumtoxin into the sphincter can be recommended. Gastrostomy can be discussed in individual cases as a last option [5].

In all cases of dysphagia, it is imperative to remember that medication sometimes cannot be properly swallowed either if they are not sufficiently dissolved or at least pulverized in a mortar. Hereby, an adaptation of medication scheme is sometimes necessary as not all PD medication can be dissolved or pulverized, for example, prolonged levodopa preparation and COMT-inhibitors need to be exchanged and additionally transdermal dopamine agonist application can be considered. The patients should in any case be in the ON state when eating (which is unfortunately not always adhered to in hospitals), as the risk of choking is far more serious in the OFF state. In PD patients with motor fluctuations and severe dysphagia, advanced therapies such as the intrajejunal application of levodopa-carbidopa intestinal gel (LCIG) via a Percutaneous endoscopic gastrostomy (PEG) can be considered. Hereby, good control of PD-specific symptoms can be ensured [24] next to enteral nutrition.

The gastrointestinal disturbances, and among them especially dysphagia, can also fluctuate, whereby these fluctuations may or may not correlate with the motor fluctuations [25].

Gastric Emptying in Parkinson's Disease

Parkinson's disease patients often complain of acid reflux [5]. This can be due to either reduced peristalsis or gastroesophageal reflux. Delayed gastric emptying in PD patients is of course undeniable [26]. In addition, a higher risk of hiatus hernias has also been described [5, 9]. Most probably, the disturbance stems from a dyscoordination between esophageal and gastric motility with the lower esophagus sphincter [5, 9].

When gastric emptying is delayed, the patients complain of epigastric pressure after meals and a feeling of satiety unexpectedly early on. In these cases, the Parkinson medication can worsen the symptoms too [5, 26]. Delayed gastric emptying induces a disturbance in resorption of levodopa (levodopa is absorbed in the small intestine) and thus seriously interferes with planning and controlling therapy. Furthermore, resorption of other compounds such as vitamins may be affected as well. Further studies are needed. This disturbance in motility is co-responsible for paroxysmal on-off-symptoms. Administering levodopa through a duodenal tube can substantially improve the symptoms of akinesia and especially fluctuations, and on-off phases can be decreased [26, 27]. We see corresponding positive effects in using soluble levodopa, transdermal application or LCIG via PEG. An essential advantage in administering levodopa preparations that do not release the active substance until reaching the small intestine cannot be expected: while any disadvantage caused by stomach acid is successfully avoided, the problems in gastric motility are not improved on.

Metoclopramide is contraindicated in the treatment of delayed gastric emptying in PD as its central effect can worsen the PD symptoms [5]. This can also induce early and late dyskinesia and drug-induced parkinsonism. Domperidone, a peripheral dopamine antagonist, can be recommended: it does not penetrate the blood–brain barrier [28] and thus lacks any central nervous effects. It can be given as adjuvant therapy in combination with levodopa because it reduces unwanted peripheral side effects of levodopa such as nausea without exerting a central influence on the PD symptoms [28]. It should be administered three times daily at a dose of 10 mg orally (caveat: QTc prolongation). In advanced stages domperidone will probably have no effect on gastric motility; long-term medication is obsolete.

Helicobacter pylori (HLO) infection in the stomach mucosal lining is likewise frequent in Parkinson patients and can induce an attenuation in levodopa effects which can however be treated [29]. If the stomach complaints are unexplained, an examination for possible HLO involvement in the stomach lining is advisable.

Furthermore, the gastrointestinal motility abnormalities could favor the occurrence of small intestinal bacterial overgrowth (SIBO) [30] which could be found in PD patients [31]. Additionally, alterations in the composition of microbiota in PD patients and its association with clinical phenotypes of the disease have been reported [32].

Constipation in Parkinson's Disease

Since first being mentioned by James Parkinson, constipation has been considered a very frequent symptom (occurring in up to 80% of patients) in PD [2, 5, 9, 11, 33, 34]. As is often the case, constipation is in fact described as the most frequent autonomic symptom [1, 3, 5]. Interestingly, healthy people presenting with constipation have shown a greater risk for subsequently developing PD [35, 36, 37]. This fits well with the studies published by Braak and co-workers [4, 6]. Constipation is now considered as one of the most relevant early signs of PD, and the frequency seems to be higher than the subjective complaints [29, 35, 37, 38, 39, 40]. The gastrointestinal tract may even play an important role in pathogenesis [4, 37], see "Brain-Gut Axis" section below.

The constipation can further develop into a megacolon, to pseudo-obstruction or volvulus [5]. A megacolon usually remains asymptomatic, with the exception of the one symptom of constipation, although an ileus and the consequent surgery [5] and a colon perforation have been described. It is interesting, though at the same time surprising, that even in spite of presenting with severe constipation, patients seldom report this problem spontaneously, which indicates that it is most probably underdiagnosed [40].

As causes for the constipation, medication, reduced physical movement, a reduced muscle tone in the diaphragm and abdominal musculature, and reduced intake of fibers and liquids have been advanced [5]. From the earliest studies onwards, anticholinergic agents have, in particular, been related to severe constipating effects, even describing the development of megacolon.

Constipation in PD is definitely disease-related [40]. It was described long before any specific therapy had been found [2, 5], and many studies of as yet non-treated patients were able to demonstrate delayed transit [5, 9]. It is much more likely

the case that in PD patients a delayed transit plays an intrinsic and prominent role and that constipation can be additionally worsened by the medical treatment itself [5].

Most probably the underlying causes for the delayed transit are degenerative changes involving Lewy bodies located centrally as well as from the upper esophagus to the rectum in the Plexus myentericus Auerbach and the Plexus submucosus Meissner and in the intermediolateral nucleus [6, 7, 8]. Additionally, anismus, a failure of normal relaxation and involuntary contractions of the anal sphincters during defecation (extremely rare!) can lead to "outlet" constipation [5].

A rather simple method in support of diagnostic work involves administering radiopaque markers (ROM) (Figure 13.2) as a gold standard diagnostic test [5]. Abdominal X-rays are taken at defined time intervals to identify the retained numbers of ingested ROMs in order to calculate a colon transit time. As an alternative method, a gamma camera can be used to track the movements of radioisotope test meals or capsules at specified time points for quantitative evaluation of scintigraphic colon transit times [41]. As guidance, it is also useful to ask the patient, for example, to eat poppy seed cake and then to note when the poppy seeds are excreted.

There is no gold standard method to assess outlet constipation, but defecography is widely preferred. It involves the installation of barium in the rectum and subjects are asked to empty it during recording of a cinematic film [42]. Anorectal dysfunction can also be assessed by external anal sphincter electromyography, balloon distension and expulsion test, and anorectal manometry [43].

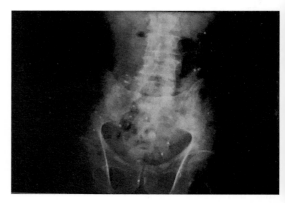

Figure 13.2 Colonic transit time with radiopaque markers (white spots in the entire colon) in a PD patient.

Up to now there is no structured guideline in the management of constipation. A fiber-rich diet, psyllium as a bulk laxative, stool softener, and sufficient liquid intake have high therapeutic value in constipation, but regular physical exercise and physical therapy are beneficial as well [5]. Removal of aggravating factors, like anticholinergics, should be considered [5]. Unfortunately, these measures are useful only in mild to moderate cases. In many cases, a colonic transit of more than seven days is demonstrated and no improvement of colonic transit can be shown by the different therapeutic options due to the upper threshold. In this case additional medication needs to be given. An effect of domperidone in the upper gastrointestinal tract has not been shown for cases of constipation [5].

Stimulants such as bisacodyl, sodium picosulfate, and Senna are safe and helpful [44]. Besides stimulant laxatives and osmotic laxatives are recommendable. The best success to date is achieved with macrogol [45, 46, 47]. Lactulose is burdened with flatulence [5]. There are also positive data on the use of probiotics and probiotic fibers [44].

There are as of yet still no studies on the effects of modern prokinetic agents such as, for example, serotonin (5-HT4) agonists, like mosapride [48]. In the meantime, prucaloprid [49] has been approved for severe constipation and may be administered in PD patients, although specific studies in this population are still lacking.

Some new drugs like relamorelin (ghrelin agonist) [34], chloride channel activators like linaclotide, lubiprostone, and plenacanatide [38, 50, 51] are in discussion.

In cases of anismus (which is extremely rare) we recommend injections of botulinumtoxin [5].

Brain–Gut Axis

There has been considerable and in fact intense debate for a number of years now as to whether the intestine could be the site of pathogenesis for PD [52, 53], whereby the discussion has been essentially influenced by the work of Braak and co-workers [4, 6]. This research group describes the presence of Lewy bodies or SNCA (Synuclein Alpha) -positive aggregates in the enteric nervous system (ENS). The studies even suggest a possible primary role of the affliction in the ENS before that in the CNS. This suggestion is interestingly compatible with the clinical observation that GIT dysfunction precedes motor symptoms by years. This would plausibly localize the onset of the process in the peripheral nervous system with an ascending progression from the ENS to the CNS [4, 6, 7, 12]. Evidence from epidemiological studies and animal models support this hypothesis. As such, constipation as a prodromal non-motor symptom of PD is meanwhile widely accepted [38, 54, 55] as well as being considered a risk factor for developing PD (up to 4.5-fold dependent on the number of bowel movements per day) [35]. Different groups could show that chronic oral or direct intragastral administration of rotenone in mice induced SNCA accumulation, selective nigrostriatal dopaminergic neurodegeneration, partly even asymmetrically, and motor deficits comparable to those in PD [56, 57, 58, 59].

It is highly interesting that the olfactory bulb and the ENS are the only nervous system structures that are directly and constantly exposed to environmental substances through inhalation or ingestion, thereby representing gateways from the environment to the nervous system. These observations are consistent with the Braak staging showing SNCA in the dorsal motor nucleus of the vagus nerve (DMNV), the olfactory bulb, the ENS (Figure 13.3), and the submandibular gland [4, 6, 7, 52]. The demonstration of a cell-to-cell transfer of SNCA in both in-vitro as well as in-vivo models (in PD patients with transplantations) thus offers good support for the postulated series within the SNCA aggregation beginning in the intestine, progressing to the nucleus of the vagus nerve in the brainstem and finally into the midbrain (the so-called propagation) [6]. The postulated propagation via the vagus nerve is supported by findings in animal studies as well as large epidemiological studies. In animals it could be observed that hemivagotomy stopped progression of PD-like pathology from ENS to the central DMNV [60, 61] as well as a time-dependent active transport of SNCA via the vagal nerve after SNCA injection into the intestinal wall of rats [62]. Recently, bidirectional routes of propagation has been proven in monkeys by striatal inoculation of Lewy bodies from Parkinson patients with propagation to the ENS and enteric inoculation of Lewy bodies from Parkinson patients with propagation to the ZNS.

Furthermore, in humans it was observed that patients who underwent truncal vagotomy were at

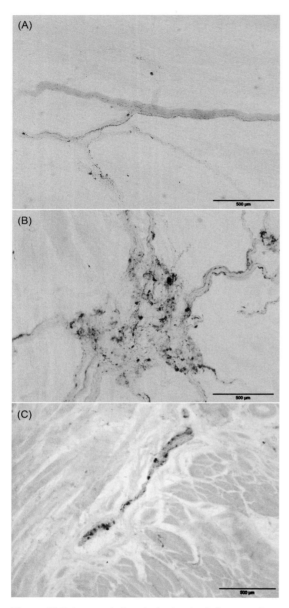

Figure 13.3 Lewy pathology in the Auerbach (intramural) plexus of the ENS in sporadic PD. (A) Aggregated α-synuclein in single axons within fiber bundles interconnecting the ganglia of the gastric cardia: 65-year-old male, Hoehn & Yahr 3, with stage 3 brain pathology. (B) Severe lesions in the gastric cardia: 78-year-old female with disease duration of 11 years, Hoehn & Yahr 4, stage 5 brain pathology. (C) Lewy bodies in the distal esophagus (*at left*, longitudinal musculature; *at right*, circular musculature): 71-year-old female with disease duration of 10 years, Hoehn & Yahr 5, stage 5 brain pathology. Syn-1 (1:2000; Clone number 42; BD Biosciences, Eysins, Switzerland) immunoreactions in tangential (A, B) and transversal (C) cryosections of 100 μm thickness. (For the color version, please refer to the plate section.)

(Reproduced with kind permission of Dr. Kelly Del Tredici-Braak, Ulm, Germany)

lower risk of developing PD [63, 64] but these findings have been questioned [65].

Microbiome

The human body contains a multiple of its own genome in the genetic information contained in the living microorganisms residing within its own confines (the so-called microbiome). The number of genes encoded in the gut metagenome is approximately 150 times larger than that of the human genome [66]. With the concept of the brain-gut-axis, the characterization of the human intestinal microbiome gains mounting relevance for viewing the pathogenesis of neurodegenerative diseases and, in particular, the Parkinson syndrome. Although methodologies and cohort sizes differed, the currently available studies showed reproducible or consistent results in terms of PD-specific alterations to the intestinal bacteria. By applying metagenomic sequencing procedures, it is even possible to distinguish PD cases from healthy individuals at a very early disease stage by means of individually modified microbiota [67]. Among others, microbiota that are associated with an altered intestinal barrier or immune function were significantly over- or under-represented. However, the association between microbiome and neuroinflammation still remains hypothetical [68, 69, 70]. There may even be a prodromal microbiome, as a comparable microbial shift is also found in patients with REM sleep behavior disorder (RBD) [71]. This is especially interesting as RBD is both a prodromal NMS in PD [54] and idiopathic RBD converts in > 75% to a neurodegenerative synucleinopathy such as PD [72, 73, 74]. In relation to this connection, there is at present discussion as to whether or not both retrograde and anterograde sequences exist as well as PNS-first and CNS-first variants [75]. Recently, it has been tried to provide evidence for these two variants of Parkinson's disease in humans by multi-modal imaging studies.

On this topic, it is relevant that many factors influence the microbial components of the gastrointestinal tract, particularly for the Parkinson syndrome. Retrospectively, it cannot be clarified whether the altered microbiome is the cause or the result of the gastrointestinal motility disturbance when severe constipation is experienced. Gut dysbiosis and SIBO have been found in PD patients [76] and can increase intestinal permeability causing excessive stimulation of the innate immune system and systemic inflammation, a mechanism involved in the initiation of SNCA deposits [77, 78]. Hereby, SNCA expression in the GI tract would reflect an immune defense mechanism [79] which is further supported by the finding that SNCA has the capability to trigger T cell responses that may also potentiate neurodegeneration [80].

If the microbiome played a pathogenetic role, then considerable differences should be observed between the populations in different continents simply due to variations in their diets, which however have not been found. In addition, evaluating the microbiome in patients undergoing treatment is only of limited use in as much as both levodopa and the other Parkinson medications influence the intestinal flora. Nonetheless it is imperative to examine just which role the microbiome is playing and what influence a targeted diet could possibly have [67, 81].

References

1. Jost WH. Autonome Regulationsstörungen beim Parkinson Syndrom. Fortschr Neurol Psychiatrie 1995; **63**: 194–205.

2. Parkinson J. *An Essay on the Shaking Palsy.* Sherwood, Neely, and Jones; 1817.

3. Barone P, Antonini, A, Colosimo C, et al. The PRIAMO study: a multicenter assessment of nonmotor symptoms and their impact on quality of life in Parkinson's disease. Mov Disord 2009; **24**: 1641–1649.

4. Braak H, Rüb U, Gai WP, Del Tredici K. Idiopathic Parkinson's disease. Possible routes by which vulnerable neuronal types may be subject to neuroinvasion by an unknown pathogen. J Neural Transm 2003; **110**: 517–536.

5. Jost WH. Gastrointestinal motility problems in patients with Parkinson's disease: effects of antiparkinsonian treatment and guidelines for management. Drugs Aging 1997; **10**: 249–258.

6. Braak H, Del Tredici K. Potential pathways of abnormal tau and α-synuclein dissemination in sporadic Alzheimer's and Parkinson's diseases. Cold Spring Harb Perspect Biol 2016; **8**. DOI: 10.1101/cshperspect.a023630

7. Stokholm MG, Danielsen EH, Hamilton-Dutoit SJ, Borghammer P. Pathological α-synuclein in gastrointestinal tissues from prodromal Parkinson disease patients. Ann Neurol 2016; **79**: 940–949.

8. Den Hartog Jager WA, Bethlem J. The distribution of Lewy bodies in the central and autonomic nervous system in idiopathic paralysis agitans. J Neurol Neurosurg Psychiatry 1960; **23**: 283–290.

9. Fasano A, Visanji NP, Liu LW, et al. Gastrointestinal dysfunction in Parkinson's disease. Lancet Neurol 2015; **14**: 625–639.

10. Wakabayashi, K, Takahashi H, Ohama E, Takeda S, Ikuta F. Lewy bodies in the visceral autonomic nervous system in Parkinson's disease. Adv Neurol 1993; **60**: 609–612.

11. Adler CH, Beach TG. Neuropathological basis of nonmotor manifestations of Parkinson's disease. Mov Disord 2016; **31**: 1114–1119.

12. Braak H, de Vos RAI, Bohl J, Del Tredici K. Gastric a-synuclein immunoreactive inclusions in Meissner's and Auerbach's plexuses in cases staged for Parkinson's disease related brain pathology. Neurosci Lett 2006; **396**: 67–72.

13. Jost WH, Bäumer T, Laskawi R, et al. Therapy of sialorrhea with botulinum neurotoxin. Neurol Ther 2019; **8**: 554–563.

14. Arbouw ME, Movig KL, Koopmann M, et al. Glycopyrrolate for sialorrhea in Parkinson disease: a randomized, double-blind, crossover trial. Neurology 2010; **74**: 1203–1207.

15. Isaacson SH, Ondo W, Jackson CE, et al. Safety and efficacy of rimabotulinumtoxinB for treatment of sialorrhea in adults: a randomized clinical trial. JAMA Neurol 2020. DOI: 10.1001/jamaneurol.2019.4565

16. Jost WH, Friedman A, Michel O, et al. SIAXI: placebo-controlled, randomized, double-blind study of incobotulinumtoxinA for sialorrhea. Neurology 2019; **92**: e1982–e1991.

17. Jost WH, Friedman A, Michel O, et al. Long-term incobotulinumtoxinA treatment for chronic sialorrhea: efficacy and safety over 64 weeks. Parkinsonism Rel Disord 2020; **70**: 23–30.

18. Pflug C, Bihler M, Emich K, et al. Critical dysphagia is common in Parkinson disease and occurs even in early stages: a prospective cohort study. Dysphagia 2018; **33**: 41–50.

19. Suiter DM, Leder SB. Clinical utility of the 3-ounce water swallow test. Dysphagia 2008; **23**: 244–250.

20. Leder SB, Suiter DM, Green BG. Silent aspiration risk is volume-dependent. Dysphagia 2011; **26**: 304–309.

21. Hughes TA, Wiles CM. Neurogenic dysphagia: the role of the neurologist. J Neurol Neurosurg Psychiatry 1998; **64**: 569–572.

22. Langmore SE. Evaluation of oropharyngeal dysphagia: which diagnostic tool is superior? Curr Opin Otolaryngol Head Neck Surg 2003; **11**: 485–489.

23. Suttrup I, Warnecke T. Dysphagia in Parkinson's disease. Dysphagia 2016; **31**: 24–32.

24. Olanow CW, Kieburtz K, Odin P, et al. Continuous intrajejunal infusion of levodopa-carbidopa intestinal gel for patients with advanced Parkinson's disease: a randomised, controlled, double-blind double-dummy study. Lancet Neurol 2014; **13**: 141–149.

25. Storch A, Schneider CB, Wolz M, et al. Nonmotor fluctuations in Parkinson disease: severity and correlation with motor complications. Neurology 2013; **80**: 800–809.

26. Thomaides T, Karapanayiotides T, Zoukos Y, et al. Gastric emptying after semi-solid food in multiple system atrophy and Parkinson's disease. J Neurol 2005; **252**: 1055–1059.

27. Kurlan R, Rubin AJ, Miller C, et al. Continuous intraduodenal infusion of levodopa for resistant on-off fluctuations in parkinsonism. Ann Neurol 1985; **18**: 139.

28. Parkes JD. Domperidone and Parkinson's disease. Clin Neuropharmacol 1986; **9**: 517–532.

29. Pierantozzi M, Pietroiusti A, Brusa L, et al. Helicobacter pylori eradication and l-dopa absorption in patients with PD and motor fluctuations. Neurology 2006; **66**: 1824–1829.

30. Barboza JL, Okun MS, Moshiree B. The treatment of gastroparesis, constipation and small intestinal bacterial overgrowth syndrome in patients with Parkinson's disease. Expert Opin Pharmacother 2015; **16**: 2449–2464.

31. Tan AH, Mahadeva S, Thalha AM, et al. Small intestinal bacterial overgrowth in Parkinson's disease. Parkinsonism Rel Disord 2014; **20**: 535–540.

32. Scheperjans F, Aho V, Pereira PA, et al. Gut microbiota are related to Parkinson's disease and clinical phenotype. Mov Disord 2015; **30**: 350–358.

33. Knudsen K, Krogh K, Østergaard K, Borghammer P. Constipation in Parkinson's disease: subjective symptoms, objective markers, and new perspectives. Mov Disord 2017; **32**: 94–105.

34. Parkinson Study Group. A randomized trial of relamorelin for constipation in Parkinson's disease (MOVE-PD): trial results and lessons learned. Parkinsonism Relat Disord 2017; **37**: 101–105.

35. Abbott RD, Petrovitch H, White LR, et al. Frequency of bowel movements and the future risk of Parkinson's disease. Neurology 2001; **57**: 456–464.

36. Svensson E, Henderson VW, Borghammer P, et al. Constipation and risk of Parkinson's disease: a Danish population-based cohort study. Parkinsonism Relat Disord 2016; **28**: 18–22.

37. Stirpe P, Hoffman M, Badiali D, Colosimo C. Constipation: an emerging risk factor for Parkinson's disease? Eur J Neurol 2016; **23**: 1606–1613.

38. Savica R, Carlin JM, Grossardt BR, et al. Medical records documentation of constipation preceding Parkinson disease: a case-control study. Neurology 2009; **73**: 1752–1758.

39. Cersosimo MG, Raina GB, Pecci C, et al. Gastrointestinal manifestations in Parkinson's disease: prevalence and occurrence before motor symptoms. J Neurol 2013; **260**: 1332–1338.

40. Gage H, Kaye J, Kimber A, et al. Correlates of constipation in people with Parkinson's. Parkinsonism Relat Disord 2011; **17**: 106–111.

41. Lundin E, Graf W, Garske U, et al. Segmental colonic transit studies: comparison of a radiological and a scintigraphic method. Colorectal Dis 2007; **9**: 344–351.

42. Agachan F, Pfeifer J, Wexner SD. Defecography and proctography. Results of 744 patients. Dis Colon Rectum 1996; **39**: 899–905.

43. Jost WH, Schrank B, Herold A, Leiß O. Functional outlet obstruction: anismus, spastic pelvic floor syndrome, and dyscoordination of the voluntary sphincter muscles. Scand J Gastroenterol 1999; **34**: 449–453.

44. Barichella M, Pacchetti C, Bolliri C, et al. Probiotics and prebiotic fiber for constipation associated with PD. Neurology 2016; **87**: 1274–1280.

45. Zesiewicz TA, Sullivan KL, Arnulf I, et al. Practice parameter: treatment of nonmotor symptoms of Parkinson disease: report of the quality standards subcommittee of the American Academy of Neurology. Neurology 2010; **74**: 924–931.

46. Bushmann M, Dobmeyer SM, Leeker L, et al. Swallowing abnormalities and their response to treatment in Parkinson's disease. Neurology 1989; **39**: 1309–1314.

47. Zangaglia R, Martignoni E, Glorioso M, et al. Macrogol for the treatment of constipation in Parkinson's disease. A randomized placebo-controlled study. Mov Disord 2007; **22**: 1239–1244.

48. Liu Z, Sakakibara R, Odaka T, et al. Mosapride citrate, a novel 5-HT4 agonist and partial 5-HT3 antagonist, ameliorates constipation in parkinsonian patients. Mov Disord 2005; **20**: 680–686.

49. Freitas ME, Alqaraawi A, Lang AE, Liu LWC. Linaclotide and prucalopride for management of constipation in patients with parkinsonism. Mov Disord Clin Pract 2018; **5**: 218–220.

50. Bassotti G, Usai Satta P, Bellini M. Plecanatide for the treatment of chronic idiopathic constipation in adult patients. Expert Rev Clin Pharmacol 2019; **12**: 1019–1026.

51. Ondo WG1, Kenney C, Sullivan K, et al. Placebo-controlled trial of lubiprostone for constipation associated with Parkinson disease. Neurology 2012; **78**: 1650–1654.

52. Klingelhoefer L, Reichmann H. Pathogenesis of Parkinson disease – the gut-brain axis and environmental factors. Nat Rev Neurol 2015; **11**: 625–636.

53. Scheperjans F, Derkinderen P, Borghammer P. The gut and Parkinson's disease: hype or hope? J Park Dis 2018; **8**: S31–S39.

54. Berg D, Postuma RB, Adler CH, et al. MDS research criteria for prodromal Parkinson's disease. Mov Disord 2015; **30**: 1600–1611.

55. Schrag A, Horsfall L, Walters K, et al. Prediagnostic presentations of Parkinson's disease in primary care: a case-control study. Lancet Neurol 2015; **14**: 57–64.

56. Pan-Montojo F, Anichtchik O, Dening Y, et al. Progression of Parkinson's disease pathology is reproduced by intragastric administration of rotenone in mice. PLoS One 2010; **5**: e8762.

57. Inden M, Kitamura Y, Takeuchi H, et al. Neurodegeneration of mouse nigrostriatal dopaminergic system induced by repeated oral administration of rotenone is prevented by 4-phenylbutyrate, a chemical chaperone. J Neurochem 2007; **101**: 1491–1504.

58. Tasselli M, Chaumette T, Paillusson S, et al. Effects of oral administration of rotenone on gastrointestinal functions in mice. Neurogastroenterol Motil 2013; **25**: e183–e193.

59. Yuan YH, Yan WF, Sun JD, et al. The molecular mechanism of rotenone-induced α-synuclein aggregation: emphasizing the role of the calcium/GSK3β pathway. Toxicol Lett 2015; **233**: 163–171.

60. Ling EA, Shieh JY, Wen CY, et al. The dorsal motor nucleus of the vagus nerve of the hamster: ultrastructure of vagal neurons and their responses to vagotomy. J Anat 1987; **152**: 161–172.

61. Pan-Montojo F, Schwarz M, Winkler C. Environmental toxins trigger PD-like progression via increased alpha-synuclein release from enteric neurons in mice. Sci Rep 2012; **2**: 898. DOI: 10.1038/srep00898

62. Holmqvist S, Chutna O, Bousset L, et al. Direct evidence of Parkinson pathology spread from the gastrointestinal tract to the brain in rats. Acta Neuropathol 2014; **128**: 805–820.

63. Svensson E, Horváth-Puhó E, Thomsen RW, et al. Vagotomy and subsequent risk of Parkinson's disease. Ann Neurol 2015; **78**: 522–529.

64. Liu B, Fang F, Pedersen NL, et al. Vagotomy and Parkinson disease: a Swedish register-based matched-cohort study. Neurology 2017; **88**: 1996–2002.

65. Tysnes OB, Kenborg L, Herlofson K, et al. Does vagotomy reduce the risk of Parkinson's disease? Ann Neurol 2015; **78**: 1011–1012.

66. Qin J, Li R, Raes J, et al. A human gut microbial gene catalogue established by metagenomic sequencing. Nature 2010; **464**: 59–65.

67. Bedarf JR, Hildebrand F, Goeser F, et al. Das Darm-Mikrobiom bei der Parkinson-Krankheit. Nervenarzt 2019; **90**: 160–166.

68. Seguella L, Sarnelli G, Esposito G. Leaky gut, dysbiosis, and enteric glia activation: the trilogy behind the intestinal origin of Parkinson's disease. Neural Regen Res 2020; **15**: 1037–1038.

69. Borghammer P, Van den Berge N. Brain-first versus gut-first Parkinson's disease: a hypothesis. J Park Dis 2019; **9**: S281–S295.

70. Bedarf JR, Hildebrand F, Coelho LPF, et al. Functional implications of microbial and viral gut metagenome changes in early stage L-DOPA-naïve Parkinson's disease patients. Genome Med 2017; **9**: 39.

71. Heintz-Buschart A, Pandey U, Wicke T, et al. The nasal and gut microbiome in Parkinson's disease and idiopathic rapid eye movement sleep behavior disorder. Mov Disord 2018; **33**: 88–98.

72. Iranzo A, Fernández-Arcos A, Tolosa E, et al. Neurodegenerative disorder risk in idiopathic REM sleep behavior disorder: study in 174 patients. PLoS One 2014; **9**: e89741. DOI: 10.1371

73. Postuma RB, Iranzo A, Högl B, et al. Risk factors for neurodegeneration in idiopathic rapid eye movement sleep behavior disorder: a multicenter study. Ann Neurol 2015; **77**: 830–839.

74. Schenck CH, Boeve BF, Mahowald MW. Delayed emergence of a parkinsonian disorder or dementia in 81% of older males initially diagnosed with idiopathic REM sleep behavior disorder (RBD): 16 year update on a previously reported series. Sleep Med 2013; **14**: 744–748.

75. Sampson TR, Debelius JW, Thron T, et al. Gut microbiota regulate motor deficits and neuroinflammation in a model of Parkinson's disease. Cell 2016; **167**: 1469–1480.

76. Hill-Burns EM, Debelius JW, Morton JT, et al. Parkinson's disease and Parkinson's disease medications have distinct signatures of the gut microbiome. Mov Disord 2017; **32**: 739–749.

77. de Vos WM, de Vos EA. Role of the intestinal microbiome in health and disease: from correlation to causation. Nutr Rev 2012; **70**(Suppl 1): S45–S56.

78. Visanji NP, Brooks PL, Hazrati LN, Lang AE. The prion hypothesis in Parkinson's disease: Braak to the future. Acta Neuropathol Commun 2013; **1**: 2. DOI: 10.1186/2051-5960-1-2

79. Stolzenberg E, Berry D, Yang D, et al. A role for neuronal alpha-synuclein in gastrointestinal immunity. J Innate Immun 2017; **9**: 456–463.

80. Sulzer D, Alcalay RN, Garretti F, et al. T cells from patients with Parkinson's disease recognize α-synuclein peptides. Nature 2017; **546**: 656–661.

81. Jackson A, Forsyth CB, Shaikh M, et al. Diet in Parkinson's disease: critical role for the microbiome. Front Neurol 2019; **10**: 1245.

82. Horsager et al. Brain 2020 143; 3077–3088 Brain-first versus body-first PD: a multimodal imaging case-control study.

Sexual Dysfunction in Parkinson's Disease

Gila Bronner and Tanya Gurevich

Introduction

Parkinson's disease (PD) is an age-related neuro-degenerative multisystem progressive disorder belonging to the α-synucleinopathy spectrum, with well-known and widely reported motor symptoms, such as tremor, rigidity, bradykinesia, and postural instability, and with highly prevalent and previously often neglected non-motor symptoms (NMS) [1], such as pain, depression, anxiety, sleep disturbances, cognitive dysfunction, and many others, that may precede the motor symptoms [2]. Sexual dysfunction (SD) is usually included in the category of autonomic NMS in PD, even though its etiology is multifactorial and involves interaction with other motor and NMS of PD [3–5]. Patients with PD rated SD twelfth out of 24 most bothersome symptoms of their disease [6], but SD remains an underrated non-motor feature of PD despite its high frequency and severe impact on the patient's quality of life [7, 8].

Epidemiology of Sexual Dysfunction in Parkinson's Disease

Sexual dysfunction may be present in PD patients for a very long time, even appearing in the "pro-dromal" stage of the disease. A prospective cohort health study of 32,616 non-PD men found an association between erectile dysfunction (ED) and the risk of developing PD in the future [9]. The ED subsequently increases after the diagnosis and the initiation of PD treatment and worsens along the disease course [10, 11]. Up to 79% of men with PD experience ED, ejaculation problems, and difficulties achieving orgasm. Up to 75% of women with PD and multiple system atrophy report sexual problems, such as vaginal dryness, decreased libido, and difficulties reaching orgasm [8, 11, 12].

The findings of studies on the main factors contributing to SD in PD are controversial.

A recent retrospective study of 53 consecutive patients found that PD negatively influences patients' sexuality independently of the patient's age, disease duration, or disease severity [10]. However, other studies found associations between SD and PD duration, advancing Hoehn and Yahr stage [13], as well as age, female gender, lower education, higher Beck Depression Inventory scores, and depression (but not antidepressant therapy) associated with decreased sexual desire [12]. Other studies found that young PD patients were significantly more dissatisfied with their sexual life, especially male patients who were unemployed and complained of ED or premature ejaculation (PE) [14].

Sexual dysfunction in PD may be divided into three main categories: 1) decreased sexuality characterized by ED and ejaculatory problems in men, vaginal dryness and decreased libido in women, and difficulties achieving orgasm in both [4, 11, 15]; 2) sexual preoccupation behaviors (SPBs), which include increased interest in sex and compulsive hypersexual behavior [16]; 3) sexual problems as a side effect of medical treatments (e.g. antidepressants, dopamine) and other comorbidities (cardiovascular, diabetes, etc.), which can cause either hyposexuality or hypersexuality [8].

Sexual Function and Sexual Response Cycle

It is well recognized that sexual function is a multifaceted bio-psycho-social process that depends on coordinated function of the neurological, vascular, and endocrine systems. It can be altered by aging, psychosocial and physical factors. The interplay of all these factors has an important role in sexual functioning of each person and his/her partner [3]. Any alteration in this delicate structure may lead to sexual problems in both.

It is unclear whether pathological findings in the specific brain regions may directly explain sexual symptoms [17]. Hypothalamic dysfunction was considered as being responsible for decreased sexuality in PD (libido and ED) via altered dopamine-oxytocin pathways, which normally promote libido and erection, as well as by neuropathy of parasympathetic fibers due to phosphorylated α-synuclein deposits in the sacral parasympathetic nucleus, pelvic plexus, pelvic ganglia [18], and nerve fibers of gonadal tissue [19].

From the pathophysiological aspect, PD may weaken the sexual response cycle. For example, decreased dopamine activity induces dysphoria and withdrawal-like conditions [20]. Incentives and expectation of reward diminish due to inability to maintain arousal (e.g. ED) and achieve satisfying orgasm, as well as by partnership difficulties and altered intimacy [21]. Both men and women with PD report reduced intimate communication since PD diagnosis (especially caressing or showing affection) [22]. Reduced sensations due to neurological changes as well as depression and distractions (thoughts about the illness, difficulties with concentration, memories of previous sexual failures) reduce the ability to respond positively to sexual stimuli [21]. Pain can further increase sexual distraction and disturb desire, arousal, and orgasm [23]. Impaired mobility worsens the ability to caress and hug a partner, to effectively stimulate (the partner or oneself), to move into positions for intercourse, to maintain pelvically steady thrusts, or to maintain a required level of arousal and erection [21]. Hypomimia and hypophonia can disturb couple communication and convey a message of indifference and lack of affection. Depressed mood, which commonly accompanies PD, is a major determinant of SD in men and women, negatively affecting desire, arousal, and orgasm [5]. Additional NMS, such as sleep disturbances, may lead to bed separation, thus decreasing opportunities for intimate and sexual activities. A lowered self-image due to changed appearance, unpleasant body odors, excessive sweating, drooling, incontinence, and gait disturbances can make patients feel less attractive. Moreover, the side effects of medication may inhibit sexual pleasure [3–5] whereupon the brain's appraisal of sexual stimuli is negatively affected during the sexual response cycle. Disappointing outcomes for PD patients and their partners reportedly decrease future motivation for any intimate or sexual activity [21].

Gender-Specific Effects on Sexual Life among Parkinson's Disease Patients

Decreased Sexual Function in Women with Parkinson's Disease

Data on the epidemiology of SD in women in the general population as well as in women with PD are sparse. The female sexual response involves neurotransmitter-mediated vascular and nonvascular smooth muscle relaxation resulting in increased pelvic blood flow, vaginal lubrication, and clitoral and labial engorgement. Furthermore, the response is affected by psychological, social, and relationship factors [24]. Women with PD report decreased sexual activity (78%), arousal and lubrication problems (87.5%), low desire (50%), and orgasmic difficulties (75%) [8, 25]. They complain of vaginal tightness, urinary incontinence during sex, sexual dissatisfaction, and low self-image as a sexual partner. Age, depression, apathy, and anxiety were identified as positive predictors of SD severity [5, 26]. Surprisingly, disease duration, UPDRS part III score, Hoehn and Yahr stage, and antiparkinsonian medication did not show significant predictive value [10, 26]. Urinary incontinence, which is characteristic in women with PD, is associated with stigma, fear, embarrassment, and shame, and negatively impacts desire and sexual function in women with PD, but not in men [13]. In support groups, women expressed concerns over their body and sexual image, and their distress about being unattractive [27, 28].

Beyond the multiple physiological causes of SD in PD, catastrophizing (a negative coping style) accompanied by high levels of pain, anxiety, and sleep disturbances contribute significantly to the frequency of SD, especially among women [29, 30]. Only few reports have addressed issues concerning femininity and reproductive health in young female PD patients. Rubin (2007) [31] reported worsening of menstrual symptoms (increased pre-menstrual symptoms, pain, and excessive bleeding), especially in those with advanced disease.

Decreased Sexual Function in Men with Parkinson's Disease

The high estimates of ED, orgasmic, and ejaculatory disorders may explain sexual dissatisfaction among men with PD [32, 33]. ED is the most studied SD in men with PD, reported in 60–80% of male patients [8, 14, 25, 34, 35]. The frequency of ED is higher in PD patients compared with healthy age-matched controls (60.4% and 37.5%, respectively) [36]. The risk of ED reportedly increased with age and advancing Hoehn-Yahr stage [8, 14, 25, 34, 35]. Men with PD use multiple medications which may contribute to ED.

Men with PD also considered motor symptoms as comprising a more substantial reason for their sexual dissatisfaction [5]. Such an association is entirely reasonable, since motor function is essential for touching, stimulating, moving into sexual positions, and maintaining pelvically steady thrusts during intercourse [21].

Difficulties reaching orgasm may represent a secondary dysfunction and be the result of an inability to achieve or maintain an erection [10]. Orgasmic dysfunction in men with PD was accompanied with fear of disappointing their partner, avoidance of sexual activities, withdrawal from a relationship, and even thoughts of separation from their partner [10]. This is an additional burden imposed on male PD patients who cope with both motor and non-motor challenges.

Psychogenic causes (anxiety, depression, and stress) can also contribute to ED and require appropriate treatment [37]. Apathy and decreased desire, which are reported by 59% of men with PD, can be explained by depressed mood and anxiety [3].

Testosterone deficiency may play an important role in decreased desire. Androgen deficiency is thought to be responsible for various age-associated conditions, such as the lack of energy, physical weakness, cognitive impairment, depression, and decreased vitality and libido [38]. Testosterone deficiency was found in 47% of male PD patients, and it was significantly correlated with their reported apathy, independently from PD stage and severity [39]. Treatment with testosterone may lead to the relief of some symptoms [38], however, no improvement in motor manifestations and NMS was found in a double-blind placebo-controlled study of 30 PD patients treated with testosterone [40].

Premature ejaculation (PE) was reported in a range of 40.6% to 51.4% of men with PD [8] compared to a prevalence of 23% among men without PD [41]. A recent study described eight cases of PD patients with new-onset PE that was characterized in all of them by a dramatically shortened intravaginal ejaculation latency (ejaculating before vaginal penetration or immediately after), hampering sexual intercourse [15]. PE appeared in these eight men after the initiation of anti-parkinsonian treatment consisting of levodopa and dopamine as well as non-dopaminergic drugs (rasagiline and amantadine). This suggests that PE may not necessarily be related to the disease itself but to the pharmacologic interventions [15]. Frequent spontaneous ejaculations secondary to rasagiline taken in combination with levodopa therapy were described in a 65-year-old man [42]. These ejaculations occurred without an erection and without being engaged in any sexually stimulating activity, and they disappeared when rasagiline was discontinued. It should be noted that there are no publications on sexual problems of lesbian, gay, bi-sexual, and transgender patients with PD, and the authors have no experience with this group of patients.

Sexual Preoccupation Behaviors and Increased Sexuality in Parkinson's Disease

Increased sexuality involves various types of behaviors in which patients seem to be overly interested in and preoccupied by sex. Little is known about the neurological control of human sexual behavior, and these behaviors generally cause embarrassment and anger of partners, caregivers, and healthcare providers (HCPs). SPBs have different etiologies, and the precise type of SPB needs to be identified in order to provide an appropriate intervention [16]. SPBs are not defined as a disease symptom but rather as a "bad and unacceptable behavior," creating negative reactions (even punishment) by caregivers and HCPs [4]. Therefore, it is essential to educate all of the relevant individuals involved in the PD patient's care about the various SPBs and their interventions.

Four types of SPBs have been described in PD [16]. The first and most prevalent is sexual desire discrepancy, seen mainly in men, which has a negative impact on partners. The gap in sexual desire between the couple can be created due to two conflicting situations: one is a restored sexual desire after the initiation of antiparkinsonian therapy with dopaminergic agents in patients [43], and the other is a concomitant decrease of sexual desire in the partners associated with burden and depression [44]. The second SPB refers to the presence of SD (mainly problems with erection and orgasm). Fears of not being able to fulfil sexual expectations of their partners [10] may drive male PD patients to repeatedly try to have sexual intercourse and achieve a satisfactory experience. In addition, they often discuss sex with their HCPs in search of professional advice. This intensive pursuit is misperceived as a compulsive sexual desire when, in fact, they want professional treatment for ED and/or orgasmic problems, or a referral to specialists in sexual medicine and sex therapy. A short explanation of the nature of this behavior may reduce the level of stress of both the patient and the partner and contribute to better quality of the couple's relationship [45].

The most devastating SPB is hypersexuality (HS) or compulsive sexual behavior (CSB), which is a part of impulse control disorders (ICDs) in PD. ICDs comprise a class of psycho-behavioral disorders (e.g. pathological gambling, CSB, pathological buying, eating disorder, punding, or lobbyism), often associated with dopamine agonist treatment [46]. ICDs were identified in 13.7–28% and CSB was reported by 3.5–7.2% of them [47]. Young age, male gender, and dopamine agonist treatment were reported as being risk factors for the occurrence of CSB in PD patients [46]. HS creates distress and evokes anger in partners, family, and HCPs. It should be distinguished from the other SPBs and promptly treated [45]. When assessing HS, one should bear in mind the following associated features: a recent augmentation of antiparkinsonian medications (particularly dopamine agonists), dopamine dysregulation syndrome, history of drug and alcohol abuse, concomitant psychiatric problems (depression, psychosis), and concurrent ICDs (gambling, shopping, eating) [48]. Male gender, novelty seeking, risk-taking behavior, and low levels of agreeableness are also associated with HS in PD [49].

The fourth SPB is restless genital syndrome (ReGS, previously named persistent genital arousal disorder), which is quite rare [50]. This uncommon sexual complaint was reported mainly by women, and it is characterized by a severe and disabling discomfort in the genital area, accompanied by burning sensations and pain and occurring without sexual desire. It is associated with spontaneous orgasms, feelings that orgasm is about to happen, and feelings that orgasmic release is needed to reduce the pain, but the discomfort is not relieved by achieving orgasm [50]. Two underlying micro-pathological mechanisms may explain the etiology of ReGS: genital small fiber sensory neuropathy and dysfunctional arteriovenous shunting and erythromelalgia. In PD, the genital discomfort has been attributed to the wearing-off of non-motor fluctuations and dopaminergic denervation [51]. Three cases of ReGS in women with PD have been published. The patients complained of typical ReGS symptoms that were exacerbated during rest at night and improved by walking [52–54]. One woman experienced successive orgasms occurring every few minutes in the preceding four months [54]. The uncomfortable genital sensations improved after treatments with a low dose of a dopamine agonist in one case, clonazepam and pramipexole in another case, and haloperidol later switched to paliperidone in the third case. When women with ReGS try to alleviate their pain by rubbing their genitals, they are mistakenly considered as hypersexual. Assessment and management of ReGS demands a multidisciplinary approach, including pelvic floor physiotherapy and stress reduction interventions.

Effects of Medical Treatments and Other Comorbidities on Sexual Function in Parkinson's Disease

Sexual problems in PD can be associated with a coexisting illness, various medical treatments, as well as PD medications and therapies [55]. ED shares common risk factors with cardiovascular disease, obesity, smoking, hypercholesterolemia, metabolic syndrome, diabetes, and radical prostatectomy [56]. Furthermore, medications used to treat the comorbidities, such as hydrochlorothiazide, beta-blockers, 5α-reductase inhibitors and many others, may contribute to SD in PD patients [11]. Medications used to treat NMS (depression, anxiety, agitation, insomnia, and psychosis) are commonly associated with decreased sexual desire, ED, delayed ejaculation, female anorgasmia, and rarely associated with retrograde ejaculation, painful ejaculation, and priapism [57]. Kummer et al. (2009) [12] observed that decreased interest in sex was not, however, associated with antidepressant therapy. As such, the loss of libido resulting from depression may be effectively treated, and HCPs should be encouraged to assess these symptoms in their patients. Finally, patients with PD who develop psychotic or nighttime behaviors may be treated with atypical antipsychotics [58], which are frequently associated with male SD (delayed ejaculation).

It is important to bear in mind that the negative effects of medications on sexual function often create clinical dilemmas: should we treat the NMS in PD patients or rather prevent the occurrence of SD as a result of treatment? Such decisions are challenging and require a personalized approach that includes consulting the patients and their partners. Our clinical experience is that some patients report a positive increase in sexual desire and sexual well-being associated with dopaminergic therapy, but this subject has not been adequately studied. Studies on the role of the dopaminergic system recognize dopamine as a pro-sexual neurotransmitter that is important for motor function and general arousal [59]. The resumption of sexual activity in 8% of PD patients following treatment with levodopa was reported by Yahr and Duvoisin back in 1972, and those authors suggested that it was the beneficial effect of the drug on motor function. Other studies have suggested that dopaminergic therapy may increase sexual behavior by inhibiting prolactin secretion (eradicating the antilibidinal effect) or by increasing the plasma level of oxytocin (producing erectogenic effects) [59, 60]. Some studies describe spontaneous erections among patients on dopamine agonist treatment (including ropinirole and apomorphine) [43], spontaneous ejaculations secondary to rasagiline [42], and undesired spontaneous female orgasm following the initiation of pramipexole as well as ropinirole therapy, all of which disappeared when they were discontinued [61].

Hypersexuality and delusional jealousy may be considered non-motor side effects of dopamine agonist therapy in PD [62]. Delusional jealousy, characterized by the false absolute certainty of the infidelity of a partner, either disappeared or was reduced in severity after decrease of PD medications. We know from our clinical experience that it is not always possible to stop medication, even though its negative effect on sexual function is obvious. The strong interplay between SD, PD, and other medical conditions suggests that the evaluation of sexual complaints of patients can have considerable diagnostic significance and sometimes provide clues to other serious physical or emotional issues.

Sexuality and Advanced Therapies in Parkinson's Disease

Subthalamic deep brain stimulation (STN-DBS) is an established surgical treatment with motor symptom benefits and improved quality of life for a well-defined group of PD patients [63]. There is inconsistent evidence on the impact DBS has on sexual function in PD. In a recent study by Dulski et al. [63], improvement of sexual symptoms, quality of life, and other NMS were most prominent in the first 6 months after STN-DBS, after which it diminished slightly (but still better than before surgery) after 12 months. In another study, female patients experienced no change in sexual functioning, while male patients younger than 60 years reported slight but significant increase in sexual satisfaction [64]. This gender difference can be explained by the fact that men's satisfaction is more dependent on their motor abilities than women's [5, 21, 33].

Some reports demonstrated an association between HS and DBS [65, 66]. A prospective study of Merola et al. [65] compared the presurgical and postsurgical prevalence of ICDs and dopamine dysregulation syndrome in 150 consecutive PD STN-DBS-treated patients. There was an overall trend for reduction in ICBs with significant improvement in HS over an average follow-up of 4.3 ± 2.1 years. Another study followed 30 PD patients post-successful bilateral STN-DBS and found significant hypersexual behavior in five younger-onset PD patients (age < 60 years) [66]. HS appeared a few days after the implant and lasted a few months, after which it gradually disappeared spontaneously. HS following STN-DBS for PD was described in two cases. One involved a 70-year-old man whose wife complained of his hypersexual behavior, which continued for almost four years and abruptly stopped without any intervention, and the other involved a 58-year-old woman who often forced herself into her husband's room to demand sex and also exposed herself to other males in the family and demanded sex. Her behavior continued for five years and was finally controlled by Clozapine [67].

The effect of continuous infusion of levodopa-carbidopa intestinal gel (LCIG) treatment on sexuality has not been investigated in depth, but one study found persistent improvement over 60 weeks in various NMS domains, including sleep/fatigue, attention/memory, gastrointestinal tract, and sexual function [68].

Apomorphine, a dopamine agonist, is widely used in PD as a rescue treatment for OFF periods and as a continuous dopaminergic stimulation treatment [69, 70]. Due to its ability to cause penile erections, apomorphine was used for improving erectile function in PD as well as non-PD men [71–73]. The combination of improved motor symptoms, restored desire, and positive effect on erectile function makes apomorphine an optional therapeutic approach for both PD and ED. Open discussion with both the PD patient and the partner is recommended before the initiation of apomorphine therapy in order to enable them to understand the potential sexual changes [74]. A retrospective analysis of 28 advanced PD patients found that continuous apomorphine pump therapy had a lower proclivity to trigger or exacerbate ICDs than oral dopamine agonists [75]. Those authors suggest that it is likely to be attributed to a more tonic stimulation of striatal dopamine receptors leading to desensitization, but it could also be attributed to a different pharmacological profile of apomorphine compared with orally active dopamine agonists. Therefore, they proposed that apomorphine can be considered as a treatment option in patients who have developed disabling ICDs while on oral agonist therapy and whose motor handicap cannot be controlled adequately on L-dopa alone.

The Effect of Parkinson's Disease on the Partner's Sexuality

Several studies found that SD in one partner affects the SD of the other, and that it should therefore be considered a couple issue [76, 77], since sexual problems and dissatisfaction in PD patients are paralleled in their partners [14, 44, 78]. The most affected couples were those in which the PD patient was the man. While 65% of male patients and 52% of their female partners reported moderate to severe sexual problems, only 34% of the female PD patients and none of their partners reported comparable difficulties

[14]. In another study, sexual function of 17 female partners of male PD patients was severely compromised in arousal, orgasm, and desire [79]. The increased burden with disease progression and the increased depression in the caregiver partners can explain this sexual deterioration among spouses and partners of PD patients [44, 78].

There are other changes that negatively affect sexual life, such as reduced opportunities for intimacy due to separate beds related to sleep disturbances, and reduced attractiveness of the patients (abnormal movements, sloppy dressing, masked faces, excessive sweating, and drooling) [4]. Since caregiver-partners take a major role in the management and support of PD patients, it is essential to evaluate their needs and difficulties in matters of relationship intimacy and sexuality. We encourage HCPs to actively promote discussions with both partners and plan specific interventions that may improve intimate and sexual relationships, leading to better quality of life [32].

Discussing Sexual Issues in Parkinson's Disease

The first challenge is a proactive initiation of "sex talk" designed to evaluate patients' as well as partners' sexual needs and concerns [80]. HCPs can contribute by providing information about the effects of the disease and the treatments on sexual functioning, for example, "patients may experience reduced genital sensations, problems in concentration, and reduced motivation to have sex." HCPs can add that these changes can disrupt arousal, orgasmic, erectile, and lubrication function. While such explanations do not offer any practical solution, they provide a logical link between the neurophysiological changes to sexual results, thus reducing stress in couples coping with PD [81, 82]. HCPs may use the "Open Sexual Communication" module to initiate a conversation during routine follow-up and to evaluate sexual issues raised by patients and partners [83]. A simple way to open "sex talk" is by commenting: "You may be unaware, but PD affects the sexual life of many patients. When you wish, we can talk about your sexual concerns. I can also refer you to a specialist." Specialists dealing with sexual problems include urologists, gynecologists, psychiatrists, endocrinologists, sex therapists, and marriage counsellors [83]. Practical solutions, such as a phosphodiesterase type 5 inhibitor (PDE5-I) for ED, making changes in the patient's medication regimen, or suggesting lubricants for vaginal dryness may be most helpful.

Healthcare professionals quite often feel that they are not sufficiently well trained and refrain from talking about sex [84]. However, there is no need to be an expert in sexual medicine or sex therapy to provide meaningful information and care. Just inquiring about sexual problems, enabling patients (or partners) to share their sexual concerns, providing some explanations to reduce anxiety, adjusting PD medications, giving practical tips, or referring to experts, is exactly what most patients need [81]. In addition, patients are grateful when they receive acknowledgment of their basic right to have sexual feelings and enjoy intimate closeness, despite their progressive disease. Handling sexual problems by means of an interdisciplinary approach and raising sexual issues in staff meetings will encourage HCPs to handle these problems more frequently, effectively, and professionally.

Treatment Modalities for Sexual Dysfunction

A personalized approach should be employed when dealing with sexual problems. Specific individual and couple needs should be considered since there is no "one size fits all."

Various modalities for the treatment of SD in neurological diseases are available [11, 82, 85]. Oral medications for SD treatment are preferred for PD patients, since injections and other devices require manual abilities and fine motor skills.

Erectile dysfunction is one of the most common conditions affecting middle-aged and older men, including male PD patients [37]. Sildenafil citrate, a PDE5-I, reportedly improved ED in men with PD, enabling them to achieve and maintain erection [86]. Sildenafil citrate was also efficacious in the treatment of ED in depressed elderly men with PD [34]. Importantly, PDE5-I is contraindicated in nitrate users and may be used with caution in patients with orthostatic hypotension due to severe risk of hypotension [55]. Another important aspect must be emphasized: effective male sexual outcomes of PDE5-I-use require subjective sexual excitement and arousal. Since reduced desire is common among PD patients [8], the efficacy of PDE5-I may be decreased as well [82]. A possible slow gastric function (one of the NMS) may delay the absorption of the medication, and patients who use PDE5-I should be instructed to wait longer (approximately 2–3 hours) than the usual recommended time (1 hour) before attempting intercourse [87].

In cases of failure to treat ED with PDE5-I, direct injections into the penile cavernosal tissue of prostaglandin E1 alone or a mixture of prostaglandin E1 with papaverine, phentolamine, and/or vasoactive intestinal polypeptide, can be effective [88]. Patients must be assessed by urologists and be instructed not to increase dosage without supervision. Spouses/partners should be involved in the process since motor restrictions may impede the ability of the patient to inject directly into his penis. One viable alternative could be the use of apomorphine due to its pro-erectile effect. Sublingual apomorphine tablets were approved by the European Medicine Agency in 2001 and marketed under the name Uprima, although nausea, dizziness, and hypotension were relatively common adverse events [71, 72]. Vacuum pump devices for ED treatment are safe and well-tolerated, and patients with autonomic dysfunction can easily get used to them [89]. A final option for ED treatment, when other interventions fail, are the implantable inflatable prostheses [37], and men are quite often satisfied with the results of penile protheses surgeries.

Premature ejaculation can be treated with selective serotonin reuptake inhibitors (such as dapoxetine), or with topical anesthetics used to extend intravaginal ejaculation latency time [56]. However, our clinical experience is that these medications are not effective in PD patients with newly occurring sudden early ejaculation associated with PD medications [15].

As mentioned earlier, testosterone insufficiency may accompany PD and contribute to low desire, absent sleep-associated erections, and delayed ejaculation [40]. Testosterone insufficiency may be easily treated in PD by a daily dose of transdermal testosterone gel, with subsequent improvement of apathy, energy level, enjoyment in life, decreased libido, and ED [40].

Therapeutic options for the treatment of female sexual dysfunction are limited, not only in PD patients, but in the general population as well [90]. In cases of dyspareunia, it is recommended to temporarily avoid penile-vaginal penetration and treat the pain. The only approved and available medication for female sexual pain is local or systemic estrogen. It may be prescribed to treat cases of dyspareunia from vulvovaginal atrophy due to estrogen deficiency. Alternatively, vaginal lubricants and moisturizers can be used during intercourse. Referring women for further pelvic floor physiotherapy may also contribute to sexual pain reduction [82]. Women can gain additional therapeutic value from individual or couple sexual psychotherapy.

Treatment of Sexual Preoccupation Behaviors

We recommend that HCPs discuss SPBs with patients and their partners both together and separately. Effective assessment must include features associated with HS, among them an increase/change of antiparkinsonian medications, dopamine dysregulation syndrome, drug or alcohol abuse history, concomitant psychiatric problems or impulse control disorders, novelty seeking, and risky behavior [48, 49]. Medication adjustments such as reduction or discontinuation of dopamine agonists, and/or the use of advanced treatments such as DBS or LCIG are essential considerations in the management of HS [45]. DBS and LCIG indirectly improve ICDs in PD, including HS [91]. Effective treatment of HS requires an interdisciplinary approach. Education of patients, partners, and caregivers is crucial [45], and it should include discussions on issues of sexual health risks due to hypersexual behaviors (e.g. sexually transmitted diseases, AIDS), as well as legal consequences due to sexual harassment [92].

There is no evidence-based treatment for ReGS [50], although there is a description of one woman with PD who was successfully treated with dopamine agonists [53]. Effective treatment requires an interdisciplinary approach, including psychotherapy, pharmacologic intervention, pelvic floor physiotherapy, stress reduction, as well as couple and sex therapy.

Integration of Novel Technologies in Sex Therapy for Parkinson's Disease

Rapidly growing new technologies are revolutionizing the field of mental health [93], including virtual reality (VR) and video games, which are powerful tools for providing clients with new learning experiences for benefiting their psychological well-being. Virtual reality has emerged as a viable helpful tool in a variety of disorders, with the most robust evidence when used as exposure therapy for patients with anxiety disorders, substance use disorders, and a distraction technique for patients with acute pain requiring an uncomfortable therapeutic procedure [94]. Meta-analyses have indicated that VR is an efficacious tool that compares favorably to comparison conditions, and that it has lasting effects that generalize to the real world. VR can help learners with disabilities expand their knowledge, skills, and attitudes in ways that would not have been possible otherwise. It enables them to engage in learning activities relatively free from the limitations imposed by their disability, and to do so in complete safety. VR also helps create empathy and expand knowledge about people with disabilities in others by helping them experience disabilities through simulated environments. VR interventions in stroke patients become a popular alternative to rehabilitation and led to significant improvements compared to conventional rehabilitation [95]. VR significantly reduced pain compared to other therapeutic interventions in hospitalized patients [96]. VR also offers promising interventions in sex therapy, particularly for the treatment of SD in which pain or anxiety play a significant etiological role. Future research is needed to determine the effectiveness of these technologies in PD patients [93].

The use of Serious Games in the health domain is expanding. Research confirms that they can be adapted to elderly people with mild cognitive impairment and dementia, and can be employed for several purposes, including treatment, stimulation, rehabilitation, and improving well-being [97]. Little evidence is available to date on the efficacy of these new and sophisticated video games specifically designed for supporting people with neurodegenerative disorders, such as PD. Future research should focus on technologies that can reduce motor and NMS that affect sexual function (e.g. anxiety, pain, concentration difficulties, and motor limitations).

Conclusion

The increased awareness of well-being and quality of life issues has led to the recognition of the contribution of sexual function and satisfaction among PD patients. A growing body of knowledge based on recent publications on SD provides an opportunity for HCPs to offer proper treatment and advice to PD patients and their partners. However, beyond this accumulation of knowledge, it is important to overcome the understandable and natural discomfort in discussing SD among the other NMS with PD patients and their caregiver partners. We call upon HCPs to take a courageous step forward by implementing specialized "neurosexological" services into clinical practice by initiating educational activities and developing new therapeutic opportunities to promote their sexual well-being.

References

1. Shulman LM, Taback RL, Rabinstein AA, et al. Non-recognition of depression and other non-motor symptoms in Parkinson's disease. Park Relat Disord 2002; **8**: 193–197.

2. Seppi K, Weintraub D, Coelho M, et al. The Movement Disorder Society evidence-based medicine review update: treatments for the non-motor symptoms of Parkinson's disease. Mov Disord 2011; **26**: S42–80.

3. Basson R, Rees P, Wang R, et al. Sexual function in chronic illness. J Sex Med 2010; **7**: 374–388.

4. Bronner G, Aharon-Peretz J, Hassin-Baer S. Sexuality in patients with Parkinson's disease, Alzheimer's disease, and other dementias. Handb Clin Neurol 2015; **130**: 297–323.

5. Kotková P, Weiss P. Psychiatric factors related to sexual functioning in patients with Parkinson's disease. Clin Neurol Neurosurg 2013; **115**: 419–424.

6. Politis M, Wu K, Molloy S, et al. Parkinson's disease symptoms: the patient's perspective. Mov Disord 2010; **25**: 1646–1651.

7. Bhattacharyya KB, Rosa-Grilo M. Sexual dysfunctions in Parkinson's disease: an underrated problem in a much-discussed disorder. Int Rev Neurobiol 2017; **134**: 859–876.

8. Bronner G, Royter V, Korczyn AD, et al. Sexual dysfunction in Parkinson's disease. J Sex Marital Ther 2004; **30**: 95–105.

9. Gao X, Chen H, Schwarzschild MA, et al. Erectile function and risk of Parkinson's disease. Am J Epidemiol 2007; **166**: 1446–1450.

10. Buhmann C, Dogac S, Vettorazzi E, et al. The impact of Parkinson's disease on patients' sexuality and relationship. J Neural Transm 2017; **128**: 983–996.

11. Palma JA, Kaufmann H. Treatment of autonomic dysfunction in Parkinson disease and other synucleinopathies. Mov Disord 2018; **33**: 372–390.

12. Kummer A, Cardoso F, Teixeira AL. Loss of libido in Parkinson's disease. J Sex Med 2009; **6**: 1024–1031.

13. Wermuth L, Stenager E. Sexual aspects of Parkinson's disease. Semin Neurol 1992; **12**: 125–127.

14. Brown RG, Jahanshahi M, Quinn N, et al. Sexual function in patients with Parkinson's disease and their partners. J Neurol Neurosurg Psychiatry 1990; **53**: 480–486.

15. Bronner G, Israeli-Korn S, Hassin-Baer S, et al. Acquired premature ejaculation in Parkinson's disease and possible mechanisms. Int J Impot Res 2018; **30**: 153–157.

16. Bronner G, Hassin-Baer S, Gurevich T. Sexual preoccupation behavior in Parkinson's disease. J Parkinsons Dis 2017; **7**: 175–182.

17. Coon EA, Cutsforth-Gregory JK, Benarroch EE. Neuropathology of autonomic dysfunction in synucleinopathies. Mov Disord 2018; **33**: 349–358.

18. Wakabayashi K, Takahashi H. Neuropathology of autonomic nervous system in Parkinson's disease. Eur Neurol 1997; **38**(Suppl 2): 2–7.

19. Garrido A, Aldecoa I, Gelpi E, et al. Aggregation of alpha synuclein in the gonadal tissue of two patients with Parkinson disease. JAMA Neurol 2017; **74**: 606–607.

20. Ikemoto S, Yang C, Tan A. Basal ganglia circuit loops, dopamine and motivation: a review and enquiry. Behav Brain Res 2015; **290**: 17–31.

21. Basson R. Human sexual response. Handb Clin Neurol 2015; **130**: 11–18.

22. Beier KM, Luders M, Boxdorfer SA. Sexuality and partnership aspects of Parkinson's disease: results of an empirical study of patients and their partners. Fortschr Neurol Psychiatr 2000; **68**: 564–575.

23. Ambler N, Williams AC, Hill P, et al. Sexual difficulties of chronic pain patients. Clin J Pain 2001; **17**:138–145.

24. Berman JR, Adhikari SP, Goldstein I. Anatomy and physiology of female sexual function and dysfunction: classification, evaluation, and treatment options. Eur Urol 2000; **38**: 20–29.

25. Koller WC, Vetere-Overfield B, Williamson A, et al. Sexual dysfunction in Parkinson's disease. Clin Neuropharmacol 1990; **13**: 461–463.

26. Varanda S, Ribeiro da Silva J, Costa AS, et al. Sexual dysfunction in women with Parkinson's disease. Mov Disord 2016; **31**: 1685–1693.

27. Posen J, Moore O, Tassa DS, et al. Young women with PD: a group work experience. Soc Work Health Care 2000; **32**: 77–91.

28. Schartau E, Tolson D, Fleming V. Parkinson's disease: the effects on womanhood. Nurs Stand 2003; **17**: 33–39.

29. Thomtén J, Lundahl R, Stigenberg K, et al. Fear avoidance and pain catastrophizing among women with sexual pain. Womens Health 2014; **10**: 571–581.

30. Lerman SF, Bronner G, Cohen OS, et al. Catastrophizing mediates the relationship between non-motor symptoms and quality of life in Parkinson's disease. Disabil Health J 2019; **12**: 673–678.

31. Rubin SM. Parkinson's disease in women. Dis Mon 2007; **53**: 206–213.

32. Hand A, Gray WK, Chandler BJ, et al. Sexual and relationship dysfunction in people with Parkinson's disease. Parkinsonism Relat Disord 2010; **16**: 172–176.

33. Bronner G, Cohen OS, Yahalom G, et al. Correlates of quality of sexual life in male and female patients with Parkinson disease and their partners. Parkinsonism Relat Disord 2014; **20**(10): 1085–1088.

34. Raffaele R, Vecchio I, Giammusso B, et al. Efficacy and safety of fixed-dose oral sildenafil in the treatment of sexual dysfunction in depressed patients with idiopathic Parkinson's disease. Eur Urol 2002; **41**: 382–386.

35. Safarinejad MR, Taghva A, Shekarchi B, et al. Safety and efficacy of sildenafil citrate in the treatment of Parkinson-emergent erectile dysfunction: a double-blind, placebo-controlled, randomized study. Int J Impot Res 2010; **22**: 325–335.

36. Singer C, Weiner WJ, Sanchez-Ramos J. Autonomic dysfunction in men with Parkinson's disease. Eur Neurol 1992; **32**: 134–140.

37. Mobley DF, Khera M, Baum N. Recent advances in the treatment of erectile dysfunction. Postgrad Med J 2017; **93**: 679–685.

38. Seidman SN, Weiser M. Testosterone and mood in aging men. Psychiatr Clin North Am 2013; **36**: 177–182.

39. Ready RE, Friedman J, Grace J, et al. Testosterone deficiency and apathy in Parkinson's disease: a pilot study. J Neurol Neurosurg Psychiatry 2004; **75**: 1323–1326.

40. Okun MS, Fernandez HH, Rodriguez RL, et al. Testosterone therapy in men with Parkinson disease: results of the TEST-PD study. Arch Neurol 2006; **63**: 729–735.

41. Porst H, Montorsi F, Rosen RC, et al. The Premature Ejaculation Prevalence and Attitudes (PEPA) survey: prevalence, comorbidities, and professional help-seeking. Eur Urol 2007; **51**: 816–823.

42. Chuang RS, Lang AE. Rasagiline-induced spontaneous ejaculation. Mov Disord 2009; **24**: 2160–2161.

43. Pohanka M, Kanovsky P, Bares M, et al. Pergolide mesylate can improve sexual dysfunction in patients with Parkinson's disease: the results of an open, prospective, 6-month follow-up. Eur J Neurol 2004; **11**: 483–488.

44. Grün D, Pieri V, Vaillant M, et al. Contributory factors to caregiver burden in Parkinson disease. Am Med Dir Assoc 2016; **17**: 626–632.

45. Bronner G, Hassin-Baer S. Exploring hypersexual behavior in men with Parkinson's disease: is it compulsive sexual behavior? J Parkinsons Dis 2012; **2**: 225–234.

46. Weintraub D, Koester J, Potenza MN, et al. Impulse control disorders in Parkinson disease: a cross-sectional study of 3090 patients. Arch Neurol 2010; **67**: 589–595.

47. El Otmani H, Mouni FZ, Abdulhakeem Z, et al. Impulse control disorders in Parkinson disease: a cross-sectional study in Morocco. Rev Neurol 2019; **175**: 233–237.

48. Moore TJ, Glenmullen J, Mattison DR. Reports of pathological gambling, hypersexuality, and compulsive shopping associated with dopamine receptor agonist drugs. JAMA Intern Med 2014; **174**: 1930–1933.

49. Sachdeva J, Harbishettar V, Barraclough M, et al. Clinical profile of compulsive sexual behaviors and paraphilia in Parkinson's disease. J Parkinsons Dis 2014; **4**: 665–670.

50. Facelle TM, Sadeghi-Nejad H, Goldmeier D. Persistent genital arousal disorder: characterization, etiology, and management. J Sex Med 2013; **10**: 439–450.

51. Lefaucheur R, Berthelot L, Sénant J, et al. Acute genital pain during non-motor fluctuations improved by apomorphine. Mov Disord 2013; **28**: 687–688.

52. Sawamura M, Toma K, Unai Y, et al. A case of Parkinson's disease following restless genital sensation. Rinsho Shinkeigaku 2015; **55**: 266–268 [in Japanese].

53. Aquino CC, Mestre T, Lang AE. Restless genital syndrome in Parkinson disease. JAMA Neurol 2014; **71**: 1559–1561.

54. Fountoulakis KN, Tegos T, Goulis DG, et al. Treatment of a female patient with persistent

genital arousal and Parkinson's disease with paliperidone. Aust N Z J Psychiatry 2017; **51**: 98–99.

55. Meco G, Rubino A, Caravona N, et al. Sexual dysfunction in Parkinson's Disease. Parkinsonism Relat Disord 2008; **14**: 451–456.

56. Hatzimouratidis K, Amar E, Eardley I, et al. Guidelines on male sexual dysfunction: erectile dysfunction and premature ejaculation. Eur Urol 2010; **57**: 804–814.

57. Serretti A, Chiesa A. Sexual side effects of pharmacological treatment of psychiatric diseases. Clin Pharmacol Ther 2011; **89**: 142–147.

58. Connolly BS, Lang AE. Pharmacological treatment of Parkinson disease: a review. JAMA 2014; **311**: 1670–1683.

59. Paredes RG, Agmo A. Has dopamine a physiological role in the control of sexual behavior? A critical review of the evidence. Prog Neurobiol 2004; **73**: 179–226.

60. Kruger TH, Hartmann U, Schedlowski M. Prolactinergic and dopaminergic mechanisms underlying sexual arousal and orgasm in humans. World J Urol 2005; **23**: 130–138.

61. Kaut O, Asmus F, Paus S. Spontaneous unwelcome orgasms due to pramipexole and ropinirole. Mov Disord 2012; **27**: 1327–1328.

62. Kataoka H, Sugie K. Delusional jealousy (Othello Syndrome) in 67 patients with Parkinson's disease. Front Neurol 2018; **9**: 129.

63. Dulski J, Schinwelski M, Konkel A, et al. The impact of subthalamic deep brain stimulation on sleep and other non-motor symptoms in Parkinson's disease. Parkinsonism Relat Disord 2019; **64**: 138–144.

64. Castelli L, Perozzo P, Genesia ML, et al. Sexual well-being in parkinsonian patients after deep brain stimulation of the subthalamic nucleus. J Neurol Neurosurg Psychiatry 2004; **75**: 1260–1264.

65. Merola A, Romagnolo A, Rizzi L, et al. Impulse control behaviors and subthalamic deep brain stimulation in Parkinson disease. J Neurol 2017; **264**: 40–48.

66. Romito LM, Raja M, Daniele A, et al. Transient mania with hypersexuality after surgery for high frequency stimulation of the subthalamic nucleus in Parkinson's disease. Mov Disord 2002; **17**: 1371–1374.

67. Doshi P, Bhargava P. Hypersexuality following subthalamic nucleus stimulation for Parkinson's disease. Neurol India 2008; **56**: 474–476.

68. Standaert DG, Rodriguez RL, Slevin JT, et al. Effect of levodopa-carbidopa intestinal gel on non-motor symptoms in patients with advanced Parkinson's disease. Mov Disord Clin Pract 2017; **4**: 829–837.

69. Drapier S, Eusebio A, Degos B, et al. Quality of life in Parkinson's disease improved by apomorphine pump: the OPTIPUMP cohort study. J Neurol 2016; **263**: 1111–1119.

70. Jenner P, Katzenschlager R. Apomorphine – pharmacological properties and clinical trials in Parkinson's disease. Parkinsonism Relat Disord 2016; **33**(Suppl 1): S13–S21.

71. Dula E, Keating W, Siami PF, et al. Efficacy and safety of fixed-dose and dose-optimization regimens of sublingual apomorphine versus placebo in men with erectile dysfunction. The Apomorphine Study Group. Urol 2000; **56**: 130–135.

72. Perimenis P, Markou S, Gyftopoulos K, et al. Efficacy of apomorphine and sildenafil in men with nonarteriogenic erectile dysfunction. A comparative crossover study. Andrologia 2004; **36**: 106–110.

73. Colzi A, Turner K, Lees A. Continuous subcutaneous waking day apomorphine in the long-term treatment of levodopa induced interdose dyskinesias in Parkinson's disease. J Neurol Neurosurg Psychiatry 1998; **64**: 573–576.

74. Bowron A. Practical considerations in the use of apomorphine injectable. Neurology 2004; **62**(6 Suppl 4): S32–S36.

75. Barbosa P, Lees AJ, Magee C, et al. A retrospective evaluation of the frequency of impulsive compulsive behaviors in Parkinson's disease patients treated with continuous waking day apomorphine pumps. Mov Disord Clin Pract 2016; **4**: 323–328.

76. Jiann BP, Su CC, Tsai JY. Is female sexual function related to the male partners' erectile function? J Sex Med 2013; **10**: 420–429.

77. Elran E, Bronner G, Uziel N, et al. The impact of vaginal penetration difficulties on the sexual functioning of women and their male partners. Eur J Contracept Reprod Health Care 2014; **19**: 352–358.

78. Wielinski CL, Varpness SC, Erickson-Davis C, et al. Sexual and relationship satisfaction among persons with young-onset Parkinson's disease. J Sex Med 2010; **7**(4 Pt 1): 1438–1444.

79. Yu M, Roane DM, Miner CR, et al. Dimensions of sexual dysfunction in Parkinson disease. Am J Geriatr Psychiatry 2004; **12**: 221–226.

80. Stevenson RWD. Sexual medicine: why psychiatrists must talk to their patients about sex. Can J Psychiatry 2004; **49**: 673–677.

81. Rutte A, van Oppen P, Nijpels G, et al. Effectiveness of a PLISSIT model intervention in patients with type 2 diabetes mellitus in primary care: design of a cluster-randomised controlled trial. BMC Fam Pract 2015; **16**: 69.

82. Basson R, Bronner G. Management and rehabilitation of neurologic patients with sexual dysfunction. Handb Clin Neurol 2015; **130**: 415–434.

83. Bronner G. Practical strategies for the management of sexual problems in Parkinson's disease. Parkinsonism Relat Disord 2009; **15** (Suppl 3): S96–S100.

84. Dyer K, das Nair R. Why don't healthcare professionals talk about sex? A systematic review of recent qualitative studies conducted in the United Kingdom. J Sex Med 2013; **10**: 2658–2670.

85. Bronner G, Gurevich T. Management of neurogenic sexual dysfunction. In: Nair KPS, Gonzalez-Fernandez M, Panicker JN, (eds.). *Neurorehabilitation Therapy and Therapeutics.* Cambridge University Press; 2019, 224–235.

86. Zesiewicz TA, Helal M, Hauser RA. Sildenafil citrate (viagra) for the treatment of erectile dysfunction in men with Parkinson's disease. Mov Disord 2000; **15**: 305–308.

87. Pfeiffer RF. Gastrointestinal dysfunction in Parkinson's disease. Lancet Neurol 2003; **2**: 107–116.

88. Costa P, Potempa AJ. Intraurethral alprostadil for erectile dysfunction: a review of the literature. Drugs 2012; **72**: 2243–2254.

89. Rocinante M. Living with autonomic failure. Clin Auton Res 2008; **18**: 48–51.

90. Allahdadi KJ, Tostes RC, Webb RC. Female sexual dysfunction: therapeutic options and experimental challenges. Cardiovasc Hematol Agents Med Chem 2009; **7**: 260–269.

91. Catalan MJ, De Pablo-Fernandez E, Villanueva C, et al. Levodopa infusion improves impulsivity and dopamine dysregulation syndrome in Parkinson's disease. Mov Disord 2013; **28**: 2007–2010.

92. Bronner G, Korczyn AD. The role of sex therapy in the management of Parkinson's disease patients. Mov Disord Clin Pract 2018; **5**: 6–13.

93. Lafortune D, Dion L, Renaud P. Virtual reality and sex therapy: future directions for clinical research. J Sex Marital Ther 2019; **4**: 1–17.

94. Maples-Keller JL, Bunnell BE, Kim SJ, et al. The use of virtual reality technology in the treatment of anxiety and other psychiatric disorders. Harv Rev Psychiatry 2017; **25**: 103–113.

95. Iruthayarajah J, McIntyre A, Cotoi A, et al. The use of virtual reality for balance among individuals with chronic stroke: a systematic review and meta-analysis. Top Stroke Rehabil 2017; **24**: 68–79.

96. Spiegel B, Fuller G, Lopez M, et al. Virtual reality for management of pain in hospitalized patients: a randomized comparative effectiveness trial. PLoS One 2019; **14**: e0219115.

97. Manera V, Ben-Sadoun G, Aalbers T, et al. Recommendations for the use of serious games in neurodegenerative disorders: 2016 Delphi Panel. Front Psychol 2017; **8**: 1243.

Chapter 15

Sleep Disturbances in Parkinson's Disease

Cristian Falup-Pecurariu, Ștefania Diaconu, Maria-Lucia Muntean

Introduction

Non-motor symptoms (NMS) are important features in Parkinson's disease (PD). Sleep disturbances have a high prevalence among NMS and affect quality of life of PD patients [1]. In this chapter we will describe the most important features of the main sleep disorders encountered in PD.

Excessive Daytime Sleepiness

Definition

Excessive daytime sleepiness (EDS) is characterized by drowsiness and inability to remain fully awake during daytime. PD patients often report chronic sleepiness during the day, which is clinically difficult to be distinguished from fatigue. Episodes of sudden onset of sleep might be considered a specific feature of EDS and are characterized by a sudden and irresistible drive to sleep during passive or active situations. First described as "sleep attacks," this term is still employed today. However, its use is discouraged. Some of the episodes are preceded by a compelling desire to sleep, but in most cases patients fall asleep without any warning sign. These unpredictable episodes of sudden onset sleep are of outmost importance as they may occur in dangerous circumstances – for example while driving [2, 3].

Epidemiology

Large cross-sectional studies on PD patients have shown that almost one-third reported EDS: 29% out of 1,625 patients in France [4], 34.1% out of 1,221 patients in China [5]. EDS was correlated with age, male gender, cognitive decline, and severity of the motor features [5, 6]. Studies belonging to the Parkinson's Progression Markers Initiative (PPMI) suggest that EDS is more common in PD patients compared to controls, with a tendency to increase over time [7]. Furthermore, there might be a strong association between EDS and swallowing difficulties [8].

Pathophysiology

The etiology of EDS is multifactorial. The arousal systems in the hypothalamus and brainstem are affected and this may explain the EDS in PD. DaTscan studies found presynaptic dopaminergic impairments in the basal ganglia in PD patients affected by EDS [7]. Other suggested pathogenic mechanisms were related to the reduced dopaminergic activity in the caudate nucleus as demonstrated with SPECT imaging [9] or microstructural changes within the white matter leading to reduced connectivity in the fornical area and cerebellar peduncles [10]. One recent study suggests that the increased expression of phosphodiesterease 4 (PDE 4) in the caudate, hypothalamic and limbic areas is associated with EDS in PD [11].

An important cause of daytime sleepiness is the administration of PD medication. Levodopa and dopamine agonists were the most frequently incriminated [12].

Specific Features in Parkinson's Disease

The presence of daytime sleepiness and sudden onset of sleep resembles the clinical picture of narcolepsy, which is characterized in addition by loss of postural tone induced by strong emotions (cataplexy), hypnagogic hallucinations, and sleep paralysis [13]. In PD patients, studies have shown varied results of the hypocretin levels in the cerebral spinal fluid – low [14] or normal [15], while the reduction of hypocretin-producing cells by the hypothalamus was correlated with the neurodegenerative process – and thus, with the progression of PD [16].

Assessment

The most used and straightforward tool is the Epworth Sleepiness Scale (ESS), a simple screening test including eight active or passive situations in which the patient evaluates the chance of dozing. A score of more than ten is considered suggestive for abnormal sleepiness during the daytime. This scale was validated for assessment of EDS in PD patients [17]. The Stanford Sleepiness Scale (SSS) measures sleepiness at the time of the assessment, using a scale ranging from 0 to 7 [18]. The multiple sleep latency test (MSLT) is used as an objective method to evaluate daytime sleepiness. Polysomnographic (PSG) studies failed to find a correlation between ESS and objective measurement parameters, even if the total sleep time, sleep efficiency, and REM sleep were reduced in PD patients [19].

Treatment

Optimization of antiparkinsonian treatment is the main approach; the doses of dopamine agonists (DAs) should be reduced or another DA should be tried [20]. Light therapy was found to improve EDS in PD patients [21]. Modafinil, methylphenidate, and sodium oxybate, the main therapeutic options proposed in narcolepsy, were also tried for PD patients with EDS and were found to have a positive effect on daytime sleepiness [22, 23, 24]. The main pharmacological treatment options for EDS and for other sleep disorders are summarized in Table 15.1.

Insomnia

Definition

Inability to initiate or to maintain sleep, also associating early awakenings and reduced sleep quality overnight [25].

Epidemiology

Cohort studies have shown that insomnia is the most common sleep disorder in PD. Its prevalence is 25–80% [26]. Insomnia becomes more prevalent and severe as the disease advances, and the main associated factors are depression, motor complications, autonomic dysfunction, and fatigue [27], [28], [29].

Pathophysiology

The main causes for insomnia are the neurodegenerative process, inadequate sleep habits, the discomfort created by the akinesia, tremor, and stiffness, the association with depression, and the side effects of various antiparkinsonian drugs [30]. Among medication, the dopamine agonists, selegiline, and trihexyphenidyl can trigger insomnia as a side effect [31].

Specific Features in Parkinson's Disease

Sleep maintenance insomnia in PD is multifactorial. PD patients with insomnia have shorter latency of REM sleep onset compared with those without insomnia [32]. The subtypes of insomnia may have a fluctuating course over time in PD – for instance the occurrence of maintenance insomnia has a tendency to increase as the disease advances [33]. Compared to controls, PD patients with declared insomnia had altered sleep architecture, reduced total sleep time, and reduced sleep efficiency as revealed by PSG recordings [34].

Assessment

Thorough history combined with a sleep diary is helpful to assess the type, frequency, and severity of the symptoms and also the possible causes (behavioral habits and associated factors that contribute to insomnia). Actigraphy is useful to determine the activity during daytime and nighttime and might provide some information regarding behavioral habits and also some sleep parameters (like total sleep time, sleep efficiency), but it cannot distinguish accurately the transition between wakefulness to sleep stages [35].

Treatment

Correction of inadequate sleep habits, cognitive behavioral treatment [36], and bright light therapy [37] are among the first-line non-pharmacological treatments that should be tried. Regarding medical treatment, melatonin [38] and eszopiclone [39] were among the medications commonly used to improve insomnia in PD (but their effect was not demonstrated in large trials). Doxepin (10 mg) was also found to improve insomnia in PD patients [40]. Dopamine agonists (especially transdermal rotigotine) could improve sleep quality during the nighttime by controlling motor symptoms [41].

Table 15.1 Common pharmacological agents used for treating sleep disorders in Parkinson's disease [22, 23, 24, 26, 31, 38, 41, 43, 60, 63, 84, 85, 94, 95, 96]

Substance	Sleep disorders type	Medication, dose/ comments	Main side effects
Dopamine agonists	Insomnia	Rotigotine Apomorphine	• EDS • Hallucinations • Dopamine dysregulation syndrome • Impulse control disorder • Visual hallucinations
	RLS	• Pramipexole: 0.25–0.75 mg/day • Ropinirole: 0.78–4.6 mg/day • Rotigotine: 2–3 mg/day	Same as above + augmentation
Modafinil	EDS	200 mg/day	Dizziness, Palpitations
Sodium oxybate	EDS	3–9 g/day	• Dizziness • Asthenia • Sleep apnea
α2δ ligands	RLS	• Gabapentin encarbil: 1,200 mg/day • Pregabalin: 150–450 mg/day • Gabapentin: 800 mg/day	• Dizziness • Somnolence
Opioids (oxycodone/ naloxone)	RLS	5/2.5–40/20 mg/day	• Addiction • Sleep-related respiratory difficulties
Opioids (tramadol)	RLS	50–200 mg/day	• Sedation • Nausea • Sleep apnea
Opioids (methadone)	RLS	5–20 mg/day	• Sedation • Nausea • Sleep apnea • Prolonged QT interval
Atypical antipsychotics (Quetiapine)	Insomnia	12.5–50 mg	• Exacerbation of RLS • Sleepiness • Prolonged QT syndrome
Nonbenzodiazepinic hypnotics (eszopiclone)	Insomnia	2–3 mg bedtime	• Unpleasant taste • Headache • Dyspepsia • Pain
Benzodiazepines (clonazepam)	RBD	0.5–2 mg bed-time	• Gait instability • Dizziness • Somnolence • Urinary incontinence
Melatonin	RBD	3–9 mg bed-time	• Somnolence • Headache • Fatigue
	Insomnia	3–50 mg bed-time	

Abbreviations: sc: subcutaneous; EDS: excessive daytime sleepiness; RBD: rapid eye movement (REM) sleep behavior disorder; RLS: restless legs syndrome.

Restless Legs Syndrome

Definition

According to the International Restless Legs Syndrome Study Group (IRLSSG) criteria, the symptoms of restless legs syndrome (RLS) (an urge to move the legs associated with unpleasant sensations such as paresthesias and dysesthesias) occur during rest or inactivity, mostly during evening or nighttime, are usually relieved by voluntary movements, and are not better explained by other disorders [42]. Periodic limb movements of sleep (PLMS) are defined by involuntary movements, such as partial flexion of the legs, which may co-occur in almost 90% of patients with RLS [43].

Epidemiology

A recent meta-analysis of 28 studies regarding RLS in PD concluded the pooled prevalence of RLS is 14%. Eleven studies revealed that RLS is more prevalent in PD compared to healthy controls (3.8–21.3% versus 2.3–10%) [44]. Longitudinal studies have shown that the prevalence of RLS increases with the course of PD and is associated with worse sleep quality [45].

Pathophysiology

Restless legs syndrome and PD may share same common pathophysiological pattern, related to the dopaminergic depletion – but even for idiopathic RLS, the precise pathophysiological mechanism has still not been identified [46]. The impairment of iron metabolism – as suggested by abnormal iron concentration in the substantia nigra – may contribute to oxidative damage and to progressive dopamine neurodegeneration and may explain the co-occurrence of these pathologies [47].

Specific Features in Parkinson's Disease

Restless legs syndrome and PLMS induce daytime sleepiness and impair sleep by inducing difficulty in sleep initiation and nocturnal sleep fragmentation, due to an increased number of awakenings or microarousals [48, 49]. RLS in PD is associated with older age at onset, disease severity, depression, anxiety, dysautonomic features, and poor nutritional status [45, 50, 51]. Serum ferritin levels in most cases of idiopathic RLS were found to be low. In PD patients the results were contradictory: some studies found no differences regarding serum ferritin concentration between PD patients with and without RLS [52]; on the other hand, a recent meta-analysis concluded that lower serum ferritin levels were associated with RLS in PD patients [47].

Assessment

Diagnosis of RLS is made on the clinical review of the IRLSSG criteria, with careful exclusion of the various mimics. The measurement of serum ferritin levels can be useful. Several scales were developed in order to evaluate the symptoms and the severity of RLS. The International Restless Legs Scale (IRLS) [53] and the newly developed self-assessment version (sIRLS) [54] are used to quantify the severity of the disease and also the therapeutic response. Other assessment scales are the RLS-6 scale [55] and the 12 self-assessment items of Kohnen Restless Legs Syndrome-Quality of Life questionnaire (KRLS-QoL) [56]. The suggested immobilization test was validated as an objective method to analyze RLS in PD patients, as it combines the assessment of perceived discomfort and the objective leg movements during one hour of immobilization before sleep [57].

Treatment

Dopamine agonists are beneficial for patients suffering with both PD and RLS, even if there is no data for a standard treatment of RLS in these patients [58]. Pramipexole, ropinirole, or transdermal rotigotine were recommended as first-line therapy for RLS [43]. DA were also efficient in reducing PLMS during the nighttime, according to a small study involving 19 drug-naive PD patients [59]. The approved α2δ ligand is gabapentin enacarbil, but gabapentin and pregabalin could also be tried [43]. Recent guidelines indicate α2δ ligands (gabapentin enacarbil) as first-line therapy for idiopathic RLS instead of DA [60]. Gabapentin enacarbil is a calcium channel ligand with well-sustained plasma levels which was proved to alleviate the symptoms of RLS and also the sleep disturbances related with RLS [61]. In severe refractory cases, opioids like oxycodone-naloxone or methadone should be considered [43, 62]. Even if treatment with oral or intravenous iron is efficient in idiopathic RLS, there is no sufficient evidence to support its beneficial effect in PD [63]. The efficacy of subthalamic nucleus stimulation in PD patients with RLS is controversial, but some recent studies report positive results [50].

Sleep-Related Breathing Disorders

Definition

The most frequently encountered sleep-related breathing disorder (SBD) in PD is obstructive sleep apnea (OSA), but the spectrum of SBD can include central apnea, mixed apnea, sleep-related hypoventilation, and hypoxemia during sleep. The cessation of breathing during sleep and snoring can be observed by the bed partner, but the patient usually complains of sleepiness during the daytime and unrefreshing sleep [64].

Epidemiology

The prevalence of OSA varies between 21% and 62% [65, 66]. According to one study, snoring was found to be more prevalent in patients with PD (40.5%) compared to healthy controls (35.5%). OSA was also more common in the PD/parkinsonism group [67].

Pathophysiology

The tendency of collapse of the upper-airway muscles is the main pathological mechanism involved in the development of OSA. In the general population, high body mass index (BMI) is an important risk factor for OSA, but the majority of PD patients are not obese and BMI is not associated with severity of OSA [68].

Specific Features in Parkinson's Disease

Polysomnographic studies in PD patients with OSA revealed less time spent in stage 3 of NREM sleep, higher awakening index, and higher desaturation index compared to PD patients without OSA [66].

Assessment

Screening for OSA can be done using the following tools: Multivariable Apnea Prediction (MAP) Index, Berlin Questionnaire, and STOP-Bang Questionnaire [18]. For the confirmation and classification of SBD, polygraphic or polysomnographic studies are mandatory. The total number of events/hour is measured and is used to establish the severity of SBD [25, 64].

Treatment

Continuous positive airway pressure (CPAP), the main therapy indicated in the general population, has beneficial effects on PD patients as well. Clinical data show that CPAP improves not only the severity of OSA, but also the motor dysfunction over time [69]. Mandibular advancement devices were suggested in the treatment of OSA in PD patients, with higher adherence rates than CPAP, but larger randomized studies are needed for confirmation [70].

Rapid Eye Movement Sleep Behavior Disorder

Definition

Rapid eye movement sleep behavior disorder (RBD) is a sleep disorder characterized by loss of normal muscle atonia during rapid eye movement (REM) sleep with recurrent dream enactment and excessive motor activity [71]. In PD patients, RBD can occur years before the motor clinical symptoms appear and thus could be considered a preclinical biomarker for the disease.

The symptoms are mostly described by the bed partners of the patients and include movements and/or vocalizations, which are in most cases the expression of dreams. If a patient awakens during one such episode, they can mostly recall the content of the dream, which is often threatening or violent, with the patient fighting or trying to defend themself. The movements are jerky, abrupt, or can sometimes mimic physiological movements. These movements can sometimes be very disturbing [72]. The vocalizations vary from murmuring and laughing or crying to screaming or short speeches, where all the words can be understood [73].

Epidemiology

Rapid eye movement sleep behavior disorder is reported to occur between 15% and 51% of PD patients [74, 75]. Male patients with PD have a higher prevalence [76].

Pathophysiology

The degeneration of nuclei in the medulla oblongata and pontine tegmentum is most probably responsible for the occurrence of RBD [71].

Lesions in the pontine sublaterodorsal nucleus lead to disappearance of the inhibition of the alpha-motoneurons [77]. Furthermore, a disturbance of the flip-flop switch between the REM-on and REM-off structures might be involved [78].

Specific Features in Parkinson's Disease

Rapid eye movement sleep behavior disorder could occur at the onset of the neurodegenerative process. In a large multicentric study, patients with idiopathic RBD showed a conversion rate to an overt neurodegeneration of 6.3% per year, 73% of them converting in 12 years [79]. The only variable proven to differentiate between conversion to dementia or parkinsonism first was cognition itself [79].

Assessment

The diagnosis of RBD is made according to the International Classification of Sleep Disorders (ICSD)-3 criteria published in 2014 [25]. There are four criteria:

1) Episodes of sleep-related vocalization and/or complex motor behaviors
2) These behaviors are documented by PSG to occur during REM sleep
3) Polysomnographic recording demonstrates REM sleep without atonia (RWA)
4) The disturbance is not better explained by another sleep disorder, mental disorder, medication, or substance abuse.

Polysomnography is mandatory for the diagnosis of RBD and is necessary in order to quantify RWA. Polysomnographic electromyographic (EMG) analysis has also the advantage of high night to night stability, compared to the very variable clinical manifestation of dream enactment. Different criteria are used to quantify RWA on PSG, analyzing different muscles and differentiating between tonic and phasic motor activity [80]. The Sleep Innsbruck Barcelona (SINBAR) Group used the 3s- epochs and performed multiple investigations in order to determine the minimal combination of EMG channels/muscle registrations needed to have a proper RBD diagnosis. Measuring the muscle activity in chin and upper limbs seems to be the most reliable combination for defining RBD [81].

During the videopolysomnogram (vPSG) it can be noticed that in these patients REM sleep with atonia (RWA) is preserved [82]. PLMS could occur in all sleep stages in PD patients. However, it has been shown that PD patients with RBD feature a higher number of PLMS than PD patients without RBD [76].

Screening for Rapid Eye Movement Sleep Behavior Disorder

Videopolysomnogram requires specialized personnel and a special setting, thus being quite expensive and not always available. Screening questionnaires are a cheap and time-saving method to look for RBD.

Severity of Rapid Eye Movement Sleep Behavior Disorder

The severity of RBD can be assessed during the vPSG. The RBD severity scale (RBDSS) developed by Sixel-Döring and colleagues [83] evaluates motor behavior and vocalizations during vPSG monitoring.

Treatment

The most used medications are clonazepam and melatonin. For clonazepam different studies exist which have demonstrated the efficacy of doses between 0.5 and 2 mg [84]. Melatonin doses used were between 3 and 9 mg [85].

Mechanical protection can be used to minimize injuries during violent RBD episodes, for example, mattresses near the bed or mechanical barrier between bed partners.

Specific Considerations: Sleep Fragmentation and Other Sleep Disturbances

The multiple interruptions of sleep, frequent awakenings and difficulties falling back to sleep, disturb the normal sleep architecture, contribute to poor sleep quality, and induce sleepiness during daytime [86]. Several factors are causative for sleep fragmentation, including PD severity, nocturnal akinesia, rigidity, nocturia, PLMS, hallucinations, or OSA [67, 87].

Two useful scales to evaluate sleep characteristics in PD are the Parkinson's Disease Sleep Scale (PDSS-2) [88] and the Scales for Outcomes in Parkinson's Disease (SCOPA-SLEEP) [89]. For the assessment of nocturnal hypokinesia, PSG represents the best option. The global evaluation of sleep quality can be realized through the Pittsburg Sleep Quality Index (PSQI) [90].

The pharmacological treatment of sleep fragmentation implies conducting effective management of PD severity and also assuring an adequate dopamine concentration during the nighttime to avoid nocturnal hypokinesia. Considering this, long-acting dopamine agonists (DA) and sustained-release levodopa might be beneficial [91], including their positive effect on RLS and PLMS [31]. Continuous subcutaneous apomorphine infusion was proved to reduce nighttime motor sleep symptoms and to improve insomnia in advanced PD [92]. Deep brain stimulation (DBS) was found to improve quality and sleep efficiency [93].

Conclusions

Sleep disturbances are highly prevalent NMS in PD patients. They significantly impact on quality of life.

Careful patient history and clinical examination are important to define the types of sleep disturbances. Observations obtained from bed partners could offer valuable information for rapid eye movement sleep behavior disorders. Specific questionnaires and scales, actigraphy, and polysomnography are important instruments in screening and assessing PD patients with sleep complaints.

References

1. Chaudhuri KR, Healy DG, Schapira AH. National Institute for Clinical Excellence. Non-motor symptoms of Parkinson's disease: diagnosis and management. Lancet Neurol 2006; 5(3): 235–245.

2. Maestri M, Romigi A, Schirru A, et al. Excessive daytime sleepiness and fatigue in neurological disorders. Sleep Breath 2019; 24(2): 413–424.

3. Knie B, Mitra MT, Logishetty K, Chaudhuri KR. Excessive daytime sleepiness in patients with Parkinson's disease. CNS Drugs 2011; 25(3): 203–212.

4. Ghorayeb I, Loundou A, Auquier P, et al. A nationwide survey of excessive daytime sleepiness in Parkinson's disease in France. Mov Disord 2007; 22(11): 1567–1572.

5. Xiang YQ, Xu Q, Sun QY, et al. Clinical features and correlates of excessive daytime sleepiness in Parkinson's disease. Front Neurol 2019; 10: 121.

6. Yoo SW, Kim JS, Oh YS, Ryu DW, Lee KS. Excessive daytime sleepiness and its impact on quality of life in de novo Parkinson's disease. Neurol Sci 2019; 40(6): 1151–1156.

7. Amara AW, Chahine LM, Caspell-Garcia C, et al. Parkinson's Progression Markers Initiative. Longitudinal assessment of excessive daytime sleepiness in early Parkinson's disease. J Neurol Neurosurg Psychiatry 2017; 88(8): 653–662.

8. Marano M, Gupta D, Motolese F, et al. Excessive daytime sleepiness is associated to the development of swallowing impairment in a cohort of early stage drug naïve Parkinson's disease patients. J Neurol Sci 2019; 410: 116626.

9. Yousaf T, Pagano G, Niccolini F, Politis M. Excessive daytime sleepiness may be associated with caudate denervation in Parkinson disease. J Neurol Sci 2018; 387: 220–227.

10. Ashraf-Ganjouei A, Kheiri G, Masoudi M, et al. White matter tract alterations in drug-naïve Parkinson's disease patients with excessive daytime sleepiness. Front Neurol 2019; 10: 378.

11. Wilson H, Pagano G, Niccolini F, et al. The role of phosphodiesterase 4 in excessive daytime sleepiness in Parkinson's disease. Parkinsonism Relat Disord 2019; 77: 163–169.

12. Sobreira-Neto MA, Pena-Pereira MA, Sobreira EST, et al. Factors related to excessive sleepiness in patients with Parkinson's disease. Neurol Res 2019; 41(3): 227–233.

13. Bassetti CLA, Adamantidis A, Burdakov D, et al. Narcolepsy – clinical spectrum, aetiopathophysiology, diagnosis and treatment. Nat Rev Neurol 2019; 15(9): 519–539.

14. Drouot X, Moutereau S, Nguyen JP, et al. Low levels of ventricular CSF orexin/hypocretin in advanced PD. Neurology 2003; 61(4): 540–543.

15. Overeem S, van Hilten JJ, Ripley B, et al. Normal hypocretin-1 levels in Parkinson's disease patients with excessive daytime sleepiness. Neurology 2002; 58(3): 498–499.

16. Thannickal TC, Lai YY, Siegel JM. Hypocretin (orexin) and melanin concentrating hormone loss and the symptoms of Parkinson's disease. Brain 2008; 131(Pt 1): e87.

17. Hagell P, Broman JE. Measurement properties and hierarchical item structure of the Epworth

Sleepiness Scale in Parkinson's disease. J Sleep Res 2007; **16**(1): 102–109.

18. Kurtis MM, Balestrino R, Rodriguez-Blazquez C, Forjaz MJ, Martinez-Martin P. A review of scales to evaluate sleep disturbances in movement disorders. Front Neurol 2018; **9**: 369.

19. Shpirer I, Miniovitz A, Klein C, et al. Excessive daytime sleepiness in patients with Parkinson's disease: a polysomnography study. Mov Disord 2006; **21**(9): 1432–1438.

20. Calandrella A, Albanese A. Management of sleep disorders in Parkinson's disease. In: Gálvez-Jiménez NG, Fernandez HH, Espay AJ, Fox SH, (eds.). *Parkinson's Disease: Current and Future Thrapeutics and Clinical Trials*. Cambridge University Press; 2016, 151–161.

21. Videnovic A, Klerman EB, Wang W, et al. Timed light therapy for sleep and daytime sleepiness associated with Parkinson disease: a randomized clinical trial. JAMA Neurol 2017; **74**(4): 411–418.

22. Lou JS, Dimitrova DM, Park BS, et al. Using modafinil to treat fatigue in Parkinson disease: a double-blind, placebo-controlled pilot study. Clin Neuropharmacol 2009; **32**(6): 305–310.

23. Büchele F, Hackius M, Schreglmann SR, et al. Sodium oxybate for excessive daytime sleepiness and sleep disturbance in Parkinson disease: a randomized clinical trial. JAMA Neurol 2018; **75**(1): 114–118.

24. Devos D, Krystkowiak P, Clement F, et al. Improvement of gait by chronic, high doses of methylphenidate in patients with advanced Parkinson's disease. J Neurol Neurosurg Psychiatry 2007; **78**(5): 470–475.

25. Darien I. *The International Classification of Sleep Disorders*, 3rd ed. American Academy of Sleep Medicine; 2014.

26. Wallace DM, Wohlgemuth WK, Trotti LM, et al. Practical evaluation and management of insomnia in Parkinson's disease: a review. Mov Disord Clin Pract 2020. DOI: 10.1002/mdc3.12899

27. Chung S, Bohnen NI, Albin RL, et al. Insomnia and sleepiness in Parkinson disease: associations with symptoms and comorbidities. J Clin Sleep Med 2013; **9**(11): 1131–1137.

28. Zhu K, van Hilten JJ, Marinus J. The course of insomnia in Parkinson's disease. Parkinsonism Relat Disord 2016; **33**: 51–57.

29. Kay DB, Tanner JJ, Bowers D. Sleep disturbances and depression severity in patients with Parkinson's disease. Brain Behav 2018; **8**(6): e00967.

30. Sobreira-Neto MA, Pena-Pereira MA, Sobreira EST, et al. High frequency of sleep disorders in Parkinson's disease and its relationship with quality of life. Eur Neurol 2017; **78**(5–6): 330–337.

31. Loddo G, Calandra-Buonaura G, Sambati L, et al. The treatment of sleep disorders in Parkinson's disease: from research to clinical practice. Front Neurol 2017; **8**: 42.

32. Shafazand S, Wallace DM, Arheart KL, et al. Insomnia, sleep quality, and quality of life in mild to moderate Parkinson's disease. Ann Am Thorac Soc 2017; **14**(3): 412–419.

33. Tholfsen LK, Larsen JP, Schulz J, Tysnes OB, Gjerstad MD. Changes in insomnia subtypes in early Parkinson disease. Neurology 2017; **88**(4): 352–358.

34. Yong MH, Fook-Chong S, Pavanni R, Lim LL, Tan EK. Case control polysomnographic studies of sleep disorders in Parkinson's disease. PLoS One 2011; **6**(7): e22511.

35. Maglione JE, Liu L, Neikrug AB, et al. Actigraphy for the assessment of sleep measures in Parkinson's disease. Sleep 2013; **36**(8): 1209–1217.

36. Lebrun C, Gély-Nargeot MC, Rossignol A, Geny C, Bayard S. Efficacy of cognitive behavioral therapy for insomnia comorbid to Parkinson's disease: a focus on psychological and daytime functioning with a single-case design with multiple baselines. J Clin Psychol 2019. DOI: 10.1002/jclp.22883

37. Martino JK, Freelance CB, Willis GL. The effect of light exposure on insomnia and nocturnal movement in Parkinson's disease: an open label, retrospective, longitudinal study. Sleep Med 2018; **44**: 24–31.

38. Dowling GA, Mastick J, Colling E, et al. Melatonin for sleep disturbances in Parkinson's disease. Sleep Med 2005; **6**(5): 459–466.

39. Menza M, Dobkin RD, Marin H, et al. Treatment of insomnia in Parkinson's disease: a controlled trial of eszopiclone and placebo. Mov Disord 2010; **25**(11): 1708–1714.

40. Rios Romenets S, Creti L, Fichten C, et al. Doxepin and cognitive behavioural therapy for insomnia in patients with Parkinson's disease – a randomized study. Parkinsonism Relat Disord 2013; **19**: 670–675.

41. Fei L, Zhou D, Ding ZT. The efficacy and safety of rotigotine transdermal patch for the treatment of sleep disorders in Parkinson's disease: a meta-analysis. Sleep Med 2019; **61**: 19–25.

42. Allen RP, Picchietti DL, Garcia-Borreguero D, et al. International Restless Legs Syndrome Study Group. Restless legs syndrome/Willis-Ekbom disease diagnostic criteria: updated International

Restless Legs Syndrome Study Group (IRLSSG) consensus criteria – history, rationale, description, and significance. Sleep Med 2014; **15**(8): 860–873.

43. Gonzalez-Latapi P, Malkani R. Update on restless legs syndrome: from mechanisms to treatment. Curr Neurol Neurosci Rep 2019; **19**(8): 54.

44. Yang X, Liu B, Shen H, et al. Prevalence of restless legs syndrome in Parkinson's disease: a systematic review and meta-analysis of observational studies. Sleep Med 2018; **43**: 40–46.

45. Moccia M, Erro R, Picillo M, et al. A four-year longitudinal study on restless legs syndrome in Parkinson disease. Sleep 2016; **39**(2): 405–412.

46. Munhoz RP, Constantino MCL, Silveira-Moriyama L. The Parkinson's disease and restless legs syndrome/Willis-Ekbom disorder link: evidence, biases and clinical relevance. Arq Neuropsiquiatr 2019; **77**(1): 47–54.

47. Li K, Liu B1, Wang F, et al. Decreased serum ferritin may be associated with increased restless legs syndrome in Parkinson's disease (PD): a meta-analysis for the diagnosis of RLS in PD patients. Int J Neurosci 2019; **129**(10): 995–1003.

48. Happe S, Trenkwalder C. Movement disorders in sleep: Parkinson's disease and restless legs syndrome. Biomed Tech 2003; **48**(3): 62–67.

49. Covassin N, Neikrug AB, Liu L, et al. Clinical correlates of periodic limb movements in sleep in Parkinson's disease. J Neurol Sci 2012; **316**(1–2): 131–136.

50. Alonso-Navarro H, García-Martín E, Agúndez JAG, Jiménez-Jiménez FJ. Association between restless legs syndrome and other movement disorders. Neurology 2019; **92**(20): 948–964.

51. Fereshtehnejad SM, Shafieesabet M, Shahidi GA, Delbari A, Lökk J. Restless legs syndrome in patients with Parkinson's disease: a comparative study on prevalence, clinical characteristics, quality of life and nutritional status. Acta Neurol Scand 2015; **131**(4): 211–218.

52. Muntean ML, Sixel-Döring F, Trenkwalder C. Serum ferritin levels in Parkinson's disease patients with and without restless legs syndrome. Mov Disord Clin Pract 2015; **2**(3): 249–252.

53. Walters AS, LeBrocq C, Dhar A, et al. International Restless Legs Syndrome Study Group. Validation of the International Restless Legs Syndrome Study Group rating scale for restless legs syndrome. Sleep Med 2003; **4**(2): 121–132.

54. Sharon D, Allen RP, Martinez-Martin P, et al. International RLS Study Group. Validation of the self-administered version of the international

Restless Legs Syndrome study group severity rating scale – The sIRLS. Sleep Med 2019; **54**: 94–100.

55. Kohnen R, Martinez-Martin P, Benes H, et al. Rating of daytime and nighttime symptoms in RLS: validation of the RLS-6 scale of restless legs syndrome/Willis-Ekbom disease. Sleep Med 2016; **20**: 116–122.

56. Kohnen R, Martinez-Martin P, Benes H, et al. Validation of the Kohnen Restless Legs Syndrome-Quality of Life instrument. Sleep Med 2016; **24**: 10–17.

57. De Cock VC, Bayard S, Yu H, et al. Suggested immobilization test for diagnosis of restless legs syndrome in Parkinson's disease. Mov Disord 2012; **27**(6): 743–749.

58. You S, Jeon SM, Do SY, Cho YW. Restless legs syndrome in Parkinson's disease patients: clinical features including motor and nonmotor symptoms. J Clin Neurol 2019; **15**(3): 321–327.

59. Puligheddu M, Figorilli M, Aricò D, et al. Time structure of leg movement activity during sleep in untreated Parkinson disease and effects of dopaminergic treatment. Sleep Med 2014; **15**: 816–824.

60. Wanner V, Garcia Malo C, Romero S, Cano-Pumarega I, García-Borreguero D. Non-dopaminergic vs. dopaminergic treatment options in restless legs syndrome. Adv Pharmacol 2019; **84**: 187–205.

61. Ahmed M, Hays R, Steven Poceta J, et al. Effect of gabapentin enacarbil on individual items of the international restless legs study group rating scale and post-sleep questionnaire in adults with moderate-to-severe primary restless legs syndrome: pooled analysis of 3 randomized trials. Clin Ther 2016; **38**: 1726–1737.

62. Silber MH, Becker PM, Buchfuhrer MJ, et al. The appropriate use of opioids in the treatment of refractory restless legs syndrome. Mayo Clin Proc 2018; **93**(1): 59–67.

63. De Cock VC. Therapies for restless legs in Parkinson's disease. Curr Treat Options Neurol 2019; **21**(11): 56.

64. Foldvary-Schaefer NR, Waters TE. *Sleep-Disordered Breathing*. Continuum; 2017, 1093–1116.

65. Béland SG, Postuma RB, Latreille V, et al. Observational study of the relation between Parkinson's disease and sleep apnea. J Parkinsons Dis 2015; **5**(4): 805–811.

66. Sobreira-Neto MA, Pena-Pereira MA, Sobreira EST, et al. Obstructive sleep apnea and Parkinson's disease: characteristics and associated factors. Arq Neuropsiquiatr 2019; **77**(9): 609–616.

67. Crosta F, Desideri G, Marini C. Obstructive sleep apnea syndrome in Parkinson's disease and other parkinsonisms. Funct Neurol 2017; **32**(3): 137–141.

68. Bahia CMCS, Pereira JS2, Lopes AJ. Laryngopharyngeal motor dysfunction and obstructive sleep apnea in Parkinson's disease. Sleep Breath 2019; **23**(2): 543–550.

69. Meng L, Benedetti A, Lafontaine AL, et al. Obstructive sleep apnea, CPAP therapy and Parkinson's disease motor function: a longitudinal study. Parkinsonism Relat Disord 2019; **70**: 45–50.

70. Castel M, Cochen De Cock V, Léon H, Dupuy-Bonafé I. Mandibular advancement device in Parkinson's disease: a pilot study on efficacy and usability. Sleep Med 2019; **66**: 78–81.

71. Boeve BF, Silber MH, Saper CB, et al. Pathophysiology of REM sleep behaviour disorder and relevance to neurodegenerative disease. Brain 2007; **130**(Pt 11): 2770–2788.

72. De Cock VC. Recent data on rapid eye movement sleep behavior disorder in patients with Parkinson disease: analysis of behaviors, movements, and periodic limb movements. Sleep Med 2013; **14**(8): 749–753.

73. Boeve BF. REM sleep behavior disorder: updated review of the core features, the REM sleep behavior disorder-neurodegenerative disease association, evolving concepts, controversies, and future directions. Ann N Y Acad Sci 2010; **1184**: 15–54.

74. Gagnon JF, Bédard MA, Fantini ML, et al. REM sleep behavior disorder and REM sleep without atonia in Parkinson's disease. Neurology 2002; **59**(4): 585–589.

75. Mollenhauer B, Trautmann E, Sixel-Döring F, et al. DeNoPa Study Group. Nonmotor and diagnostic findings in subjects with de novo Parkinson disease of the DeNoPa cohort. Neurology 2013; **81**(14): 1226–1234.

76. Sixel-Döring F, Trautmann E, Mollenhauer B, Trenkwalder C. Associated factors for REM sleep behavior disorder in Parkinson disease. Neurology 2011; **77**(11): 1048–1054.

77. Krenzer M, Anaclet C, Vetrivelan R, et al. Brainstem and spinal cord circuitry regulating REM sleep and muscle atonia. PLoS One 2011; **6**(10): e24998.

78. Lu J, Sherman D, Devor M, Saper CB. A putative flip-flop switch for control of REM sleep. Nature 2006; **441**(7093): 589–594.

79. Postuma RB, Iranzo A, Hu M, et al. Risk and predictors of dementia and parkinsonism in idiopathic REM sleep behaviour disorder: a multicentre study. Brain 2019; **142**(3): 744–759.

80. Lapierre O, Montplaisir J. Polysomnographic features of REM sleep behavior disorder: development of a scoring method. Neurology 1992; **42**(7): 1371–1374.

81. Frauscher B, Iranzo A, Gaig C, et al. SINBAR (Sleep Innsbruck Barcelona) Group. Normative EMG values during REM sleep for the diagnosis of REM sleep behavior disorder. Sleep 2012; **35**(6): 835–847.

82. Iranzo A, Santamaría J. Severe obstructive sleep apnea/hypopnea mimicking REM sleep behavior disorder. Sleep 2005; **28**(2): 203–206.

83. Sixel-Döring F, Schweitzer M, Mollenhauer B, Trenkwalder C. Intraindividual variability of REM sleep behavior disorder in Parkinson's disease: a comparative assessment using a new REM sleep behavior disorder severity scale (RBDSS) for clinical routine. J Clin Sleep Med 2011; **7**(1): 75–80.

84. Howell MJ, Schenck CH. Rapid eye movement sleep behavior disorder and neurodegenerative disease. JAMA Neurol 2015; **72**(6): 707–712.

85. McGrane IR, Leung JG, St Louis EK, Boeve BF. Melatonin therapy for REM sleep behavior disorder: a critical review of evidence. Sleep Med 2015; **16**(1): 19–26.

86. Falup-Pecurariu C, Diaconu Ș. Sleep dysfunction in Parkinson's disease. Int Rev Neurobiol 2017; **133**: 719–742.

87. Bhidayasiri R, Trenkwalder C. Getting a good night sleep? The importance of recognizing and treating nocturnal hypokinesia in Parkinson's disease. Parkinsonism Relat Disord 2018; **50**: 10–18.

88. Trenkwalder C, Kohnen R, Högl B, et al. Parkinson's disease sleep scale–validation of the revised version PDSS-2. Mov Disord 2011; **26**(4): 644–652.

89. Marinus J, Visser M, van Hilten JJ, Lammers GJ, Stiggelbout AM. Assessment of sleep and sleepiness in Parkinson disease. Sleep 2003; **26**(8): 1049–1054.

90. Buysse DJ, Reynolds CF 3rd, Monk TH, Berman SR, Kupfer DJ. The Pittsburgh Sleep Quality Index: a new instrument for psychiatric practice and research. Psychiatry Res 1989; **28**(2): 193–213.

91. Bhidayasiri R, Sringean J, Thanawattano C. Sensor-based evaluation and treatment of nocturnal hypokinesia in Parkinson's disease: an evidence-based review. Parkinsonism Relat Disord 2016; **22**(Suppl 1): S127–133.

92. Fernández-Pajarín G, Sesar Á, Ares B, Castro A. Evaluating the efficacy of nocturnal continuous subcutaneous apomorphine infusion in sleep disorders in advanced Parkinson's disease: the APO-NIGHT Study. J Parkinsons Dis 2016; **6**(4): 787.

93. Sharma VD, Sengupta S, Chitnis S, Amara AW. Deep brain stimulation and sleep-wake disturbances in Parkinson disease: a review. Front Neurol 2018; 9: 697.

94. Juri C, Chaná P, Tapia J, Kunstmann C, Parrao T. Quetiapine for insomnia in Parkinson disease: results from an open-label trial. Clin Neuropharmacol 2005; 28(4): 185–187.

95. Fernández-Pajarín G, Sesar Á, Ares B, Castro A. Evaluating the efficacy of nocturnal continuous subcutaneous apomorphine infusion in sleep disorders in advanced Parkinson's disease: the APO-NIGHT Study. J Parkinsons Dis 2016; 6(4): 787–792.

96. During EH, Winkelman JW. Drug treatment of restless legs syndrome in older adults. Drugs Aging 2019; 36(10): 939–946.

Chapter 16

Musculoskeletal Disorders and Pain in Parkinson's Disease

Ovidiu-Alexandru Bajenaru

Musculoskeletal disorders and **pain in Parkinson's disease (PD)** are two complex clinically and pathophysiologically distinct problems, but a high degree of overlap exists between the pathogenesis and understanding of these two types of clinical manifestations. Although not commonly recognized as such these non-motor symptoms are quite frequent, impacting patients' quality of life. Early clinical observations [1] have noticed that both musculoskeletal disorders and pain related to these appear even in the prodromal phase, but also during definite PD manifestation, mainly by different algic syndromes determined by so-called fibromyalgia (fibrositis, tendinitis, myalgia), shoulder pain, cervicobrachialgia, ischialgia, lower back pain, and arthralgia. These probably appear indirectly as a component of PD, and seem to be significantly improved by the administration of levodopa. In PD patients with motor fluctuations, musculoskeletal pain tends to occur more often when parkinsonian disability is maximal and less frequently when disability is minimal [2].

Musculoskeletal Disorders

In population-based studies [3, 4] of PD-associated comorbid conditions, bone breaks and hip fractures appear with a higher incidence in PD patients, more frequent in those whose clinical onset was before the age of 70. Osteopathies, chondropathies, and acquired musculoskeletal deformities (according to ICD-9 classification) were also more frequent in PD patients. More recently, another prospective population-based study [5] has shown that vertebral, hip, and femoral fractures are common among PD patients, in particular, for female PD patients over 60 with osteoporosis.

Studies of posture in PD patients have emphasized severe musculoskeletal deformities, in particular spine deformities both in the sagittal (camptocormia) and the coronal plane (scoliosis and Pisa syndrome). One relatively recent study [6] in patients with confirmed PD prospectively evaluated for angles of spinal inclination in upright position, extension, and flexion using a mechanical computer-assisted, hand-held device (Spinal Mouse) with patients who underwent clinical examination and bone mineral density measurement. The degree of upright inclination correlated with age, older age at disease onset, longer disease duration, higher Unified Parkinson's Disease Rating Scale (UPDRS) motor and posture score, the presence of back-pain, and osteoporosis. Re-evaluation of posture 10–17 months after the initial assessment found a significant deterioration in forward bending and was significantly associated with disease duration, worsening of the UPDRS score, presence of vertebral fractures, and the lack of physical activity. Spine disorders in patients with PD are probably determined both by degenerative pathology and secondary to motor effects related to parkinsonism. In addition, degenerative disorders of the spine frequently associated to PD, such as spinal stenosis and sagittal instability, can further impact the quality of life of the patient. Recently it has been shown that patients with PD are at higher risk of osteoporotic vertebral compression fractures compared to controls and have elevated mortality rates [7, 8]. In patients undergoing spinal surgery, complication rates are higher in patients with PD than in those without the disease [9].

Camptocormia

Camptocormia in PD has a prevalence of 3–18%. It is progressive, presenting weeks to years after disease onset, and is strongly correlated with old age, advanced Parkinsonism, axial rigidity, postural instability, and impaired gait. Most experts consider camptocormia in PD to be a consequence of central and peripheral mechanism which both might contribute to its pathogenesis [10, 11]. Camptocormia (also known as "bent spine syndrome") is an abnormal flexion of the trunk with lumbar kyphosis appearing in standing position, increasing while walking, but disappearing in the supine position, standing against a wall or using a walking support [10]. Arbitrarily, most authors use at least 45 degrees of thoracolumbar bent to differentiate camptocormia from kyphosis of the dorsal spine.

Many PD patients with camptocormia have an associated scoliosis too. Camptocormia is not always improved by levodopa and other dopaminergic drugs, probably due to impairment of other non-dopaminergic pathways. Some earlier isolated pathological observations suggest an inflammatory myopathic mechanism of camptocormia, but the data are scarce and most experts today do not support this pathogenetic hypothesis [12, 13, 14, 15, 16]. Also, disturbances in the proprioceptive polysynaptic reflex arch have been evoked as a consequence of mechanisms of neurodegeneration in PD [17].

There is no consensus regarding the treatment of camptocormia in PD. Levodopa therapy and other dopaminergic drugs may worsen its clinical presentation, but in other cases seem to be beneficial. Deep brain stimulation (DBS) [18] and periodic botulinum toxin injections may be helpful in some cases, but controlled clinical trials are necessary. Physical neurorehabilitation must include camptocormia as a target in the treatment of PD [10, 19].

Pisa Syndrome

Pisa syndrome, manifested by lateral trunk flexion, is quite common among PD patients, with an estimated prevalence around 8.8% [20]. It seems to be more frequently associated with some specific patient features: more severe motor phenotype, ongoing combined pharmacological treatment with levodopa and dopamine agonists, gait disorders, and osteoporosis and arthrosis as comorbidities [20]. Due to its impact on posture and physical activity in daily life, it is an important clinical manifestation with implications for both drugs but mainly physical neurorehabilitation in PD.

The pathophysiology is probably multifactorial, but most of the data supports central, rather than peripheral, hypotheses (including both animal studies and clinical data showing asymmetry of basal ganglia dysfunction and abnormalities in the central integration of sensory information coming from different sources such as proprioception, vision, and the vestibular system and cognitive dysfunctions affecting the body schema perception and postural control) [20, 21]. The pathophysiology of this syndrome is far from clear and further research is needed.

An interesting study has shown that abnormal subjective visual vertical perception, associated with postural imbalance and unilateral electromyography (EMG) hyperactivity of paraspinal muscles, is an independent contributor to Pisa syndrome [22]. Some clinicians consider Pisa syndrome to be a form of trunk dystonia, but criteria for dystonia phenomenology (such as an absence of sensory ticks) are missing [23].

Some pathological muscle modifications have been described in the paravertebral muscles in PD patients with Pisa syndrome, but a possible explanation could be that atrophy through fatty degeneration might be caused by secondary mechanisms as a result of stretching stress on the muscle contralateral to the bending side [24].

The diagnosis of Pisa syndrome is based on the clinical evaluation of trunk lateral displacement, measured using different goniometric devices and a radiograph of the patient's spine while standing in the coronal and sagittal planes. A lateral flexion of at least 10 degrees is considered a criterion [25, 26]. If scoliosis is present by association of vertebral rotation, it does not disappear in supine position [20, 27, 28]. Very frequently, these patients complain of back pain [26], which may impact on both quality of life and the motor impairment (due to adoption of compensatory postures to minimize the pain perception). There is general consensus related to Pisa syndrome, but pharmacological and neurorehabilitation have to be included in the management of these patients to improve their quality of life [20, 29].

Osteoporosis

Osteoporosis is common in PD. PD patients with musculoskeletal pain often have low bone mineral density and are at risk of developing osteoporosis.

For this reason, PD patients with musculoskeletal pain and other risk factors related to low bone mineral density are candidates for screening of osteoporosis [4, 30, 31].

The cause of osteoporosis in PD is not completely clear, but different suspected mechanisms of accelerated bone loss in PD appear to play key roles, including weight loss and reduced mobility. Antiparkinsonian drugs, particularly levodopa, may also be associated with decreased bone mineral density as a result of hyperhomocysteinemia. Other nutritional deficiencies, such as vitamins D, B12, folate, or vitamin K may also play a role [32, 33, 34].

Currently there is no guideline consensus related to osteoporosis management in PD but some evidence supports updating guidelines globally concerning the management of PD, which presently fail to adequately address bone health and therefore impacts severely the quality of life of patients with PD [35]. Osteoporosis represents a quite severe but often unrecognized non-motor feature of PD. Only when it becomes complicated with bone fractures, spinal deformities, and different forms of musculoskeletal pain and/or starts to seriously affect quality of life will it come to the attention of the treating physician.

Shoulder Complaints

Shoulder complaints appear to be more frequent in PD patients than in non-PD controls [36]. In an ultrasonographic study [36] the authors found that tendon tearing was the most common abnormal finding, most frequently involving the supraspinatus tendon. The most severely affected patients were found to have experienced a longer duration of the disease. Also, adhesive capsulitis was significantly frequent and correlated with higher scores for rigidity. In a recent study [37] shoulder pathology seems to be determined by the postural alteration observed in PD, due to anterior tilt of the scapula, occurring with the increment of thoracic kyphosis. This skeletal modification determines a subacromial impingement, and the rigidity of the shoulder causes further alteration in the posture, and so on.

"Frozen shoulder syndrome" is a common musculoskeletal disorder of idiopathic PD at the origin of long-term pain and physical disability. An ultrasonographic study of PD patients with this syndrome has shown thickness of bicipital effusion and tendon thickness of the subscapularis and supraspinatus, and these manifestations correlated with mean ipsilateral UPDRS III and its tremor, rigidity, and bradykinesia subscores [38]. **Elbow joint** impairment in PD has also been studied in relation to rigidity. Another study [39] has shown that parkinsonian rigidity has variable properties depending on the elbow joint angle, which is detected at the distal phase of elbow extension.

Pain in Parkinson's Disease

Pain in Parkinson's disease is associated with all stages of PD evolution and o is often a troublesome symptom. Even James Parkinson mentioned in the first description of the disease that pain is an early symptom during its evolution [40], and recently, using the King's Parkinson's Disease Pain Scale [41], an increase in frequency and severity of pain has been correlated to the progression of PD, postural instability and gait difficulty motor subtypes, mood alterations, and sleep/fatigue disturbances. In a survey [42] the average prevalence of pain in PD was approximately 40%. In early-stage PD, pain was rated as the most bothersome non-motor symptom, ranked after the three motor symptoms (slowness, tremor, and stiffness), while in advanced PD, pain was perceived as the sixth most troublesome symptom. In a study evaluation of the worldwide prevalence of pain in PD [43], according to different regional reports between 2006 and 2011, prevalence ranged from 40% (Asia) to more than 80% (UK and Norway). At the same time it is surprising that in the most recent practice standards, pain is not mentioned in the treatment guidelines for non-motor symptoms of PD [44]. In a recent review [45] it has been emphasized that in PD, pain is one of the most common and troublesome non-motor symptoms, which can appear at any time during the disease, even before the diagnosis of PD. Due to the different forms of pain described in PD and the different study methodologies used in research, as we shall show in this chapter, there is no consensus on the definition and criteria of pain in PD, and no uniformity in therapeutic recommendations, which are generally based on dopaminergic drugs and opiate analgesics.

The clinical features and topography of pain in PD are not homogenous, so we cannot identify only one type of well-defined pain related to this disease. For example the painful syndromes in 388 consecutive parkinsonian patients of the Lausanne Movement Disorders Registry [46] identified the following subtypes of painful syndromes: 269 (67%) had sensory or painful syndromes; 94% of patients had **muscular pain** (stiffness: 85%; cramps, pseudo-cramps, spasms: 3%; various types of myalgia: 7%); 51% had **osteo-ligamentar "rheumatologic" pain** (articular: 23%; periarticular: 3%; spinal: 31%) while less frequent (8% of patients) the painful syndromes were less defined and had localized neurogenic features (paresthesia: 6%; dysesthesia <1%; burning sensation: 2%; itching <1%; ill-defined discomfort: 6%, and a feeling of local heaviness: 1%). As to the topography, the same registry report shows also a significant variety: segmental (86%), axial (54%), radicular or pseudo-radicular (14%), distal (4%), anorectal and visceral distribution (less frequently); restless legs or akathisia were occasional (10%) while headaches and facial pain were less frequent (1%). This analysis also showed that painful syndromes are found in two-thirds of patients with PD and the most frequent form of pain is of muscular origin, followed by osteo-articular and neurogenic painful syndromes.

Musculoskeletal pain in the setting of PD may result from a combination of factors, including rigidity, arthralgic pain, skeletal deformity, and mechanical factors. One-third of patients experience pain in relation to motor fluctuations; more than one-quarter among these painful syndromes were present at the beginning of the disease and 3% of them resolved during the development of the disease. A very interesting observation was that about one-third (34%) of these cases were clearly linked with motor fluctuations, the majority occurring in the "off" phase, emphasizing the fact that pain is in these cases a secondary manifestation of the clinical features of the disease. Musculoskeletal pain in the setting of PD probably results from a combination of factors, including rigidity, arthralgic pain, skeletal deformity, and mechanical factors, while no correlation with age, gender, duration or stage of disease, levodopa equivalent dose, depression, insomnia, or autonomic dysfunction was obvious.

Based on many such clinical observations, some classifications of painful and unpleasant sensations in PD have been proposed, which more or less overlap. One such classification [47] categorizes pain in PD into the following subtypes: musculoskeletal, radicular/neuropathic, pain related to dystonia, central or primary pain, and akathisia. The musculoskeletal pain may manifest as aching, cramping, arthralgic and myalgic sensations in joints and muscles, and at the physical examination may be accompanied by the usual rheumatologic signs seen in such situations associated and exacerbated by the neurologic signs typical for parkinsonism such as rigidity, stiffness and fluctuations and improvement by levodopa therapy. Radicular and central/primary pain are both subtypes of neuropathic pain (peripheral in the radicular type, and central neuropathic pain in the other). In radicular and peripheral neuropathic pain, distribution is in the territory of one root or nerve, often associated with motor and/or objective sensory signs in the same distribution. Sometimes this type of pain may be determined by a root or nerve entrapment, and the diagnosis has to be completed by standard neuroelectrophysiological examination. The central/primary neuropathic pain in PD is much more complex and it may be subjectively perceived as different forms of sensation: burning, tingling, formication, sometimes relentless and difficult to define in quality, with a different topography than in the case of peripheral neuropathic pain; in other cases the pain may be of a dysautonomic type with different visceral sensations (although internal diagnostic studies reveal no abnormality) as dyspnea, abdominal pain, gastroesophageal reflux and feeling hot and flushed, consistent with non-motor "off" symptoms and has temporal fluctuations related to levodopa therapy, as a non-motor fluctuation, not related to the motor PD signs or a visceral lesion. These features suggest a central dopaminergic dysfunction as its cause and based on this, also the therapeutic symptomatic solutions. Central pain in PD is presumed to be a direct consequence of the disease itself, and not the result of dystonia, rigidity, or a musculoskeletal cause. There are several reports of unusual pain syndromes involving the face, head, pharynx, epigastrium, abdomen, pelvis, rectum, and genitalia – all areas in which painful dystonia or musculoskeletal conditions are unlikely or implausible. Pain of central origin may have a relentless, obsessional, distressing quality that overshadows the patients' other parkinsonian symptoms [48]. The pain accompanying dystonia in PD is explained by forceful muscle contractions and is related to the different times when dystonia may appear in PD patients treated with levodopa: early morning dystonia, off dystonia, biphasic dystonia (beginning-of-dose and end-of-dose), peak-dose dystonia. Very rarely dystonia may also appear as a clinical manifestation of non-treated PD. This type of pain in PD may improve significantly with the dose adjustment of levodopa and the treatment of motor fluctuations, including device-added therapies (such as LCGI pump or apomorphine injections) and the treatment of dystonia itself (with botulinum toxin or subthalamic DBS, if it is the case). Akathisia is also classified by this author in the group of pain syndromes and manifests as a subjective sense of restlessness, often accompanied by an urge to move [49].

A recent proposed classification of non-motor subtypes in PD [50] identified, among six main subtypes, one where the main feature is lower limb pain. This phenotypic subtype has the following features: it is more frequent in males than in females, is present across all age groups in moderate to advanced PD, pain manifests in the anterior proximal aspect of lower limbs and is subjectively described as internal pain, it is not responsive to physiotherapy but it is responsive to opiates, and has no relationship to non-motor fluctuations, but has a high association with non-motor symptoms burden as measured by NMSS. The characterization of this subtype has been facilitated by a recently published validated scale for pain in PD, "King's Parkinson's Disease Pain Scale" [51], allowing the exclusion of secondary pain in PD as far as possible.

In spite of such a great variety of pain subtypes existing within PD, these classifications, based on their clinical descriptions, are quite useful because they allow a practical approach for their management, and this approach has to be done in relation to motor symptoms and clinical neurologic, rheumatologic, and eventually orthopedic examination, but also in relation to dopaminergic treatment [52, 53]. Painful symptoms in PD should be considered in relation to the cardinal symptoms of tremor, rigidity, akinesia, dystonia, and akathisia that occur in PD. It is important to note whether antiparkinsonian medications induce, exacerbate, or relieve PD-associated pain. Pain caused by dystonia can be diagnosed when there is visible twisting, cramping, posturing of the painful extremity or body part. Primary

parkinsonian pain, unrelated to a disturbance in motor function, is presumed to be of central origin, and may be inferred partly by its clinical features, and partly through exclusion of other causes. Painful symptoms tend to worsen in PD patients who are off medication. For many individuals pain sensations occur in strict relation to the motor fluctuations of the disease and are designated non-motor fluctuations. Akathisia, while not painful, is intensely unpleasant, and represents a distinctive symptom that occurs in PD. Painful sensations often have a visceral character, such as abdominal bloating or chest wall tightening; non-motor painful sensations may have an autonomic origin in some patients.

As we may notice, the pathophysiology of painful manifestations in PD may be related to the two main types of pain: nociceptive (which in this disease is directly related to the motor symptoms and the secondary musculoskeletal disorders) and neuropathic (resulting from an abnormal nociceptive information processing, due to lesions on the neural peripheral and central neural structures and pathways related to nociception, in the case of PD also determined by the disease itself or its complications). Previous clinical and neuroimaging studies [54] have reported lowered pain thresholds and abnormal activations of nociceptive areas in PD [55]. Also, it is known that levodopa administration raises pain thresholds and decreases hyperactivation in the nociceptive brain areas, reducing pain perception [56]. The neurophysiology of pain perception in PD is not well understood. From the neurophysiology studies related to pain, we know that this is a very complex sensation which implies more aspects: nociception, pain perception itself, suffering to pain and a reactive pain behavior. These intricate processes are subserved by different neural pathways and structures, which may be subdivided into a lateral pain pathway responsible for nociception transmission and a very complex medial pathway functioning by nociceptive processing at different hierarchical organized neuronal networks implying both ascending and descending pathways in the entire central nervous system, including not only multiple brain cortical areas but also the basal ganglia, more thalamic nuclei, substantia nigra, the limbic system, and many brainstem nuclei [57]. Basal ganglia probably perform an important gating role for nociceptive information within the striatum and limbic system, before this information reaches consciousness, having interconnections with the cortical-basal ganglia-thalamic networks involved in mediating motivation and emotional drive and goal-directed behaviors [47, 58]. In these complex processes dopamine, together with substance P and endogenous opioids modulate the subjective pain perception by increasing the pain threshold, while in the absence of dopaminergic activity pain may be related to widespread abnormal activation of the sensory cortex in response to painful stimuli. Along the same lines, the medial pain pathway is also associated with the autonomic nervous system, which via the limbic system modulates the affective and cognitive responses to pain, explaining the observed autonomic reflexes and affective behavioral responses in these patients [47, 58].

Also non-dopaminergic mechanisms may be implicated in pain perceptions in patients with PD, as some other studies suggest [59, 60, 61, 62]. Glutamate, serotonin, and norepinephrine may also be pain modulators due to their effect on descending pain pathways in relation to the influence of depression on pain perception. In some of the above cited studies there was a significant association between pain and depression scores in these patients. Furthermore, the administration of duloxetine, a selective serotonin and epinephrine reuptake inhibitor, improves central pain in PD. In an anatomical and functional study [63] of persistent pain in PD, associated changes with supraspinal structures have been noticed, in particular, related to frontal, prefrontal, and insular areas in nociceptive modulation and accumbens–hippocampus disconnection.

Some evidence also supports the possibility of peripheral nervous system participation in painful manifestations of PD [64, 65, 66, 67, 68, 69, 70]. Among these potential mechanisms, it was speculated that nociceptor neurodegeneration may be an early pathologic event in PD. Also, some histological evaluations from skin biopsies in these patients have shown evidence of cutaneous denervation at the level of the epidermal nerve fibers and Meissner corpuscles versus control subjects. A decrease in the density of non-myelinated nerve fibers has also been reported in the sural nerves of PD patients [70]. An interesting recent observation is that pain showed a moderate association with nocturnal sleep dysfunction in PD [71] and musculoskeletal pains, in particular, and the best

predictors for this correlation were co-existing depression and anxiety.

Despite the important impact of pain on PD patients' quality of life, there is no specific therapeutic approach for this clinical manifestation in such patients. In an attempt to evaluate a potential therapeutic option, a controlled double blind therapeutic trial has been designed to assess the effect of oxycodone on pain in patients in various stages of PD [69]. A total of 210 patients with various stages of PD have been included, experiencing pain of various causes, who have been screened by a numerical rating scale over the week before randomization and enrolled if they had severe pain. A total of 252 patients were assessed for eligibility, 50 were excluded for a variety of reasons, and a total of 202 patients were randomized to either prolonged-release oxycontin versus placebo, though the authors had planned to enroll a total of 210 patients in various stages of PD experiencing pain due to a variety of causes. An 11-point numerical rating scale was used, commencing on week 1 before randomization. Ninety-three were randomized to oral prolonged-released oxycodone-naloxone versus 109 to placebo and followed for 16 weeks with a primary endpoint of a mean average 24-hours pain score change at 16 weeks. At the end of the study period there was no significant difference between the two groups. However, a post-hoc analysis showed that the percentage of patients with severe pain decreased from baseline to 16 weeks for all pain types in both treatment groups, and this decrease was significant in patients with severe musculoskeletal PD pain (King's Parkinson's Disease Pain Scale domain 1), in whom oxycodone improved pain compared with placebo (p = 0.023). Similar results were seen in the post-hoc analyses for severe nocturnal pain (King's Parkinson's Disease Pain Scale domain 4, p = 0.010). The King's Parkinson's Disease Pain Scale [51] is nowadays an internationally validated reliable scale for grade rating of various phenotypes of pain in PD. This scale has been shown in different studies to be able to explore the distribution of the diverse subtypes of pain in PD and to be associated with health-related quality of life [72].

The different therapeutic observations reported in the literature offer some general therapeutic principles [49, 71], taking into account the pain subtype. Pain associated with levodopa-related dystonia may respond to manipulation of dopaminergic medication. Dopaminergic therapy may also improve musculoskeletal pain related to rigidity and akinesia, as well as akathisia in PD. Botulinum toxin injections can be effective for treatment of painful focal dystonia. Pain and dysesthesia have been reported to improve with subthalamic DBS in a significant number of cases, independent of the motor effect, with a decrease in pain intensity between 40% and over 80%, lasting up to 24 months after surgery [72]. Subthalamic stimulation produced significant improvement of overall pain related to PD in patients with advanced PD, and the efficacy continued for at least 1 year (musculoskeletal pain and dystonic pain responded well to this therapeutic procedure, but patients with back pain – a type of somatic pain – and radicular/peripheral neuropathic pain originating from spinal disease have a potential risk for postoperative deterioration of their pain).

The treatment of presumed central pain in PD is challenging, especially if dopaminergic agents, the first line of therapy for this disabling problem, are not effective, while conventional analgesics, opiates, tricyclics, and atypical neuroleptics, including clozapine, may be helpful. In patients with severe musculoskeletal PD pain and severe nocturnal pain, prolonged oxycodone significantly improved pain compared with placebo (as shown in the PANDA trial). Peripheral nerve blockade does not abolish pain, supporting the notion that parkinsonian pain originates in the central nervous system.

References

1. Gonera EG, van 't Hof M, Berger HJC, van Weel C, Horstink MWIM. Symptoms and duration of the prodromal phase in Parkinson' s disease. Mov Disord 1997; 12(6): 871–876.

2. Goetz CG, Tanner CM, Levy M, Wilson RS, Garron DC. Pain in Parkinson's disease. Mov Disord 1986; 1: 4549.

3. Leibson CL, Maraganore DM, Bower JH, et al. Comorbid conditions associated with Parkinson's disease: a population-based study. Mov Disord 2006; 21(4): 446–455.

4. Ezzatian-Ahar S, Schwarz P, Pedersen SW. Osteoporosis often occurs in Parkinson's disease patients. Ugeskr Laeger 2014; 176(36): V03140145.

5. Park SB, Chung CK, Lee JY, Lee JY, Kim J. Risk factors for vertebral, hip, and femoral fractures among patients with Parkinson's disease: a 5-year follow-up in Korea. J Am Med Dir Assoc 2019; 20 (5): 617–623.

6. Khlebtovsky A, Djaldetti R, Rodity Y, et al. Progression of postural changes in Parkinson's disease: quantitative assessment. J Neurol 2017; 264(4): 675–683.

7. Galbusera F, Bassani T, Stucovitz E, et al. Surgical treatment of spinal disorders in Parkinson's disease. Eur Spine J 2018; 27(Suppl 1): 101–108.

8. Lee CK, Choi SK, Shin DA, et al. Parkinson's disease and the risk of osteoporotic vertebral compression fracture: a nationwide population-based study. Osteoporos Int 2018; 29 (5):1117–1124.

9. Baker JF, McClelland S 3rd, Hart RA, Bess RS. Management of spinal conditions in patients with Parkinson disease. J Am Acad Orthop Surg 2017; 25(8): e157–e165.

10. Srivanitchapoom P, Hallett M. Camptocormia in Parkinson's disease: definition, epidemiology, pathogenesis and treatment modalities. J Neurol Neurosurg Psychiatry 2016; 87(1): 75–85.

11. Lenoir T, Guedj N, Boulu P, Guigui P, Benoist M. Camptocormia: the bent spine syndrome, an update. Eur Spine J 2010; 19: 1229–1237.

12. Wrede A, Margraf NG, Goebel HH, Deuschl G, Schulz-Schaeffer WJ. Myofibrillar disorganization characterizes myopathy of camptocormia in Parkinson's disease. Acta Neuropathol 2012; 123: 419–432.

13. Bouchaud-Chabot A, Sicre J, Bardin Th, Kahn MF. Myosites focales. In: Kahn MF et al. (eds.). L'actualite´ rhumatologique. Expansion scientifique Française; 1996, 55–64.

14. Charpentier P, Dauphin A, Stojkovic T, et al. Maladie de Parkinson, camptocormie et myosite focale paraspinale. Revue Neurologique 2005; 161 (4): 459–463.

15. Cumming W, Weiser R, Teoh R, Hudgson P, Walton JN. Localized nodular myositis: a clinical and pathological variant of polymyositis. Q J Med 1977; 46(184): 531–546.

16. Heffner R, Armbrustmacher V, Eanle K. Focal myositis. Cancer 1977; 40(1): 301–306.

17. Schulz-Schaeffer WJ. Camptocormia in Parkinson's disease: a muscle disease due to dysregulated proprioceptive polysynaptic reflex arch. Front Aging Neurosci 2016; 8: 128.

18. Schulz-Schaeffer WJ, Margraf NG, Munser S, et al. Effect of neurostimulation on camptocormia in Parkinson's disease depends on symptom duration. Mov Disord 2015; 30(3): 368–372.

19. Margraf NG, Wrede A, Deuschl G, Schulz-Schaeffer WJ. Pathophysiological concepts and

treatment of camptocormia. J Parkinsons Dis 2016; **6**(3): 485–501.

20. Tinazzi M, Geroin C, Gandolfi M, et al. Pisa syndrome in Parkinson's disease: an integrated approach from pathophysiology to management. The pathogenesis of Pisa syndrome in Parkinson's disease. Mov Disord 2016; **31**(12): 1785–1795.

21. Castrioto A, Piscicelli C, Pérennou D, Krack P, Debu B. The pathogenesis of Pisa syndrome in Parkinson's disease. Mov Disord 2014; **29**(9): 1100–1107.

22. Young EH, Kunhyun K, Won-Ho C, et al. Pisa syndrome in Parkinson's disease: pathogenic roles of verticality perception deficits. Sci Rep 2018; **8** (1): 1804.

23. Albanese A, Bhatia K, Bressman SB, et al. Phenomenology and classification of dystonia: a consensus update. Mov Disord 2013; **28**(7): 863–873.

24. Tinazzi M, Juergenson I, Squintani G, et al. Pisa syndrome in Parkinson's disease: an electrophysiological and imaging study. J Neurol 2013; **260**(8): 2138–2148.

25. Doherty KM, van de Warrenburg BP, Peralta MC, et al. Postural deformities in Parkinson's disease. Lancet Neurol 2011; **10**(6): 538–549.

26. Tinazzi M, Fasano A, Geroin C, et al. Italian Pisa Syndrome Study Group. Pisa syndrome in Parkinson disease: an observational multicenter Italian study. Neurology 2015; **85**(20): 1769–1779.

27. Vrtovec T, Pernus F, Likar B. A review of methods for quantitative evaluation of spinal curvature. Eur Spine J 2009; **18**(5): 593–607.

28. Vrtovec T, Pernus F, Likar B. A review of methods for quantitative evaluation of axial vertebral rotation. Eur Spine J 2009; **18**(8): 1079–1090.

29. de Azevedo AKeC, Claudino R, Conceição JS, Swarowsky A, Santos MJd. Anticipatory and compensatory postural adjustments in response to external lateral shoulder perturbations in subjects with Parkinson's disease. PLoS ONE 2016; **11**(5): e0155012.

30. Metta V, Sanchez TC, Padmakumar C. Osteoporosis: a hidden nonmotor face of Parkinson's disease. Int Rev Neurobiol 2017; **134**: 877–890.

31. Choi SM, Kim BC, Jung HJ, . The association of musculoskeletal pain with bone mineral density in patients with Parkinson's disease. Eur Neurol 2017; **77**(3–4): 123–129.

32. Malochet-Guinamand S, Durif F, Thomas T. Parkinson's disease: a risk factor for osteoporosis. Joint Bone Spine 2015; **82**(6):406–410.

33. van den Bos F, Speelman AD, Samson M, et al. Parkinson's disease and osteoporosis. Age Ageing 2013; **42**(2):156–162.

34. Invernizzi M, Carda S, Viscontini GS, Cisari C. Osteoporosis in Parkinson's disease. Parkinsonism Relat Disord 2009; **15**(5): 339–346.

35. Lyell V, Henderson E, Devine M, Gregson C. Assessment and management of fracture risk in patients with Parkinson's disease. Age Ageing 2015; **44**(1): 34–41.

36. Seong-Beom K, Jee-Hoon R, Ji Hyun K, et al. Ultrasonographic findings of shoulder disorders in patients with Parkinson's disease. Mov Dis Volume 2008; **23**(12): 1772–1776.

37. Papalia R, Torre G, Papalia G, et al. Frozen shoulder or shoulder stiffness from Parkinson disease? Musculoskelet Surg 2019; **103**(2): 115–119.

38. Ya-Ting C, Wen-Neng C, Nai-Wen T, et al. Clinical features associated with frozen shoulder syndrome in Parkinson's disease. Parkinsons Dis 2015; **3**: 1–7.

39. Endo T, Hamasaki T, Okuno R, et al. Parkinsonian rigidity shows variable properties depending on the elbow joint angle. Parkinsons Dis 2013: 258374.

40. Parkinson J. *An Essay on the Shaking Palsy.* Sherwood, Neely, Jones; 1817.

41. Rodriguez-Violante M, Alvarado-Bolanos A, Cervantes-Arriaga A, et al. Clinical determinants of Parkinson's disease-associated pain using the King's Parkinson's Disease Pain Scale. Mov Disord Clin Pract 2017; **4**(4): 545–551.

42. Politis M, Wu K, Molloy S, et al. Parkinson's disease symptoms: the patient's perspective. Mov Disord 2010; **25**(11): 1646–1651.

43. Hong-Bo W, Zhen-Xin Z, Han W, et al. Epidemiology and clinical phenomenology for Parkinson's disease with pain and fatigue. Parkinsonism Relat Disord 2012; **18S1**: S222–S225.

44. Zesiewicz TA, Sullivan KL, Arnulf I, et al. Practice parameter: treatment of nonmotor symptoms of Parkinson disease. Report of the Quality Standards Subcommittee of the American Academy of Neurology. Neurology 2010; **74**: 924–931.

45. Antonini A, Tinazzi M, Abbruzzese G, et al. Pain in Parkinson's disease: facts and uncertainties. Eur J Neurol 2018; **25**(7): 917–e69.

46. Giuffrida R, Vingerhoets FJ, Bogousslavsky J, Ghika J. Pain in Parkinson's disease. Rev Neurol 2005; **161**(4): 407–418.

47. Ford B. Pain in Parkinson's disease. Mov Disord 2010; **25**(Suppl 1): S98–S103.

48. Beiske AG, Loge JH, Rønningen A, Svensson E. Pain in Parkinson's disease: prevalence and characteristics. Pain 2009; 141(1–2): 173–177.

49. Ha AD, Jankovic J. Pain in Parkinson's disease. Mov Disord 2012; 27(4): 485–491.

50. Sauerbier A, Jenner P, Todorova A, Chaudhuri KR. Non motor subtypes and Parkinson's disease. Parkinsonism Relat Disord 2015; 22(Suppl 1): S41–S46.

51. Chaudhuri KR, Rizos A, Trenkwalder C, et al. EUROPAR and the IPMDS Non Motor PD Study Group. King's Parkinson's disease pain scale, the first scale for pain in PD: an international validation. Mov Disord 2015; 30: 1623–1631.

52. Rana AQ, Qureshi AR, Rahman L, et al. Association of restless legs syndrome, pain, and mood disorders in Parkinson's disease. Int J Neurosci 2016; 126(2):116–120.

53. Sophie M, Ford B. Management of pain in Parkinson's disease. CNS Drugs 2012; 26(11): 937–948.

54. Schreder EJA, Swaab DF. Pain in dementia. In Aminoff MJ, Boller F, Swaab DF, Cervero F, Jensen T (eds.). Handbook of Clinical Neurology, vol. 81. Elsevier; 2006, 817–829.

55. Haber SN, Calzavara R. The cortico-basal ganglia integrative network: the role of the thalamus. Brain Res Bull 2009; 16(78(2–3): 69–74.

56. Dellapina E, Gerdelat-Mas A, Ory-Magne F, et al. Apomorphine effect on pain threshold in Parkinson's disease: a clinical and positron emission tomography study. Mov Disord 2011; 26(1): 153–157.

57. Fava M. The role of the serotonergic and noradrenergic neurotransmitter systems in the treatment of psychological and physical symptoms of depression. J Clin Psychiatry 2003; 64(Suppl 13): 26–29.

58. Ehrt U, Larsen JP, Aarsland D. Pain and its relationship to depression in Parkinson disease. Am J Geriatr Psychiatry 2009; 17(4): 269–275.

59. Djaldetti R, Yust-Katz S, Kolianov V, Melamed E, Dabby R. The effect of duloxetine on primary pain symptoms in Parkinson disease. Clin Neuropharmacol 2007; 30(4): 201–205.

60. Polli A, Weis L, Biundo R, et al. Anatomical and functional correlates of persistent pain in Parkinson's disease. Mov Disord 2016; 31(12): 1854–1864.

61. Lavreysen H, Dautzenberg FM. Therapeutic potential of group III metabotropic glutamate receptors. Curr Med Chem 2008; 15(7): 671–684.

62. Goudet C, Chapuy E, Alloui A, et al. Group III metabotropic glutamate receptors inhibit hyperalgesia in animal models of inflammation and neuropathic pain. Pain 2008; 137(1): 112–124.

63. Pertovaara A, Wei H. Dual influence of the striatum on neuropathic hypersensitivity. Pain 2008; 137(1): 50–59.

64. Chudler EH, Dong WK. The role of the basal ganglia in nociception and pain. Pain 1995; 60(1): 3–38.

65. Reichling DB, Levine JD. Pain and death: neurodegenerative disease mechanisms in the nociceptor. Ann Neurol 2011; 69(1): 13–21.

66. Nolano M, Provitera V, Estraneo A, et al. Sensory deficit in Parkinson's disease: evidence of a cutaneous denervation. Brain 2008; 131(Pt 7): 1903–1911.

67. Kanda T, Tsukagoshi H, Oda M, Miyamoto K, Tanabe H. Changes of unmyelinated nerve fibers in sural nerve in amyotrophic lateral sclerosis, Parkinson's disease and multiple system atrophy. Acta Neuropathol 1996; 91(2): 145–154.

68. Martinez-Martin P, Rizos AM, Wetmore KB, et al., on behalf of EUROPAR & MDS Non-Motor PD Study Group. Relationship of nocturnal sleep dysfunction and pain subtypes in Parkinson's disease. Mov Disord Clin Prac 2019; 6(1): 57–64.

69. Trenkwalder C, Chaudhuri KR, Martinez-Martin P, et al., PANDA study group. Prolonged-release oxycodone-naloxone for treatment of severe pain in patients with Parkinson's disease (PANDA): a double-blind, randomised, placebo-controlled trial. Lancet Neurol 2015; 14(12): 1161–1170.

70. Martinez-Martin P, Rojo-Abuin JM, Rizos A, et al. on behalf of KPPS, EUROPAR and the IPMDS Non Motor PD Study Group. Distribution and impact on quality of life of the pain modalities assessed by the King's Parkinson's disease pain scale. Parkinsons Dis 2017; 3: 8.

71. Oshima H, Katayama Y, Morishita T, et al. Subthalamic nucleus stimulation for attenuation of pain related to Parkinson disease. J Neurosurg 2012; 116(1): 99–106.

72. Mylius V, Ciampi de Andrade D, Cury RG, et al. Pain in Parkinson's disease: current concepts and a new diagnostic algorithm. Mov Dis Clin Prac 2015; 2(4): 357–364.

Cutaneous Manifestations of Parkinson's Disease

Rivka Inzelberg and Esther Azizi

In neurological clinical practice, Parkinson's disease (PD) is commonly associated with a variety of dermatological disorders, such as seborrheic dermatitis, rosacea, bullous pemphigoid, skin cancer, and melanoma, as well as sweating dysfunction. The recognition, diagnosis, and therapeutic approaches of these characteristic skin disorders affecting PD patients are important for the clinician and may even be life-saving, considering the relatively higher incidence of malignant skin tumors in PD patients.

Cutaneous Manifestations Inherent or Closely Associated with Parkinson's Disease

Seborrheic Dermatitis

Seborrheic dermatitis (SD) is a common chronic inflammatory skin disorder, affecting around 1% to 3% of the general population [1]. The lesions consist of red, well-demarcated papules and plaques appearing in sebum-rich areas, such as the scalp, face, glabella, hairline, eyebrows, nasolabial folds, ears, upper chest, and in skin folds under the arms and groin. A combination of several body regions commonly occurs. The face and scalp are the most affected areas (88% and 70% of patients with SD), followed by the chest (27%), while only 1% to 2 % involve the limbs [2]. SD of the scalp, (seborrhea capitis) is commonly associated with pruritus and dandruff. In patients with SD, the affected skin is sensitive to irritation, and exposure to sun or heat, febrile illnesses, and overly aggressive topical therapy may precipitate flares and dissemination.

Seborrhea in PD was initially described in patients with post-encephalitic and other types of parkinsonism, as shiny and greasy skin. It was further supported by several additional reports.

Recently, large database studies have focused on the SD-PD link. Neurologist-diagnosed PD cases and controls matched for age, gender, and smoking were compared in a large integrated health system database in California [3]. Medically diagnosed SD was either analyzed when occurring prior to index date, defined as the diagnosis date in PD patients (n = 2651), or at an equivalent time point in matched controls (n = 13,255). The prevalence of SD was 4% of PD patients compared to 2.5% of non-PD controls, indicating an increased risk of PD in persons with SD (OR = 1.69, 95% CI 1.36, 2.1; p < 0.001). In patients with PD, seborrheic dermatitis is a common finding, along with seborrhea. Its severity, however, is not correlated with that of the PD [4].

Concerning the timing of SD within the course of PD, SD prevalence increases after PD diagnosis, being more frequent in patients with longer than five years since diagnosis, versus recent diagnosis (OR 2.18, 95% CI 1.08–4.39; p = 0.038) and SD is more common with disease progression [5, 6]. SD risk is also relatively more common in premotor PD, five or more years prior to PD diagnosis (2.1% cases, 1.4% controls, OR = 1.42, 95% CI: 1.05–1.93, p = 0.024) [3].

The etiology of seborrhea in PD is unknown. The inter-relationship of sebum over-secretion, the growth of commensal Malassezia yeasts, and host-immune response play a role [7]. Unlike PD, non-PD controls with SD may have normal sebum production and those with excessive sebum production are often free of SD. In PD-related SD, the amount of sebaceous secretion is higher in men as compared to women, while no such gender difference is seen in SD of non-PD controls [8]. This is also paralleled by the male predilection consistently observed in PD-related SD (OR 1.72, 95% CI 1.03–2.89; p = 0.043) [4, 6, 9], while no male SD preponderance is shown in non-PD populations [9]. The amount of sebum may decrease after the initiation of levodopa [10, 11]. The quantitative reduction of sebum, whenever recorded, could not be related to the degree of neurological improvement [11].

The genus Malassezia consists of lipophilic yeasts that are part of the normal resident skin flora [12]. There is, however, no simple quantitative relationship between yeast number and severity of SD, and unaffected skin may carry a load of organisms similar to SD lesions. The facial immobility of patients with PD might result in a greater accumulation of sebum in the skin, resulting in a permissive effect on the growth of Malassezia [12]. SD may be more common in patients with other causes of immobility, such as cerebrovascular accidents. Sebum accumulation or overproduction in PD patients can facilitate the growth of Malassezia. The number of yeasts however, drops in parallel with the therapeutic benefit of antimycotic agents and rises again when SD relapses.

The role of the growth of Malassezia yeasts and their enzymatic activity in PD-related SD was recently reported [9]. High density of these yeasts and their high phosphatase and lipase activity characterize PD-related SD [9]. Antifungal agents such as Ketoconazole, which may reduce the yeasts' growth and enzymatic activity, are beneficial [7, 9]. A possible pathogenic mechanism proposed in SD pertains to the effect on saturated fatty acids released by the Malassezia lipase, as a kind of "proliferative fuel" for these yeasts. The inflammation seen in SD may be irritant, caused by toxic metabolites, lipase, and reactive oxygen species [12].

Treatment options for non-scalp and scalp SD include topical agents and shampoos that contain antifungal agents (such as Ketoconazole), anti-inflammatory agents, keratolytic agents, and calcineurin inhibitors [13, 14]. Seborrheic dermatitis tends to relapse if a maintenance regimen is not instituted. As Malassezia furfur has a slow proliferation rate, an interval of two to several weeks will pass until relapses appear. The intervals of topical therapy should follow this rhythm [12].

Rosacea

Rosacea is a chronic inflammatory condition, a common facial dermatosis, characterized by persistent facial erythema, edema, papular and pustular rash, telangiectasias and stinging. Epidemiological studies point to a possible link between rosacea and neurodegenerative diseases, namely PD and dementia [15]. Reported by a Danish longitudinal study, among 5,472,745 persons with no rosacea or PD at baseline, followed for 15 years, 68,053 of the participants developed rosacea [16]. The incidence of PD was more than twice as high in the rosacea cohort versus the non-rosacea one (adjusted incidence rate ratio (IRR) of PD 1.71, 95% CI 1.52–1.92). The study also found a two-fold increased risk of PD in persons classified as having ocular rosacea (adjusted IRR 2.03, 95% CI 1.67–2.48) [16]. Another large study also reported significantly more cases of PD in the rosacea cohort (n = 14,647) versus non-rosacea controls (n = 399,383) (OR = 1.39; 95% CI:1.04–1.85) [17].

Since rosacea is an umbrella term for different subtypes, it has been argued that special attention should be given to dissect specific types of rosacea that may be linked to PD [18, 19]. One study showed a relationship to phytomatous rosacea (adjusted IRR 1.43 (95% CI 0.54–3.83; p = 0.50) [19].

Two of the major abnormalities encountered in rosacea are "neurovascular dysregulation" and an "aberrant innate immune response," both of which can lead to cutaneous inflammation [20]. Histopathologic studies of lesional skin found an elevated expression of vascular endothelial growth factor (VEGF), CD31, and the lymphatic endothelial marker D2-40 (podoplanin), implying increased stimulation of vascular and lymphatic endothelial cells [20]. Evidence that an aberrant innate immune response also plays a role in the pathogenesis of rosacea relies on histopathologic studies of papulopustular rosacea (PPR): inflammatory changes were noted to be most pronounced near the bulge region of the pilosebaceous follicle, the site of stem cells whose expression profile overlaps with that of the innate immune system [20].

Demodex mites (folliculorum and brevis) are normally present on the face as commensals, but in rosacea, greater numbers of these mites are detected by skin surface biopsy techniques, or by dermoscopy [21]. It has been suggested that Demodex mites and their associated bacteria upregulate local proteases, thereby potentiating dysregulation of the cutaneous innate immune response [20].

The mechanisms of the association between PD and rosacea are yet speculative. An increase in matrix metalloproteinase (MMP) activity was proposed to provide a pathogenic link between the two conditions. This hypothesis stems from the fact that increased expression of MMP-1, MMP-3, and MMP-9 has been observed in skin affected by rosacea, while MMP-3 and MMP-9 have also been related to inflammatory processes in neurodegeneration. The upregulation of MMPs may thus represent the common denominator [16, 22]. Genetics may also play an important role in this association. Rosacea patients predominantly have Fitzpatrick skin types I and II [19], while PD also occurs more commonly in persons with fair skin and red hair color [23–26]. Other proposed explanations point to the microbiome–gut–brain axis related to both conditions [19, 27, 28]. A new raised concept is the "immunocompromised cutaneous district," limiting the occurrence of opportunistic skin disorders to a sectional vulnerable skin area [19, 27, 28]. It is questionable whether α-synuclein, which is abundantly deposited in PD skin [29], may contribute to any dysfunction of such an immunocompromised cutaneous district.

To clear inflammatory PPR lesions, or as indefinite maintenance therapy, topical application of either Metronidazole (0.75–1% gel or cream), 5% Sulfur cream, 2% Erythromycin solution, 1% Clindamycin combined with 5% Benzoyl Peroxide lotion may be used.

Many patients with moderate and severe PPR require repeated short-term courses of systemic antibiotic therapy (i.e. Doxycycline or Azithromycin). Some patients may remain clear of inflammatory lesions even when a single dose of an oral antibiotic is taken every other day and then relapse if the drug is discontinued. For more resistant chronic conditions, topical 1% Ivermectin cream, which has anti-inflammatory and antiparasitic properties, is a recently approved treatment for PPR. Topical tretinoin cream, or 1% pimecrolimus cream may provide additional therapeutic benefit. Low-dose isotretinoin and photodynamic therapy are alternative treatment options in patients whose lesions prove resistant to first-line therapies [30].

Skin Conditions Related to Parkinson's Disease Symptoms

Perioral Dermatitis

Perioral dermatitis seen in PD is associated with severe and intractable drooling. The cause of drooling is probably related to diminished swallowing, rather than increased production of saliva. Symptomatic treatments aim either to reduce saliva production (anticholinergics, Botulinum toxin injections, or radiotherapy to the salivary glands), or swallowing exercises to improve the quality and frequency of swallowing [31]. Topical dermacombin cream (Triamcinolone 1 mg, Nystatin 100,000 units, Neomycin base 2.5 mg, Gramycidin 0.25 mg, per g) may provide additional benefit, in case of secondary candidiasis).

Sweating Abnormalities

Sweating dysfunction, in the form of either hyperhidrosis or hypohidrosis, is part of the autonomic dysfunction seen in PD and is often associated with additional autonomic symptoms [7, 32–34]. Abnormal sweating is a common feature affecting 30% to 60% of patients, with hyperhidrosis being almost twice as common than hypohidrosis [7, 32, 34, 35].

Sweating disturbances may be asymmetrical, not related to the side of motor symptoms. They are not correlated with disease severity, but rather with additional autonomic symptoms, mainly urinary frequency and sialorrhea [32]. The timing within daily hours corresponds to off periods or on periods with dyskinesias [32, 36]. Hyperhidrosis is more common in patients with dyskinesias, with no correlation to their duration or severity [32]. Sweating abnormalities are reportedly more common in patients with young onset (<45 years) versus older onset [37]. The onset of excessive sweating within the course of PD may be premotor, appearing two to ten years prior to the onset of motor symptoms [38]. It becomes more common with disease progression [5].

Hyperhidrosis rarely affects the whole body, but rather some areas, mainly the trunk and head [32]. This distribution was proposed to be a compensatory phenomenon subsequent to thermoregulatory dysfunction in the extremities [7, 32, 39].

The mechanisms of abnormal sweating are not well understood. Off period sweating may result from insufficient central dopaminergic stimulation. Indeed, drenching sweats have been related to off periods and low blood levodopa levels [36]. Sweating associated with dyskinesias may be related to excessive physical activity [32]. The contribution of central mechanisms to sweating abnormalities is supported by observations on subthalamic (STN) deep brain stimulation (DBS) surgery. Sweating, even severe hyperhidrosis, occurs intraoperatively during DBS surgery and the exact electrode contact locations to generate and alleviate this phenomenon are still under investigation [40, 41]. Interestingly, complete disappearance of drenching sweats after STN-DBS was described in a patient [42].

The treatment of PD-related abnormal sweating has not been investigated in systematic clinical trials. Adrenergic blockers may be used for dyskinesia-related, rather than off-related sweating, however their efficacy is doubtful [32]. Botulinum toxin injections are helpful for focal, mainly axillary hyperhidrosis in the general population and have not been studied specifically in PD [43].

Iatrogenic Cutaneous Manifestations in Parkinson's Disease

Amantadine-Induced Livedo Reticularis

Livedo reticularis (LR) is an adverse event of Amantadine treatment. Morphologically, it is characterized by a violaceous, patchy, connecting network [44]. LR results from alterations in the blood flow through the cutaneous microvascular system. A cone arrangement of the cutaneous microvasculature underlies this symptom. The blood supply to the skin is through arteriolar networks. Each arteriole supplies a cone-shaped area with a base measuring from 1 to 4 cm across. The arterioles ascend perpendicularly to the skin surface and divide to form a capillary bed at the cutaneous subpapillary surface, while the supplying arteriole is at the center of the capillary bed. The venous drainage is into a subpapillary plexus

at the periphery of the bed. Thus, blood flows (like a fountain) from the central arteriole upwards and returns through the venous plexus at the periphery of the bed. At the edge of the cone, the venous plexus is more prominent and the arterial bed is diminished. Any condition that causes an augmented visibility of the venous plexus (i.e. local heating) can result in LR [44]. Vessel wall pathology and intraluminal obstruction are more likely to result in a patchy distribution of LR, depending on the underlying pathology.

The pathogenesis underlying Amantadine-induced LR is unclear. Amantadine is reported to release catecholamines from peripheral nerve storage sites, thus affecting the microvasculature of the skin [45]. This mechanism may explain the appearance of LR as a skin phenomenon and the lack of systemic vascular pathology with Amantadine use [46].

Amantadine-induced LR occurs mainly in the lower limbs, around the knees, however it may also affect the upper extremities [47, 48]. The incidence of LR during Amantadine exposure is not systematically studied, however may reach 40% of patients exposed to the drug [49–51]. Rarely, ulcers may appear, which typically resolve quickly with discontinuation [52]. LR, however, may persist weeks after Amantadine discontinuation [46, 52]. Uncomplicated LR is not considered an indication for stopping Amantadine [44]. Patient perceptions of LR and especially the presence of upper limb involvement may play significant roles in the decision to stop therapy [48].

Rotigotine Patch-Induced Application Site Reactions

A non-ergot dopamine agonist, Rotigotine is administered to PD patients as transdermal patch for 24-hour application. Its long-lasting effect and the non-invasive non-oral administration are advantageous. Application site contact dermatitis, very likely due to primary irritation, occurs in 20% to 50% of Rotigotine-exposed patients and consists of localized erythematous, swollen, pruritic patches [53–55]. These local contact dermatitis reactions are generally mild and tolerable and may lead to discontinuation of treatment in less than 8% of patients [54]. Less than 3% of exposed patients develop severe skin reactions [55].

The recommended use is to rotate daily the application site (abdomen, thigh, hip, flank, shoulder, or upper arm) and avoid the same site for 14 days [7, 53]. Washing the application site with soap and water, or baby oil, after patch removal, to eliminate any drug or adhesive, may be useful. Alcohol and other solvents (such as nail polish remover) may cause skin irritation and should not be used. Unprotected direct exposure to sunlight should be avoided until the skin heals, because it could lead to post-inflammatory hyperpigmentation [7, 53].

Skin Lesions Induced by Apomorphine Injections and Pump

Subcutaneous injection of the dopamine agonist Apomorphine is a well-established and effective treatment for PD. Due to rapid efficacy, Apomorphine injections provide a suitable option for both predictable and unpredictable off periods. Apomorphine infusion via a subcutaneous pump is indicated for advanced PD which cannot be adequately controlled with oral medication [56, 57].

The subcutaneous injections are usually well tolerated. Injection site skin reactions range from mild pruritic erythema to itchy, painful subcutaneous nodules. Subcutaneous skin nodules may occur in up to 70% of patients exposed to Apomorphine pump [56–58]. Lesions are usually of mild to moderate severity and necrotic ulcers are limited to single case reports [59]. At the pathological level the nodules are associated with panniculitis [13]. The type of panniculitis is diverse, the majority being eosinophilic, others lymphocytic, mixed, or septal [60].

Skin reactions are rarely (<1%) the cause of discontinuation [58]. Expert consensus recommendations comprise the rotation of infusion sites, adjusting delivery at an optimal angle (45–90 degrees), use of Teflon needles, practicing skin hygiene, using emollients at the infusion site, silicone gel dressings, massaging the infusion site (using a spiky rubber massage ball or vibrating device), or applying ultrasound treatment [57]. Ultrasound treatment renders the area suitable for further injections [61]. Lowering the Apomorphine dose may also be helpful since lower concentrations are associated with less common site reactions [57].

Stoma-Related Skin Lesions Associated with Levodopa/Carbidopa Intestinal Gel Administration

Levodopa/carbidopa intestinal gel (LCIG) or Duopa/Duodopa is indicated in advanced PD with fluctuations and troublesome dyskinesias [62–65]. LCIG is administered intrajejunally, through a stoma, by a percutaneous endoscopic gastrostomy (PEG)-jejunostomy (J) tube, which may cause complications. Stoma-related skin lesions include secretion, infection, abdominal cellulitis, peristomal granulation tissue, or decubitus ulcers [62, 66]. Although PEG is considered as a relatively minor surgical procedure, wound infection is the most common complication [67]. Stoma infection is common in 3% to 33% of patients following PEG-J insertion [7, 62–66, 68, 69]. This is mainly in the form of transient local infection, not necessitating discontinuation in the great majority of cases. The rate of treatment discontinuation does not exceed 1% [64, 69]. The main causes of discontinuation are associated with device-related complications and disease progression and not due to any skin lesion [69].

The insertion of a PEG tube is not considered a sterile procedure and patients vulnerable to infection may require antibiotic prophylaxis. These include old persons, those with compromised nutritional intake, immunosuppression, and underlying disease such as malignancy and diabetes [67].

Skin Lesions Induced by Pulse Generators for Deep Brain Stimulation

Deep brain stimulation is a well-established and efficacious treatment for advanced PD with fluctuations. DBS-related skin lesions are associated with implantation of foreign material causing erosions and infections. A review of 8,983 patients who underwent DBS for various indications (not solely PD), reported that infections and skin erosions were the most common hardware-related complications seen in 5.1% of patients exposed [70]. Multiple sites (16.9%) or recurrent infections (7.6%) were also reported. The internal pulse generator (IPG) pocket was the most common site (27.5%), followed by the extension cable at the level of either the post-auricular area or along the extension cable (15.7%), scalp (9.1%), and at the burr hole (intracranial leads entry) (7.5%). The most common pathogen identified from wound culture in PD was *Staphylococcus aureus*, followed by *Staphylococcus epidermidis* [70]. In patients with negative cultures, foreign body reactions should be raised as differential diagnosis [7]. Skin erosions are most commonly seen in the area of the burr–hole cap, at the connection site between the DBS lead and the extension cable, or the area of the IPG socket [71, 72]. Several surgical techniques of improvement have been proposed to prevent erosions, including C-shaped incision with dual floor burr-hole technique, sine-wave-shaped incisions, and isolating the hardware from the skin incision [71–73].

Skin Diseases Epidemiologically Linked to Parkinson's Disease

Bullous Pemphigoid

Bullous pemphigoid (BP) is an autoimmune subepidermal blistering disease that affects older people (>60 years of age) [74]. It is usually a chronic disease, with spontaneous exacerbations and remissions, which may be accompanied by significant morbidity. Many studies point to the relationship between BP and PD [75–79]. A large study conducted in Taiwan focused on comorbidities occurring prior to the diagnosis of BP (3,485 patients with BP, 17,425 matching non-BP controls). PD was significantly more common in the BP cohort versus non-BP controls (OR 3.49; 95% CI 3.05–3.98). A British study comparing 868 BP cases to 3,453 controls reached a similar conclusion concerning PD (OR 3.0; 95% CI 1.8–5.0) [77]. Smaller studies showed a similar increased risk (ranging between two and six times higher) for PD in BP cohorts, versus non-BP controls [77, 78, 80, 81].

Many studies pointed to the relationship between BP and neuropsychiatric conditions, including stroke, dementia, epilepsy, MS, and schizophrenia, even suggesting that about one-third of BP patients have a neurological disorder [74–78]. This is associated with increased mortality rates of BP patients at 1–2–3 years after BP onset (26.7%, 38.4%, and 45.7%, respectively), significantly higher than non-BP controls [82]. In BP cohorts, PD as the cause of death is significantly more common than the cause of death of non-BP controls (OR 1.85, 95% CI 1.15–2.96).

The spectrum of clinical presentations is extremely broad. Characteristically, BP is an intensely pruritic eruption with widespread blister formation. In early stages, or in atypical variants of the disease, only eczematous or urticarial lesions (either localized or generalized) are present, or just excoriations due to intense pruritus. Occasionally, patients present with just pruritus.

The "bullous" stage of BP is characterized by the development of vesicles and bullae on apparently normal or erythematous skin, together with urticarial and infiltrated papules and plaques that occasionally assume an annular or figurate pattern. The blisters are tense, up to 1–4 cm in diameter, contain a clear fluid, and may persist for several days, leaving eroded and crusted areas. Occasionally, the blister fluid becomes blood-tinged.

Diagnosis relies on immunopathological examinations, particularly direct and indirect immunofluorescence microscopy, as well as ELISA for anti-BP180/BP230 autoantibodies [83]. First-line treatment of BP consists of superpotent topical corticosteroids and/or oral corticosteroids. For "extensive" disease, defined by some authors as either >10 new blisters/day, or inflammatory lesions involving a large body surface area, a regimen of oral prednisone at a dose of 0.5–1 mg/kg/day is often recommended. This dose usually controls the disease within 1 or 2 weeks and is then progressively tapered over a period of 6–9 months, or occasionally longer. However, the use of systemic corticosteroids, especially in the elderly, is associated with significant side effects. Second-line adjunctive steroid-sparing therapy consists of Azathioprine, Mycophenolate mofetil, and/or Methotrexate [84].

The mechanisms of the BP-PD relationship are not well understood. BP is an immune-mediated disease that is associated with humoral and cellular IgG autoantibodies directed against two well-characterized self-antigens: BP antigen 180 (BP180, also known as BPAG2 or type XVII collagen) and BP antigen 230 (BP230, also referred to as the epithelial isoform of BPAG1 or BPAG1-e). These two antigens are components of the hemidesmosomes, which are adhesion complexes promoting epithelial-stromal adhesion in the basal membrane of the skin [85–87].

Three major forms of BPAG1 exist. The main central nervous system isoform of BPAG1-a and the muscle isoform of BPAG1-b are highly expressed in the brain and heart, respectively [87]. The epithelial isoform BPAG1-e is only found in the skin; BPAG1-a and BPAG1-b mRNAs are also present in the skin, but at lower levels [87]. It was proposed that because of overlapping expression patterns in the skin and sequence similarities between BPAG1-e and BPAG1-a, immune cross-reactions might exist in BP patients with neurological diseases [86]. A study showed that antibodies in the sera of persons with BP and neurodegenerative disorders could recognize BPAG1 in both the human epidermis and mouse brain. This observation raised the possibility that BPAG1 could act as a shared auto-antigen in both conditions. It is speculated that alterations in the central nervous system in the course of neurodegenerative diseases could expose the neuronal isoform of BPAG1 (BPAG1-n) which is normally protected from antibody recognition. It stabilizes the cytoskeleton of sensory neurons, and damage to neurons may promote its exposure. BPAG1-n is an alternating spliced form of the epithelial BPAG1-e, and they may cross-react. The exposure of BPAG1-n could trigger an immune reaction that, along with the immunological cross-reactions, results in the development of BP [7, 86, 87].

Cutaneous Malignant Melanoma and Non-Melanoma Skin Cancers

The epidemiological link between PD and cutaneous malignant melanoma (CMM) and non-melanoma skin cancer is consistently reported for the last decades (for reviews see [23, 88, 89]. Multiple recent meta-analyses show that CMM rates in PD cohorts are 1.3 to 2.1 times higher than expected in the general population [24, 90, 91]. The risk for CMM is higher after the diagnosis of PD, rather than before [91]. The CMM-PD co-occurrence is also reported for first- and second-degree relatives of PD and CMM patients [92–94]. Inversely, in a melanoma cohort, a study showed an increased frequency of substantia nigra hyperechogenicity and prodromal motor and non-motor features of PD [95].

Non-melanoma skin cancers also occur significantly more in PD cohorts than non-PD controls, with a relative risk of 1.2 to 2.1 in diverse studies (for review see [89, 96]). An increased risk for cutaneous basal cell carcinoma (cBCC) and not cutaneous squamous cell carcinoma (cSCC), was recently reported [97]. The high rates of CMM and other skin cancers are in contrast with the ample epidemiological evidence reporting low rates of most non-skin cancers in PD [90, 98, 99]. The mechanisms underlying the CMM-PD association are not well understood. The skin and the brain derive from the embryonal ectoderm and share the neural crest origin. Dysfunction of melanin-related enzymes, impaired autophagy, and/or genetic predisposition have been implicated [23, 88]. One common denominator to account for the complex tripartite association between hair color, CMM, and PD risk could be the disruptive variants (R alleles) in the *MC1R* gene, encoding for MC1R (melanocortin 1 receptor). Some *MC1R* variants were reported to be associated with PD risk in a few countries, and none in others; CMM risk genes were not found in genotyped PD cohorts (see reviews [23, 88]).

The appearance of phosphorylated α-synuclein in both PD-affected neurons and CMM tissue, and the intersection between genes involved in CMM and PD, suggest the involvement of common pathways in both diseases [23]. At the somatic level, 45% of metastatic CMM samples harbor at least one PD-related gene (*PARK*) mutation and 25% of these tumors, multiple *PARK* mutations [100]. At the germline level, inactivating *PARK2* mutations are more frequent in CMM cases than in CMM-free controls (OR=3.95; 95% CI 1.34–15.75) [101]. *PARK2* was also found to be associated significantly with cSCC in a GWAS study [102]. In PD patients of Ashkenazi Jewish ancestry, the most common *PARK* germline mutation is in *PARK8* (also named *LRRK2*) [103]. The *PARK8*G2019S mutation was shown to increase the risk of *LRKK2* mutation carriers with PD for some cancers, especially hormone-related ones, but not skin cancers [104–107].

The relationship between levodopa and the risk of developing CMM is debated and a causal relationship is refuted because CMM often occurs in PD before levodopa exposure and a long latency (often decades) is observed between levodopa initiation and CMM (reviewed in [7, 23,

88]). Moreover, a meta-analysis was not able to evaluate the PD-CMM association with levodopa use because of the limited number of observational or cohort studies that focused on it [91]. Still, the current European Commission's Electronic Medicines Compendium states malignant melanoma as a contraindication for levodopa therapy [108]. In daily practice, medicine is personalized and it is recommended to decide on a case-by-case basis [7]. In any case, PD patients deserve, at least once a year, whole body skin examination by a qualified dermatologist, for early detection and treatment of precancerous lesions (i.e. solar keratosis), skin cancers (cBCC/cSCC), and melanoma, a life-saving procedure.

Conclusions and Future Directions

Antemortem tissue diagnosis of α-synuclein deposits is an important focus of research for PD diagnosis. The fact that α-synuclein exists in peripheral tissues, such as the skin, salivary glands, and gastrointestinal mucosa presents opportunities for biopsy. However, the significant overlap between normal aging and PD limits diagnostic value. Of all biopsied tissues, the skin presents the best specificity profile [29]. A recent meta-analysis based on 41 case-control studies showed that anti-phosphorylated-α-synuclein antibodies have higher sensitivity 0.76 (0.69–0.82) and specificity 1 (0.98–1) versus anti-native-α-synuclein antibodies (sensitivity 0.76 (0.60–0.89); specificity 0.60 (0.43–0.74)) [29]. The location of the biopsied area, the value of multiple sites, and the standardization of immunostaining methods may increase the diagnostic value for PD and the differential diagnosis versus other types of Parkinsonism.

Systematic studies of cutaneous manifestations in PD cohorts are currently sparse. The rate of pro-active dermatological follow-up for PD patients is unknown. In Brazil, 50% of the 386 interviewed PD patients have never visited a dermatologist [6]. The spectrum of lesions comprised pigmented nevi (36.3%), seborrheic dermatitis (16.5%), rosacea (15%), BP (2%), and malignant skin neoplasms, confirmed by biopsy (2.8%). Since PD patients present a wide spectrum of skin disorders, appearing from the preclinical/premotor stage to late in the disease course, documentation of skin lesions in PD cohorts, as well as in persons at risk, such as asymptomatic mutation carriers, will be informative. Dermatological follow-up should be an integrated part of PD treatment. PD patients should be informed about their higher skin cancer risk and educated for prevention methods. These concepts require educational programs for neurologists, family physicians, dermatologists, and patients.

References

1. Ravn AH, Thyssen JP, Egeberg A. Skin disorders in Parkinson's disease: potential biomarkers and risk factors. Clin Cosmet Investig Dermatol 2017; **10**: 87–92.

2. Peyri J, Lleonart M, Grupo espanol del Estudio S. Clinical and therapeutic profile and quality of life of patients with seborrheic dermatitis. Actas Dermosifiliogr 2007; **98**(7): 476–482.

3. Tanner C, Albers K, Goldman S, et al. Seborrheic dermatitis and risk of future Parkinson's disease (PD) (S42.001). Neurology 2012; **78**(Suppl 1): S42.001–S42.

4. Martignoni E, Godi L, Pacchetti C, et al. Is seborrhea a sign of autonomic impairment in Parkinson's disease? J Neural Transm 1997; **104** (11–12): 1295–1304.

5. Antonini A, Barone P, Marconi R, et al. The progression of non-motor symptoms in Parkinson's disease and their contribution to motor disability and quality of life. J Neurol 2012; **259**(12): 2621–2631.

6. Antunes I, Purim KSM, Grande LL, et al. Dermatoses in parkinsonism: the importance of multidisciplinary follow-up. Rev Assoc Med Bras (1992) 2019; **65**(6): 791–795.

7. Skorvanek M, Bhatia KP. The skin and Parkinson's disease: review of clinical, diagnostic, and therapeutic issues. Mov Disord Clin Pract 2017; **4** (1): 21–31.

8. Fischer M, Gemende I, Marsch WC, Fischer PA. Skin function and skin disorders in Parkinson's disease. J Neural Transm 2001; **108**(2): 205–213.

9. Arsic Arsenijevic VS, Milobratovic D, Barac AM, et al. A laboratory-based study on patients with Parkinson's disease and seborrheic dermatitis: the presence and density of Malassezia yeasts, their different species and enzymes production. BMC Dermatology 2014; **14**(1): 5.

10. Burton JL, Shuster S. Effect of L-dopa on seborrhoea of parkinsonism. Lancet 1970; **2**(7662): 19–20.

11. Kohn SR, Pochi PE, Strauss JS, et al. Sebaceous gland secretion in Parkinson's disease during L-dopa treatment. J Invest Dermatol 1973; **60**(3): 134–136.

12. Reider N, Fritsch PO. Other eczematous eruptions. In: Bolognia JL SJ, Cerroni L, (eds.). *Dermatology*, 4th ed. Elsevier; 2018, 228–41.

13. Gregory R, Miller S. Parkinson's disease and the skin. Pract Neurol 2015; **15**(4): 246–249.

14. Gary G. Optimizing treatment approaches in seborrheic dermatitis. J Clin Aesthet Dermatol 2013; **6**(2): 44–49.

15. Vera N, Patel NU, Seminario-Vidal L. Rosacea comorbidities. Dermatol Clin 2018; **36**(2): 115–122.

16. Egeberg A, Hansen PR, Gislason GH, Thyssen JP. Exploring the association between rosacea and Parkinson disease: a Danish nationwide cohort study. JAMA Neurol 2016; **73**(5): 529–534.

17. Mathieu RJ, Guido N, Ibler E, et al. Rosacea and subsequent diagnosis for Parkinson's disease: a large, urban, single center, US patient population retrospective study. J Eur Acad Dermatol Venereol 2018; **32**(4): e141–e144.

18. He A, Sweren RJ, Kwatra SG. Association between rosacea and Parkinson disease. JAMA Neurol 2016; **73**(9): 1158–1159.

19. Egeberg A, Thyssen JP. Association between rosacea and Parkinson disease-reply. JAMA Neurol 2016; **73**(9): 1159–1160.

20. Powell FC, Raghallaigh SN. Rosacea and related disorders. In: Bolognia JL SJ, Cerroni L, (eds.). *Dermatology*, 4th ed. Elsevier; 2018, 604–614e1.

21. Segal R, Mimouni D, Feuerman H, Pagovitz O, David M. Dermoscopy as a diagnostic tool in demodicidosis. Int J Dermatol 2010; **49**(9): 1018–1023.

22. Wood H. Parkinson disease: new evidence for a pathogenic link between rosacea and Parkinson disease. Nat Rev Neurol 2016; **12**(5): 250–251.

23. Inzelberg R, Flash S, Friedman E, Azizi E. Cutaneous malignant melanoma and Parkinson disease: common pathways? Ann Neurol 2016; **80**(6): 811–820.

24. Liu R, Gao X, Lu Y, Chen H. Meta-analysis of the relationship between Parkinson disease and melanoma. Neurology 2011; **76**(23): 2002–2009.

25. Gao X, Simon KC, Han J, Schwarzschild MA, Ascherio A. Genetic determinants of hair color and Parkinson's disease risk. Ann Neurol 2009; **65**(1): 76–82.

26. Herrero Hernandez E. Pigmentation genes link Parkinson's disease to melanoma, opening a window on both etiologies. Med Hypotheses 2009; **72**(3): 280–284.

27. Alexoudi A, Alexoudi I, Gatzonis S. Parkinson's disease pathogenesis, evolution and alternative pathways: a review. Rev Neurol 2018; **174**(10): 699–704.

28. Alexoudi A, Alexoudi I, Gatzonis S. Association between rosacea and Parkinson disease. JAMA Neurol 2016; **73**(9): 1159.

29. Tsukita K, Sakamaki-Tsukita H, Tanaka K, Suenaga T, Takahashi R. Value of in vivo alpha-synuclein deposits in Parkinson's disease: a systematic review and meta-analysis. Mov Disord 2019; **34**(10): 1452–1463.

30. Taieb A, Ortonne JP, Ruzicka T, et al. Superiority of ivermectin 1% cream over metronidazole 0.75% cream in treating inflammatory lesions of rosacea: a randomized, investigator-blinded trial. Br J Dermatol 2015; **172**(4): 1103–1110.

31. Bloem BR, Kalf JG, van de Kerkhof PC, Zwarts MJ. Debilitating consequences of drooling. J Neurol 2009; **256**(8): 1382–1383.

32. Swinn L, Schrag A, Viswanathan R, et al. Sweating dysfunction in Parkinson's disease. Mov Disord 2003; **18**(12): 1459–1463.

33. De Pablo-Fernandez E, Tur C, Revesz T, et al. Association of autonomic dysfunction with disease progression and survival in Parkinson disease. JAMA Neurol 2017; **74**(8): 970–976.

34. Hirayama M. Sweating dysfunctions in Parkinson's disease. J Neurol 2006; **253**(Suppl 7): VII42–47.

35. Mano Y, Nakamuro T, Takayanagi T, Mayer RF. Sweat function in Parkinson's disease. J Neurol 1994; **241**(10): 573–576.

36. Sage JI, Mark MH. Drenching sweats as an off phenomenon in Parkinson's disease: treatment and relation to plasma levodopa profile. Ann Neurol 1995; **37**(1): 120–122.

37. Spica V, Pekmezovic T, Svetel M, Kostic VS. Prevalence of non-motor symptoms in young-onset versus late-onset Parkinson's disease. J Neurol. 2013; **260**(1): 131–137.

38. Pont-Sunyer C, Hotter A, Gaig C, et al. The onset of nonmotor symptoms in Parkinson's disease (the ONSET PD study). Mov Disord 2015; **30**(2): 229–237.

39. Schestatsky P, Valls-Sole J, Ehlers JA, Rieder CR, Gomes I. Hyperhidrosis in Parkinson's disease. Mov Disord 2006; **21**(10): 1744–1748.

40. Yang C, Qiu Y, Wu X, et al. Analysis of contact position for subthalamic nucleus deep brain stimulation-induced hyperhidrosis. Parkinson's Dis 2019; **2019**: 8180123.

41. Ramirez-Zamora A, Smith H, Youn Y, et al. Hyperhidrosis associated with subthalamic deep brain stimulation in Parkinson's disease: insights

into central autonomic functional anatomy. J Neurol Sci 2016; **366**: 59–64.

42. Sanghera MK, Ward C, Stewart RM, et al. Alleviation of drenching sweats following subthalamic deep brain stimulation in a patient with Parkinson's disease – a case report. J Neurol Sci. 2009; **285**(1–2): 246–249.

43. Naumann M, Dressler D, Hallett M, et al. Evidence-based review and assessment of botulinum neurotoxin for the treatment of secretory disorders. Toxicon 2013; **67**: 141–152.

44. Gibbs MB, English JC, 3rd, Zirwas MJ. Livedo reticularis: an update. J Am Acad Dermatol 2005; **52**(6): 1009–1019.

45. Grelak RP, Clark R, Stump JM, Vernier VG. Amantadine-dopamine interaction: possible mode of action in Parkinsonism. Science 1970; **169** (3941): 203–204.

46. Sladden MJ, Nicolaou N, Johnston GA, Hutchinson PE. Livedo reticularis induced by amantadine. Br J Dermatol 2003; **149**(3): 656–658.

47. Quaresma MV, Gomes AC, Serruya A, et al. Amantadine-induced livedo reticularis – Case report. An Bras Dermatol 2015; **90**(5): 745–747.

48. Rana AQ, Masroor MS. Patient perception of Levido reticularis due to amantadine. Int J Neurosci 2012; **122**(7): 363–366.

49. Shealy CN, Weeth JB, Mercier D. Livedo reticularis in patients with parkinsonism receiving amantadine. JAMA1970; **212**(9): 1522–1523.

50. Silver DE, Sahs AL. Livedo reticularis in Parkinson's disease patients treated with amantadine hydrochloride. Neurology 1972; **22** (7): 665–669.

51. Vollum DI, Parkes JD, Doyle D. Livedo reticularis during amantadine treatment. Br Med J 1971; **2** (5762): 627–628.

52. Shulman LM, Minagar A, Sharma K, Weiner WJ. Amantadine-induced peripheral neuropathy. Neurology 1999; **53**(8): 1862–1865.

53. Benitez A, Edens H, Fishman J, Moran K, Asgharnejad M. Rotigotine transdermal system: developing continuous dopaminergic delivery to treat Parkinson's disease and restless legs syndrome. Ann N Y Acad Sci 2014; **1329**: 45–66.

54. Sprenger FS, Seppi K, Poewe W. Drug safety evaluation of rotigotine. Expert Opin Drug Saf 2012; **11**(3): 503–512.

55. Sanford M, Scott LJ. Rotigotine transdermal patch: a review of its use in the treatment of Parkinson's disease. CNS Drugs 2011; **25**(8): 699–719.

56. Carbone F, Djamshidian A, Seppi K, Poewe W. Apomorphine for Parkinson's disease: efficacy and safety of current and new formulations. CNS Drugs 2019; **33**(9): 905–918.

57. Trenkwalder C, Chaudhuri KR, Garcia Ruiz PJ, et al. Expert Consensus Group report on the use of apomorphine in the treatment of Parkinson's disease – clinical practice recommendations. Parkinsonism Relat Disord 2015; **21**(9): 1023–1030.

58. Deleu D, Hanssens Y, Northway MG. Subcutaneous apomorphine: an evidence-based review of its use in Parkinson's disease. Drugs Aging 2004; **21**(11): 687–709.

59. Wojtecki L, Sudmeyer M, Schnitzler A. Multiple subcutaneous abscesses and necroses due to apomorphine pump treatment. Parkinsonism Relat Disord 2012; **18**(8): 1002.

60. Acland KM, Churchyard A, Fletcher CL, et al. Panniculitis in association with apomorphine infusion. Br J Dermatol 1998; **138**(3): 480–482.

61. Poltawski L, Edwards H, Todd A, et al. Ultrasound treatment of cutaneous side-effects of infused apomorphine: a randomized controlled pilot study. Mov Disord 2009; **24**(1): 115–118.

62. Fernandez HH, Standaert DG, Hauser RA, et al. Levodopa-carbidopa intestinal gel in advanced Parkinson's disease: final 12-month, open-label results. Mov Disord 2015; **30**(4): 500–509.

63. Olanow CW, Kieburtz K, Odin P, et al. Continuous intrajejunal infusion of levodopa-carbidopa intestinal gel for patients with advanced Parkinson's disease: a randomised, controlled, double-blind, double-dummy study. Lancet Neurol 2014; **13**(2): 141–149.

64. Devos D, French DSG. Patient profile, indications, efficacy and safety of duodenal levodopa infusion in advanced Parkinson's disease. Mov Disord 2009; **24**(7): 993–1000.

65. Antonini A, Fung VS, Boyd JT, et al. Effect of levodopa-carbidopa intestinal gel on dyskinesia in advanced Parkinson's disease patients. Mov Disord 2016; **31**(4): 530–537.

66. Saddi MV, Sarchioto M, Serra G, et al. Percutaneous endoscopic transgastric jejunostomy (PEG-J) tube placement for levodopa-carbidopa intrajejunal gel therapy in the interventional radiology suite: a long-term follow-up. Mov Disord Clin Pract 2018; **5**(2): 191–194.

67. Lucendo AJ, Friginal-Ruiz AB. Percutaneous endoscopic gastrostomy: an update on its indications, management, complications, and care. Rev Esp Enferm Dig 2014; **106**(8): 529–539.

68. Buongiorno M, Antonelli F, Camara A, et al. Long-term response to continuous duodenal

infusion of levodopa/carbidopa gel in patients with advanced Parkinson disease: the Barcelona registry. Parkinsonism Relat Disord 2015; **21**(8): 871–876.

69. Sensi M, Cossu G, Mancini F, et al. Which patients discontinue? Issues on levodopa/carbidopa intestinal gel treatment: Italian multicentre survey of 905 patients with long-term follow-up. Parkinsonism Relat Disord 2017; **38**: 90–92.

70. Jitkritsadakul O, Bhidayasiri R, Kalia SK, et al. Systematic review of hardware-related complications of deep brain stimulation: do new indications pose an increased risk? Brain Stimul 2017; **10**(5): 967–976.

71. Park YS, Kang JH, Kim HY, et al. A combination procedure with double C-shaped skin incision and dual-floor burr hole method to prevent skin erosion on the scalp and reduce postoperative skin complications in deep brain stimulation. Stereotact Funct Neurosurg 2011; **89**(3): 178–184.

72. Falowski SM, Ooi YC, Bakay RA. Long-term evaluation of changes in operative technique and hardware-related complications with deep brain stimulation. Neuromodulation 2015; **18**(8): 670–677.

73. Solmaz B, Tatarli N, Ceylan D, et al. A sine-wave-shaped skin incision for inserting deep-brain stimulators. Acta Neurochir 2014; **156**(8): 1523–1525.

74. Schmidt E, Zillikens D. Pemphigoid diseases. Lancet 2013; **381**(9863): 320–332.

75. Chou PS, Chou TC, Chang CH, Yu S, Lee CH. Chronic eczematous dermatitis in patients with neurodegenerative diseases may be an early marker of bullous pemphigoid. Med Hypotheses 2017; **103**: 86–89.

76. Chen YJ, Wu CY, Lin MW, et al. Comorbidity profiles among patients with bullous pemphigoid: a nationwide population-based study. Br J Dermatol 2011; **165**(3): 593–599.

77. Langan SM, Groves RW, West J. The relationship between neurological disease and bullous pemphigoid: a population-based case-control study. J Invest Dermatol 2011; **131**(3): 631–636.

78. Brick KE, Weaver CH, Savica R, et al. A population-based study of the association between bullous pemphigoid and neurologic disorders. J Am Acad Dermatol 2014; **71**(6): 1191–1197.

79. Foureur N, Descamps V, Lebrun-Vignes B, et al. Bullous pemphigoid in a leg affected with hemiparesia: a possible relation of neurological diseases with bullous pemphigoid? Eur J Dermatol 2001; **11**(3): 230–233.

80. Bastuji-Garin S, Joly P, Lemordant P, et al. Risk factors for bullous pemphigoid in the elderly: a prospective case-control study. J Invest Dermatol 2011; **131**(3): 637–643.

81. Casas-de-la-Asuncion E, Ruano-Ruiz J, Rodriguez-Martin AM, Velez Garcia-Nieto A, Moreno-Gimenez JC. Association between bullous pemphigoid and neurologic diseases: a case-control study. Actas Dermosifiliogr 2014; **105**(9): 860–865.

82. Cai SC, Allen JC, Lim YL, et al. Mortality of bullous pemphigoid in Singapore: risk factors and causes of death in 359 patients seen at the National Skin Centre. Br J Dermatol 2014; **170**(6): 1319–1326.

83. Bernard P, Borradori L. Pemphigoid group. In: Bolognia JL, Schaffer JV, Cerroni L, (eds.). *Dermatology*, 4th ed. Elsevier; 2018, 510–526.e2.

84. Schadt CR, Jackson SM. Glucocorticoids. In: Bolognia JL, Schaffer JV, Cerroni L, (eds.). *Dermatology*, 4th ed. Elsevier; 2018, 2186–2199.

85. Behlim T, Sharma YK, Chaudhari ND, Dash K. Dyshidrosiform pemphigoid with Parkinsonism in a nonagenarian Maharashtrian female. Indian Dermatol Online J 2014; **5**(4): 482–284.

86. Chen J, Li L, Chen J, et al. Sera of elderly bullous pemphigoid patients with associated neurological diseases recognize bullous pemphigoid antigens in the human brain. Gerontology 2011; **57**(3): 211–216.

87. Leung CL, Zheng M, Prater SM, Liem RK. The BPAG1 locus: alternative splicing produces multiple isoforms with distinct cytoskeletal linker domains, including predominant isoforms in neurons and muscles. J Cell Biol 2001; **154**(4): 691–697.

88. Bose A, Petsko GA, Eliezer D. Parkinson's disease and melanoma: co-occurrence and mechanisms. J Parkinsons Dis 2018; **8**(3): 385–398.

89. Inzelberg R, Israeli-Korn SD. The particular relationship between Parkinson's disease and malignancy: a focus on skin cancers. J Neural Transm 2009; **116**(11): 1503–1507.

90. Zhang P, Liu B. Association between Parkinson's disease and risk of cancer: a PRISMA-compliant meta-analysis. ACS Chem Neurosci 2019; **10**(10): 4430–4439.

91. Huang P, Yang XD, Chen SD, Xiao Q. The association between Parkinson's disease and melanoma: a systematic review and meta-analysis. Transl Neurodegener 2015; **4**: 21.

92. Kareus SA, Figueroa KP, Cannon-Albright LA, Pulst SM. Shared predispositions of parkinsonism

and cancer: a population-based pedigree-linked study. Arch Neurol 2012; **69**(12): 1572–1577.

93. Gao X, Simon KC, Han J, Schwarzschild MA, Ascherio A. Family history of melanoma and Parkinson disease risk. Neurology 2009; **73**(16): 1286–1291.

94. Olsen JH, Jorgensen TL, Rugbjerg K, Friis S. Parkinson disease and malignant melanoma in first-degree relatives of patients with early-onset melanoma. Epidemiology 2011; **22**(1): 109–112.

95. Walter U, Heilmann E, Voss J, et al. Frequency and profile of Parkinson's disease prodromi in patients with malignant melanoma. J Neurol Neurosurg Psychiatry 2016; **87**(3): 302–310.

96. Rugbjerg K, Friis S, Lassen CF, Ritz B, Olsen JH. Malignant melanoma, breast cancer and other cancers in patients with Parkinson's disease. Int J Cancer 2012; **131**(8): 1904–1911.

97. Lerman S, Amichai B, Weinstein G, Shalev V, Chodick G. Parkinson's disease, melanoma, and keratinocyte carcinoma: a population-based study. Neuroepidemiology 2018; **50**(3–4): 168–173.

98. Inzelberg R, Jankovic J. Are Parkinson disease patients protected from some but not all cancers? Neurology 2007; **69**(15): 1542–1550.

99. Olsen JH, Friis S, Frederiksen K, et al. Atypical cancer pattern in patients with Parkinson's disease. Br J Cancer 2005; **92**(1): 201–205.

100. Inzelberg R, Samuels Y, Azizi E, et al. Parkinson disease (*PARK*) genes are somatically mutated in cutaneous melanoma. Neurol Genet 2016; **2**(3).

101. Hu HH, Kannengiesser C, Lesage S, et al. PARKIN inactivation links Parkinson's disease to melanoma. J Natl Cancer Inst 2016; **108**(3).

102. Siiskonen SJ, Zhang M, Li WQ, et al. A genome-wide association study of cutaneous squamous cell carcinoma among European descendants. Cancer epidemiology, biomarkers and prevention: a publication of the American Association for Cancer Research, cosponsored by the American Society of Preventive Oncology. 2016; **25**(4): 714–720.

103. Inzelberg R, Hassin-Baer S, Jankovic J. Genetic movement disorders in patients of Jewish ancestry. JAMA Neurol 2014; **71**(12): 1567–1572.

104. Saunders-Pullman R, Barrett MJ, Stanley KM, et al. LRRK2 G2019S mutations are associated with an increased cancer risk in Parkinson disease. Mov Disord 2010; **25**(15): 2536–2541.

105. Agalliu I, San Luciano M, Mirelman A, et al. Higher frequency of certain cancers in LRRK2 G2019S mutation carriers with Parkinson disease: a pooled analysis. JAMA Neurol 2015; **72**(1): 58–65.

106. Inzelberg R, Cohen OS, Aharon-Peretz J, et al. The LRRK2 G2019S mutation is associated with Parkinson disease and concomitant non-skin cancers. Neurology 2012; **78**(11): 781–786.

107. Agalliu I, Ortega RA, Luciano MS, et al. Cancer outcomes among Parkinson's disease patients with leucine rich repeat kinase 2 mutations, idiopathic Parkinson's disease patients, and nonaffected controls. Mov Disord 2019; **34**(9): 1392–1398.

108. European-Commission-Medicines-Compendium. 2017. Levodopa-Carbidopa. www.medicines.org.uk/emc/medicine/9650 [last accessed January 14, 2020].

Chapter 18

Genetics of Non-Motor Symptoms of Parkinson's Disease

Konstantin Senkevich, Roy N. Alcalay, Ziv Gan-Or

Introduction – Genetics in Parkinson's Disease

Parkinson's disease (PD) has long been considered as a prototype of a sporadic disorder with little or no involvement of genetic factors. Three to four decades ago, the typical perception of genetics in PD was that "it appears unlikely that heredity is an important determinant in the development of the disorder" [1]. The discovery of *SNCA* mutations in 1997 [2] started a new era of genetic studies in PD. We now know of at least 90 independent genome-wide association study (GWAS) risk variants in 78 loci that are associated with sporadic PD [3]. Several other genes that are involved in familial, sporadic PD, or atypical forms of familial parkinsonism, have also been identified (Table 18.1).

Probably the two most frequently identified variants linked to PD are variants in *GBA* and *LRRK2*. Variants in *GBA* are found in 5–20% of PD patients [4], and *LRRK2* variants are found in 1–40% of PD patients [5], depending on ethnicity. In addition to the high prevalence of *GBA* variants in PD, this gene is of particular importance since the activity of the enzyme encoded by *GBA*, glucocerebrosidase, is reduced in a subset of patients who do not carry *GBA* variants [6, 7]. Mutations in other genes associated with familial PD, including *SNCA*, *VPS35*, *PRKN*, *PINK1*, and *PARK7*, are probably responsible for a maximum of only 1–2% of PD patients [8], with the latter three genes associated with autosomal recessive PD and found in about 15% of PD patients with age at onset < 50 [9]. The role of some suggested PD-related genes such as *CHCHD2*, *LRP10*, *DNAJC13*, *TMEM230*, and others is still not clear, as there are contradicting results regarding their association with PD [10]. Other genes, despite getting the prefix *PARK*, such as *ATP13A2* (*PARK9*), *PLA2G6* (*PARK14*), and others, are associated with atypical parkinsonism with additional symptoms that clearly distinguish them clinically from PD [11].

In recent years, numerous studies have been focused not only on identifying genes that are associated with risk for PD, but also with its symptoms. Most efforts were put into identifying genetic variants that affect motor symptoms and age at onset [12]. However, with our increased understanding of the importance of non-motor symptoms (NMS) in PD [13], the number of studies aiming to understand the genetic basis of NMS in PD has also been rapidly growing. Studying the different causes of NMS in PD is crucial for the well-being of the patients, as these symptoms often significantly affect the quality of life of the patients, as well as of their caregivers. Therefore, treating these symptoms has been defined as a top priority by the Movement Disorders Society Evidence-Based Medicine Committee [14]. The next sections will focus on the known genetic evidence for different NMS in PD.

Genetics of Sleep Disorders in Parkinson's Disease

Rapid Eye Movement Sleep Behavior Disorder

Rapid eye movement (REM)-sleep behavior disorder (RBD) is defined as a lack of muscle atonia during REM sleep and enactment of dreams [15]. RBD is one of the most important NMS of PD, for several reasons. First, individuals with idiopathic (now also termed "isolated") RBD are highly likely (more than 80% chance) to convert to PD or another synucleinopathy, within 10–12 years on average after the diagnosis of RBD [15]. Second, having RBD before or during PD is a strong risk factor for other NMS, most importantly, cognitive decline and autonomic dysfunction [15]. In recent

Table 18.1 Genes linked to PD, PD phenotype, and atypical parkinsonism

Genes associated with typical PD		Genes associated with PD in GWAS [3]	Genetic loci linked to PD phenotype, but not to PD risk	Genes associated with atypical parkinsonian syndromes
Good evidence	**Requires confirmation**			
Chr. 22q11.2 deletion, GBA, GCH1, LRRK2, PRKN, PARK7, PINK1, SMPD1, SNCA, VPS35	*ARSA, CHCHD2, DNAJC13, LRP10, NUS1, RIC3, TMEM230*	*ASXL3, BAG3, BIN3, BST1, CAB39 L, CAMK2D, CHRNB1, CNTN1, CRHR1, CRLS1, CTSB, CUEDC2, CYLD, DCAF16, DDRGK1, DLG2, DNAH17, DYRK1A, ELOVL7, FAM47E, FAM49B, FBRSL1, FCGR2A, FGD4, FGF20, FYN, GAK, GALC, GBAP1, GCH1, GPNMB, GRN, GXYLT1, HIP1 R, HLA-DRB5, IGSF9B, IP6K2, ITGA8, ITPKB, KANSL1, KCNIP3, KCNS3, KPNA1, KRTCAP2, LINC00174, LINC00693, LRRK2, MAP3K14, MAP4K4, MAPT-AS1, MBNL2, MCCC1, MED12 L, MED13, MEX3 C, MIPOL1, NEK1, NFATC2IP, NMD3, NOD2, NSF, NUCKS1, PAM, PMVK, PRSS3, RAB29, RETREG3, RIMS1, RIT2, RNF141, RPS12, RPS6KL1, SATB1, SCAF11, SCARB2, SEC23IP, SEMA4A, SETD1A, SH3GL2, SIPA1L2, SLC44A4, SNCA, SPPL2B, STK39, SYT17, TMEM163, TMEM175, TRIM40, TXNDC15, UBTF, VAMP4, VPS13 C, WNT3, ZNF608*	*APOE, BDNF COMT*	*ATP13A2, ATP6AP2, DNAJC6, FBXO7, PLA2G6, RAB39B, SYNJ1, VPS13 C*

years, genetic studies have increased our understanding of RBD, and suggested that RBD has a distinct genetic background that only partially overlaps with that of PD and dementia with Lewy bodies (DLB) [16–22].

GBA variants have been consistently associated with risk for RBD [15, 23], and they may also affect the rate of phenoconversion to neurodegenerative diseases [17, 23]. In contrast, PD-causing mutations in *LRRK2* are not associated with the development of RBD; in fact, a protective effect of a *LRRK2* haplotype has been suggested [18]. Fine mapping of the *SNCA* locus demonstrated that while there is an association with RBD at this locus, it is different from the association with PD. In RBD, the association was with 5'-associated *SNCA* variants, while the 3' variant that is associated with increased risk for PD was associated with decreased risk for RBD [22]. A recent study showed that *TMEM175*, which is a potential modifier of *GBA* [16, 24], is also associated with

RBD [16]. Variants in *MAPT* and *APOE* that are associated with risk for PD and DLB, respectively, are not associated with RBD [19, 20]. Larger studies, including direct comparisons using GWAS data, are required to fully delineate the genetic correlation between RBD, PD, and DLB.

Other Sleep Disorders

Overall, sleep-related disorders represent the most common NMS in PD. In addition to RBD, they include periodic leg movement in sleep, restless legs syndrome (RLS), obstructive sleep apnea, circadian sleep-wake cycle disruption, insomnia, fragmentation of sleep, and excessive daytime sleepiness (EDS). Whether these sleep-related disorders are part of the PD pathogenic process is still not clear. Since sleep disorders significantly affect the well-being of PD patients, providing specific and efficient treatments could dramatically improve patients' quality of life.

Restless Legs Syndrome

Restless legs syndrome (RLS) is characterized by an urge to move the legs, typically when going to sleep, usually accompanied by unpleasant sensations. RLS is frequently concomitant with insomnia, may be present in other body parts, and responds to PD medications like dopamine agonist and L-DOPA. GWAS did not demonstrate a similar genetic background between RLS and insomnia. The largest RLS GWAS has identified 12 new loci and confirmed six previously reported loci, with the strongest association at the *MEIS1* locus [25]. Genes linked to synapse formation (*NTNG1*), neuronal specification (*HOXB* cluster family and *MYT1*), axon guidance and synaptogenesis (*SEMA6D*, *PTPRD*), and neurogenesis (*MEIS2*, *TOX3*, *MEIS1*) may play an important role in RLS development [25]. *TOX3* has also been associated with PD, but with the opposite effect (decreased risk in RLS and increased risk in PD) [26]. None of the other RLS genes have been previously associated with PD [27, 28], and there is a negative genetic correlation between GWAS data from RLS and PD [25]. Studies on the prevalence of RLS in PD patients with common genetic variants such as in *GBA*, *LRRK2*, and *SNCA* are lacking. Thus, there is no clear evidence for genetic overlap between PD and RLS, yet they do co-occur. Targeting genes involved in RLS for drug development can therefore help RLS patients with or without PD.

Excessive Daytime Sleepiness

Excessive daytime sleepiness (EDS) affects about 50% of PD patients [29] and up to 20% in the general population [30]. Moreover, EDS in PD may be caused by treatment (e.g. it's a common side effect of different dopamine agonists) and other factors that are not directly related to the PD pathogenic process [31]. A recent GWAS nominated 42 loci associated with EDS, none of them has been previously associated with PD [30]. Several studies examined whether variants in different genes, such as *GBA*, *ALDH2*, *NOD2*, and *KCNS3* are associated with EDS among PD patients [32–35], yet most of them include small sample sizes and require replications.

Insomnia

Insomnia is very common in PD, reported in up to 80% of PD patients [36]. In a recent GWAS of more than one million individuals, 202 risk loci for insomnia have been identified [37]. Further *in silico* analyses highlighted the involvement of specific tissue and cell types, including expression of *SNCA* in the frontal cortex and cerebellar hemisphere [37], suggesting a potential functional link between risk for insomnia and PD. Insomnia and sleep fragmentation have also been described as a common feature in PD patients with the *LRRK2* p.G2019S mutation [5], and variants in the *ADRA2A* and *CTSB* loci were associated with lower risk for insomnia in PD patients [35].

Genetics of Cognitive Decline and Dementia in Parkinson's Disease

There is wide heterogeneity in cognitive function among PD patients. By definition, people with PD do not develop dementia within a year of motor symptoms onset (which is the definition of dementia with Lewy bodies), but cognitive impairment develops and progresses at different rates in the majority of PD patients. In part, this variability may be due to environmental factors, other comorbidities, aging, and the natural course of PD. However, genetic predisposition may also play an important role in the development of cognitive impairment [38].

Familial Parkinson's Disease Genes and Cognition in Parkinson's Disease

Cognitive decline is common in patients with *SNCA* mutations [39] and multiplications, as 56.7% of PD patients with duplications and 73.3% with triplications have developed dementia, with a mean disease duration of 9.7 and 11.3 years, respectively [40]. Common variants in the *SNCA* locus, mainly within the 5' region of *SNCA*, have been associated with cognitive decline and dementia [41, 42]. These *SNCA* 5' region variants are also associated with other synucleinopathies associated with dementia, such as RBD, DLB, and the Lewy body variant of Alzheimer's disease [22].

Two studies that applied a comprehensive neuropsychological battery have shown better cognitive function in *LRRK2*-associated PD compared to sporadic PD [43, 44]. However, other studies that used shorter cognitive tools or tested a smaller number of participants did not identify cognitive differences between carriers and non-carriers of *LRRK2* mutations [45–47]. Nevertheless, only ~20% of all reported *LRRK2*-

PD patients have received a cognitive diagnosis, i.e., mild cognitive impairment or dementia [40].

In one study, out of 25 PD patients with *PRKN* mutations who underwent full cognitive assessment, only three presented with mild cognitive impairment or dementia [40]. Similarly, other studies have reported that cognitive function in *PRKN* mutation carriers is often better than in non-carriers and can remain conserved even after a very long disease duration [48, 49]. These results suggest that cognitive decline and dementia are not common in PD patients with biallelic *PRKN* mutations. Fewer studies examined cognition in *PINK1* mutation carriers. Out of 17 patients with *PINK1* mutations, ten presented with cognitive impairment [40], suggesting that in these patients, cognitive decline may be more common than in *PRKN* patients. However, in both cases, additional studies are required to better estimate the association with dementia and cognition.

GBA

Patients with *GBA* variants have a higher risk for developing cognitive impairment and dementia, as was demonstrated in longitudinal [32, 50] and cross-sectional [51] studies. Further supporting this evidence is the observation that *GBA* mutations are also associated with dementia with Lewy bodies (DLB) [52], and that neuropathological studies of *GBA* mutation carriers show they had cortical Lewy body involvement associated with dementia [53–55]. *GBA* mutations are also associated with RBD [23], which is another strong predictor of dementia in PD [56]. A meta-analysis confirmed an increased risk of cognitive impairment in PD patients bearing *GBA* mutations [57]. The strong association between *GBA* variants and dementia merits closer follow-up on cognition and addressing it early during the disease course.

APOE, COMT, MAPT, and BDNF

The *APOE* ε4 allele is a well-known risk factor for Alzheimer's disease, while *APOE* ε2 is a protective allele [38]. The association between *APOE* ε4 and cognitive impairment in PD has been suggested in some studies, but not all [41, 58, 59]. A meta-analysis has shown that ε3/4 and ε4/4 alleles are associated with increased risk for cognitive impairment in PD [60]. These results were confirmed by a recent, large longitudinal study, where the ε4 allele, but not the ε2 allele, was associated with cognitive decline [35].

The *COMT* gene encodes for catechol-O-methyltransferase, an enzyme responsible for dopamine metabolism. The *COMT* p.V158M polymorphism, which leads to reduced COMT activity and thus higher levels of dopamine, was suggested to affect cognition in PD. However, contradicting results from several studies cast doubt on these associations [58, 61]. A recent meta-analysis revealed a lack of association between intelligence quotient (IQ) score in PD patients and p.V158M, except in subgroup analyses in the Asian population [62].

The *MAPT* gene encodes the microtubule-associated protein tau, which accumulates in Alzheimer's disease and mutated in other tauopathies [63]. The *MAPT* H1 haplotype has been associated with cognitive decline in PD in a few studies [64, 65], but a recent large-scale study did not replicate this association [58]. In patients with early-stage PD, using functional MRI, an association was demonstrated between the *MAPT* H1/H1 genotype and decreased brain activation in the medial temporal and parietal regions during memory tasks and visual-spatial tasks, but no association with the frontostriatal function was found [66, 67].

The *BDNF* gene, encoding for the brain-derived neurotrophic factor, is a ubiquitously expressed nerve growth factor, which is also involved in dopaminergic neurons maintenance. While several studies reported an association between the p.V66M variant and cognitive decline, most of the studies reported a lack of association [68].

Overall, there is convincing evidence for the association of *APOE* genotypes with cognitive decline in PD. However, considering the contradicting results for variants in *COMT*, *MAPT*, and *BDNF*, we cannot conclude whether variants in these genes are associated with cognition in PD. There are several possible explanations for the differences reported by various groups that studied these genes. Differences in potential confounders such as age, disease duration, environmental exposures, and medications may explain some of the discrepancies. Moreover, since each individual may carry different genotypes in each of these genes, as well as other genes, the interaction between multiple genetic factors may affect the results.

Psychiatric Symptoms: Anxiety, Depression, Hallucinations, Impulsive-Compulsive Behaviors

Psychiatric symptoms, along with cognitive impairment, contribute significantly to deterioration in the quality of life and disability in PD patients. Moreover, more than 60% of PD patients may suffer from symptoms of anxiety, depression, hallucinations, apathy, or obsessive-compulsive disorder [69].

Anxiety

Several studies have suggested that anxiety could be more common in *GBA*-PD than in sporadic PD [70, 71], yet other studies did not replicate this association [72, 73]. The severity of anxiety did not differ between patients with *PRKN*-associated PD and sporadic PD [74]. The frequency of anxiety also did not differ between sporadic PD and PD patients with the *LRRK2* p.G2019S mutation [40]. It was suggested that anxiety might be common in *PARK7*-associated PD patients prior to the onset of PD [75]. It is also possible that anxiety is a common feature in *PINK1*-associated PD [76–78]. Altogether, there is insufficient evidence to suggest association of specific genes and genetic variants with anxiety in PD, and much larger studies are necessary.

Depression

The risk for depression may be higher in patients with *GBA*-PD [57], and patients with severe *GBA* mutations (i.e. p.L444P, c.84insG, 370Rec) had more severe depression than carriers of mild *GBA* mutations and non-carriers [79]. Depression is common among carriers of *SNCA* mutations, and almost all reported carriers of *SNCA* triplications had depression [80]. Depression and treatment-associated behavioral disturbances have been reported in 66.7% of *PINK1*-associated PD patients [40]. Contradicting data exist about frequency and severity of depression in *PRKN*-associated PD [40, 81, 82]. Patients with *LRRK2* mutations, compared to sporadic PD, rarely develop depression [40, 43, 45]. Conflicting results on the frequency of depression among carriers of the *VPS35* p.D620N mutation have been

reported [40, 83]. A few studies suggested an association between variants in *BDNF*, *CRY1*, *TEF*, *SLC6A15*, *CNR1*, and *TPH2*, and depression in PD [84–88]. Here too, additional studies are required to conclusively determine the association between genetic variance and depression in PD.

Hallucinations

There is a wide range of PD-associated hallucinations, from hallucinations of different modalities (olfactory, auditory, tactile, gustatory, sensory) to well-structured visual hallucinations. Hallucinations are more common as PD advances and are associated with higher dose of dopaminergic treatment and with cognitive impairment. Hallucinations are more frequent among carriers of *GBA* variants, with higher prevalence in carriers of severe and biallelic *GBA* mutations [79]. Visual hallucinations are common among carriers of *SNCA* mutations and variants in the promotor region [42, 80]. The *APOE* ε4 allele has been associated with increased risk for hallucinations in Alzheimer's disease [89]. However, contradicting data exist on the association of the *APOE* ε4 allele and the risk of hallucinations in PD [90–92]. Studies on variants in *COMT*, *MAPT*, *DRD3*, *DRD4*, and *HTR2A* did not reveal any associations with hallucinations in PD [90, 93]. Contradicting reports exist on the association of polymorphisms in other genes, such as *DAT1*, *DRD2*, *DDC*, *SLC6A4*, *ACE*, *HOMER*, and *CCK* and risk for hallucinations in PD [90, 93].

Impulsive-Compulsive Behaviors

The association between impulse control disorder and PD is well validated; however, it remains unclear if it is caused by medications only (namely dopamine agonists), or by PD pathophysiology even without medication exposure. Carriers of *PRKN* mutations demonstrated a higher frequency of specific impulsive-compulsive behaviors (e.g. compulsive shopping, binge eating, and punding/hobbyism) compared to sporadic PD [94]. In addition, biallelic and heterozygous carriers of *PRKN* mutations without PD had higher obsessive-compulsive rating scores than non-carrier family members [95]. Impulsive-compulsive behaviors were also reported in a few carriers of *PINK1* mutations [96, 97]. Variants encoded by genes involved in dopamine (*DRD1*, *DRD2*, *DRD3*, *DAT1*, *DDC*), serotonin (*HTR2A*, *5HTR2A*), opioid (*OPRK1*, *OPRM1*), and glutamate (*GRIN2B*) metabolism may contribute to the increased risk of impulsive-compulsive behaviors in PD [98]. None of these variants are associated with risk for PD.

Genetics and Other Non-Motor Manifestations of Parkinson's Disease

Olfactory Function

In a recent GWAS, sense of smell was investigated among older adults, and a number of loci were suggested. Post-hoc analysis of genes previously associated with PD found that only the rs76904798 SNP in the *LRRK2* locus was associated with sense of smell in the European-American population [99]. Nevertheless, PD patients with *LRRK2* mutations have a more benign course of the disease and are less prone to develop olfactory dysfunction [100], reported in 49% of patients with the p.G2019S mutation, significantly less than in sporadic PD [100]. Patients with biallelic *PRKN* mutations also have a more preserved olfactory function compared to sporadic PD [101]. Olfactory function seems to be worse among PD patients who carry *GBA* or *SNCA* mutations compared to sporadic PD [39, 102, 103].

Autonomic Dysfunction

Dysfunction of the autonomic nervous system leads to common NMS in PD, including orthostatic hypotension, bladder dysfunction, sexual dysfunction, and constipation. Autonomic dysfunction is more common among carriers of *SNCA* mutations, and essentially all reported carriers of *SNCA* triplications had autonomic dysfunction [80]. There are contradicting data on autonomic dysfunction in *PRKN* mutation carriers, probably due to underpowered studies [82, 104]. A few studies suggested that PD patients with *GBA* mutations are more susceptible to autonomic dysfunction, mainly constipation, orthostatic hypotension, urinary dysfunction, sexual dysfunction [105], and reduced myocardial uptake of MIBG (metaiodobenzylguanidine) [106]. Variants in the *DDC* gene, coding for the

enzyme dopa decarboxylase, and in *SLC22A1*, coding for solute carrier family 22 member 1 protein, may affect the development of orthostatic hypotension due to differences in drug metabolism [107].

Pain

Pain occurs in more than 60% of PD patients and could be categorized into a number of different subtypes (musculoskeletal, dystonic, neuropathic, central, akathisia, and other) [108, 109]. Pain has a major impact on sleep and life quality. In PD patients, the common nonsynonymous p.R1150W variant in the *SCN9A* gene was associated with central and musculoskeletal pain subtypes, and a SNP in the *FAAH* gene was associated with musculoskeletal pain subtype [110, 111]. However, the *SCN9A* p.R1150W variant was not associated with PD in a subsequent study of 225 PD patients with pain syndrome and 193 PD patients without pain [112]. In the same study, the severity of pain was higher in carriers of the p.V158M and the p.A72S alleles in the *COMT* gene [112]. In *GBA*-PD patients, musculoskeletal pain (frozen shoulder syndrome) was reported more frequently as an initial symptom of PD compared to sporadic PD patients [113]. The data on genetic predisposition for pain syndrome in PD is extremely limited and thus cannot be conclusive. Future genetic studies on pain in PD should be longitudinal, include multiple clinical domains, and not be limited to a few SNPs.

Conclusion

The wealth of information on genetic risk factors for PD in the past decades resulted in many genotype-phenotype studies exploring the role of these genes in the natural history of PD. Of all the genes linked to PD risk, the most common and therefore the most studied include *LRRK2*, *GBA*, *SNCA*, and *PRKN* (Table 18.2). *SNCA* and *GBA* are associated with a more rapid cognitive decline than sporadic PD, often accompanied by many other NMS including RBD, autonomic dysfunction, and hyposmia. *PRKN* is associated with a slower cognitive progression, often without hyposmia. *LRRK2* phenotype is quite variable, somewhat milder than sporadic PD, and with a lower frequency of NMS.

Table 18.2 Non-motor symptoms in genetically associated Parkinson's disease

Gene	Cognition	Autonomic function	Olfactory	Sleep	Psychiatric	Others/comments
GBA	Cognitive decline and dementia at higher rates than sporadic PD, faster progression to dementia than in sporadic PD	Probably higher rates of autonomic dysfunction than sporadic PD	Impaired, might be more severe than in sporadic PD	Strong association with RBD	Depression, hallucinations and probably anxiety at higher rates compared to sporadic PD	Possible association with pain as a presenting symptom
LRRK2	Probably less impaired than in sporadic PD	Likely less impaired than in sporadic PD or similarly impaired. Possible reduced occurrence of gastrointestinal dysfunction	Less impaired on average than in sporadic PD.	RBD may be present, but less frequently than in sporadic PD. Protective effect has been suggested.	Anxiety may not differ from sporadic PD. Depression less common compared to sporadic PD	LRRK2 mutations have been associated with higher frequency of cancer compared to sporadic PD
PARK7 (DJ1)	Insufficient data	Insufficient data	Insufficient data	Insufficient data	Anxiety prior to disease onset could be a common feature	
PRKN (Parkin)	In earlier stages cognitive performance is similar to sporadic PD. Compared to sporadic PD, cognition is preserved in advanced PD	Often affected, but less than other EOPD patients	Mostly preserved, compared to sporadic PD	Conflicting data on RBD occurrence, more studies are needed	Similar or lower rate of anxiety and contradictory data on depression compared to sporadic PD. Possible higher rate of impulsive-compulsive behaviors	
PINK1	Cognitive decline and dementia have been reported. Comparison to sporadic PD, adjusted for disease duration, is lacking	Insufficient data	Hyposmia was reported in biallelic and heterozygous carriers	Insufficient data	Anxiety and depression prior to disease onset could be a common feature. Impulse-control issues were reported in a few cases. Possibly associated with psychosis	
SNCA	Associated with cognitive decline and dementia at higher rates than sporadic PD. Triplication > duplications and point mutations	Probably higher rates of autonomic dysfunction than in sporadic PD, especially among triplication carriers	Impaired, probably more than in sporadic PD	Often associated with RBD, usually prior to the onset of PD. Comparison to sporadic PD is not available	Depression is common, as well as visual and auditory hallucinations. Triplication > duplications and point mutations	Often, SNCA and GBA mutation carriers have a similar phenotype

Table 18.2 (cont.)

Gene	Cognition	Autonomic function	Olfactory	Sleep	Psychiatric	Others/comments
VPS35	Several cases with cognitive dysfunction were reported. Comparison to sporadic PD is not available	Several cases with urinary urgency were described. Comparison to sporadic PD is not available	Several cases with olfactory dysfunction were described. Comparison to sporadic PD is not available	Several cases with excessive daytime sleepiness were reported. Comparison to sporadic PD is not available	A few cases with hallucinations were reported. Comparison to sporadic PD is not available	Not enough information to determine any difference in non-motor symptoms compared to sporadic PD

While much data on PD phenotype have been collected in recent years, large longitudinal studies on many NMS are lacking. Clearly, large international collaborations are required to obtain sufficient numbers of mutation carriers. However, epidemiological biases may skew phenotype studies and should be monitored carefully. For example, estimating penetrance based on surveys of familial PD cases may overestimate PD risk. Exclusion of demented patients (who cannot consent to clinical research) may underestimate the phenotype severity. Genotyping healthy volunteers and cohorts of other neurological disorders may expand the phenotype associated with these genes, as was the case with *LRRK2* and *GBA* [114].

Such large-scale studies aimed at identifying genetic factors underlying NMS in PD may lead to a better understanding of the mechanisms involved, and better ability to stratify patients based on their genetic data and their risk for NMS towards future precision medicine.

References

1. Kopin IJ, Markey SP. MPTP toxicity: implications for research in Parkinson's disease. Annu Rev Neurosci 1988; **11**: 81–96.

2. Polymeropoulos MH, et al. Mutation in the alpha-synuclein gene identified in families with Parkinson's disease. Science 1997; **276**(5321): 2045–2047.

3. Nalls MA, et al. Identification of novel risk loci, causal insights, and heritable risk for Parkinson's disease: a meta-analysis of genome-wide association studies. Lancet Neurol 2019; **18**(12): 1091–1102.

4. Gan-Or Z, et al. Differential effects of severe vs mild GBA mutations on Parkinson disease. Neurology 2015; **84**(9): 880–887.

5. Healy DG, et al. Phenotype, genotype, and worldwide genetic penetrance of LRRK2-associated Parkinson's disease: a case-control study. Lancet Neurol 2008; **7**(7): 583–590.

6. Alcalay RN, et al. Glucocerebrosidase activity in Parkinson's disease with and without GBA mutations. Brain 2015; **138**(Pt 9): 2648–2658.

7. Gegg ME, et al. Glucocerebrosidase deficiency in substantia nigra of Parkinson disease brains. Ann Neurol 2012; **72**(3): 455–463.

8. Lesage S, Brice A. Parkinson's disease: from monogenic forms to genetic susceptibility factors. Hum Mol Genet 2009; **18**(R1): R48–R59.

9. Kilarski LL, et al. Systematic review and UK-based study of PARK2 (parkin), PINK1, PARK7 (DJ-1) and LRRK2 in early-onset Parkinson's disease. Mov Disord 2012; **27**(12): 1522–1529.

10. Blauwendraat C, Nalls MA, Singleton AB. The genetic architecture of Parkinson's disease. Lancet Neurol 2019; **19**(2): 170–178.

11. Correia Guedes L, et al. Are genetic and idiopathic forms of Parkinson's disease the same disease? J Neurochem 2020; **152**(5): 515–522.

12. Blauwendraat C, et al. Parkinson's disease age at onset genome-wide association study: defining heritability, genetic loci, and alpha-synuclein mechanisms. Mov Disord 2019; **34**(6): 866–875.

13. Pfeiffer RF. Non-motor symptoms in Parkinson's disease. Parkinsonism Relat Disord 2016; **22** (Suppl 1): S119–S122.

14. Seppi K, et al. Update on treatments for nonmotor symptoms of Parkinson's disease: an evidence-based medicine review. Mov Disord 2019; **34**(2): 180–198.

15. Barber TR, et al. Prodromal parkinsonism and neurodegenerative risk stratification in REM sleep behavior disorder. Sleep 2017; **40**(8).

16. Krohn L, et al. Genetic, structural, and functional evidence link TMEM175 to synucleinopathies. Ann Neurol 2020; **87**(1): 139–153.

17. Honeycutt L, et al. Glucocerebrosidase mutations and phenoconversion of REM sleep behavior disorder to parkinsonism and dementia. Parkinsonism Relat Disord 2019; **65**: 230–233.

18. Ouled Amar Bencheikh B, et al. LRRK2 protective haplotype and full sequencing study in REM sleep behavior disorder. Parkinsonism Relat Disord 2018; **52**: 98–101.

19. Li J, et al. Full sequencing and haplotype analysis of MAPT in Parkinson's disease and rapid eye movement sleep behavior disorder. Mov Disord 2018; **33**(6): 1016–1020.

20. Gan-Or Z, et al. The dementia-associated APOE epsilon4 allele is not associated with rapid eye movement sleep behavior disorder. Neurobiol Aging 2017; **49**: 218.e13–218.e15.

21. Gan-Or Z, et al. The role of the melanoma gene MC1 R in Parkinson disease and REM sleep behavior disorder. Neurobiol Aging 2016; **43**: 180. e7–180.e13.

22. Krohn L, et al. Fine-mapping of SNCA in REM sleep behavior disorder and overt synucleinopathies. Ann Neurol 2020; 2020. doi:10.1002/ana.25687

23. Krohn L, et al. GBA variants in REM sleep behavior disorder: a multicenter study. "Neurology 2020; 95(8):e1008-e1016. doi: 10.1212/WNL.0000000000010042"

24. Blauwendraat C, et al. Genetic modifiers of risk and age at onset in GBA associated Parkinson's disease and Lewy body dementia. Brain 2020; **143**(1): 234–248.

25. Schormair B, et al. Identification of novel risk loci for restless legs syndrome in genome-wide association studies in individuals of European ancestry: a meta-analysis. Lancet Neurol 2017; **16**(11): 898–907.

26. Mohtashami S, et al. TOX3 variants are involved in restless legs syndrome and Parkinson's disease with opposite effects. J Mol Neurosci 2018; **64**(3): 341–345.

27. Alonso-Navarro H, et al. Association between restless legs syndrome and other movement disorders. Neurology 2019; **92**(20): 948–964.

28. Gan-Or Z, et al. Genetic markers of Restless Legs Syndrome in Parkinson disease. Parkinsonism Relat Disord 2015; **21**(6): 582–585.

29. Knie B, et al. Excessive daytime sleepiness in patients with Parkinson's disease. CNS Drugs 2011; **25**(3): 203–212.

30. Wang H, et al. Genome-wide association analysis of self-reported daytime sleepiness identifies 42 loci that suggest biological subtypes. Nat Commun 2019; **10**(1): 3503.

31. Zhu K, van Hilten JJ, Marinus J. Course and risk factors for excessive daytime sleepiness in Parkinson's disease. Parkinsonism Relat Disord 2016; **24**: 34–40.

32. Iwaki H, et al. Genetic risk of Parkinson disease and progression: an analysis of 13 longitudinal cohorts. Neurol Genet 2019; **5**(4): e348.

33. Lin CY, et al. Effect of ALDH2 on sleep disturbances in patients with Parkinson's disease. Sci Rep 2019; **9**(1): 18950.

34. Yeung EYH, Cavanna AE. Sleep attacks in patients with Parkinson's disease on dopaminergic medications: a systematic review. Mov Disord Clin Pract 2014; **1**(4): 307–316.

35. Iwaki H, et al. Genomewide association study of Parkinson's disease clinical biomarkers in 12 longitudinal patients' cohorts. Mov Disord 2019; **34**(12): 1839–1850.

36. Chahine LM, Amara AW, Videnovic A. A systematic review of the literature on disorders of sleep and wakefulness in Parkinson's disease from 2005 to 2015. Sleep Med Rev 2017; **35**: 33–50.

37. Jansen PR, et al. Genome-wide analysis of insomnia in 1,331,010 individuals identifies new risk loci and functional pathways. Nat Genet 2019; **51**(3): 394–403.

38. Fagan ES, Pihlstrom, L. Genetic risk factors for cognitive decline in Parkinson's disease: a review of the literature. Eur J Neurol 2017; **24**(4): 561-e20.

39. Koros C, et al. Selective cognitive impairment and hyposmia in p.A53 T SNCA PD vs typical PD. Neurology 2018; **90**(10): e864–e869.

40. Piredda R, et al. Cognitive and psychiatric symptoms in genetically determined Parkinson's disease: a systematic review. Eur J Neurol 2019; **27**(2): 229–234.

41. Guella I, et al. Alpha-synuclein genetic variability: a biomarker for dementia in Parkinson disease. Ann Neurol 2016; **79**(6): 991–999.

42. Corrado L, et al. The length of SNCA rep1 microsatellite may influence cognitive evolution in Parkinson's disease. Front Neurol 2018; **9**: 213.

43. Alcalay RN, et al. Neuropsychological performance in LRRK2 G2019S carriers with Parkinson's disease. Parkinsonism Relat Disord 2015; **21**(2): 106–110.

44. Srivatsal S, et al. Cognitive profile of LRRK2-related Parkinson's disease. Mov Disord 2015; **30**(5): 728–733.

45. Alcalay RN, et al. Parkinson disease phenotype in Ashkenazi Jews with and without LRRK2 G2019S mutations. Mov Disord 2013; **28**(14): 1966–1971.

46. Alcalay RN, et al. Self-report of cognitive impairment and mini-mental state examination performance in PRKN, LRRK2, and GBA carriers with early onset Parkinson's disease. J Clin Exp Neuropsychol 2010; **32**(7): 775–779.

47. Shanker V, et al. Mood and cognition in leucine-rich repeat kinase 2 G2019S Parkinson's disease. Mov Disord 2011; **26**(10): 1875–1880.

48. Alcalay RN, et al. Cognitive and motor function in long-duration PARKIN-associated Parkinson disease. JAMA Neurol 2014; **71**(1): 62–67.

49. Hassin-Baer S, et al. Phenotype of the 202 adenine deletion in the parkin gene: 40 years of follow-up. Mov Disord 2011; **26**(4): 719–722.

50. Cilia R, et al. Survival and dementia in GBA-associated Parkinson's disease: the mutation matters. Ann Neurol 2016; **80**(5): 662–673.

51. Alcalay RN, et al. Cognitive performance of GBA mutation carriers with early-onset PD: the CORE-PD study. Neurology 2012; **78**(18): 1434–1440.

52. Bras J, et al. Genetic analysis implicates APOE, SNCA and suggests lysosomal dysfunction in the etiology of dementia with Lewy bodies. Hum Mol Genet 2014; **23**(23): 6139–6146.

53. Neumann J, et al. Glucocerebrosidase mutations in clinical and pathologically proven Parkinson's disease. Brain 2009; **132**(Pt 7): 1783–1794.

54. Clark LN, et al. Association of glucocerebrosidase mutations with dementia with lewy bodies. Arch Neurol 2009; **66**(5): 578–583.

55. Wong K, et al. Neuropathology provides clues to the pathophysiology of Gaucher disease. Mol Genet Metab 2004; **82**(3): 192–207.

56. Postuma RB, et al. Parkinson risk in idiopathic REM sleep behavior disorder: preparing for neuroprotective trials. Neurology 2015; **84**(11): 1104–1113.

57. Creese B, et al. Glucocerebrosidase mutations and neuropsychiatric phenotypes in Parkinson's disease and Lewy body dementias: review and meta-analyses. Am J Med Genet B Neuropsychiatr Genet 2018; **177**(2): 232–241.

58. Mata IF, et al. Large-scale exploratory genetic analysis of cognitive impairment in Parkinson's disease. Neurobiol Aging 2017; **56**: 211.e1–211.e7.

59. Pierzchlinska A, et al. The impact of Apolipoprotein E alleles on cognitive performance in patients with Parkinson's disease. Neurol Neurochir Pol 2018; **52**(4): 477–482.

60. Pang S, et al. Meta-analysis of the relationship between the APOE gene and the onset of Parkinson's disease dementia. Parkinsons Dis 2018; 2018: 9497147.

61. Bialecka M, et al. Association of COMT, MTHFR, and SLC19A1(RFC-1) polymorphisms with homocysteine blood levels and cognitive impairment in Parkinson's disease. Pharmacogenet Genomics 2012; **22**(10): 716–724.

62. Tang C, et al. Meta-analysis of the effects of the catechol-O-methyltransferase Val158/108 met polymorphism on Parkinson's disease susceptibility and cognitive dysfunction. Front Genet 2019; **10**: 644.

63. Gao YL, et al. Tau in neurodegenerative disease. Ann Transl Med 2018; **6**(10): 175.

64. Goris A, et al. Tau and alpha-synuclein in susceptibility to, and dementia in, Parkinson's disease. Ann Neurol 2007; **62**(2): 145–153.

65. Seto-Salvia N, et al. Dementia risk in Parkinson disease: disentangling the role of MAPT haplotypes. Arch Neurol 2011; **68**(3): 359–364.

66. Winder-Rhodes SE, et al. Association between MAPT haplotype and memory function in patients with Parkinson's disease and healthy aging individuals. Neurobiol Aging 2015; **36**(3): 1519–1528.

67. Nombela C, et al. Genetic impact on cognition and brain function in newly diagnosed Parkinson's disease: ICICLE-PD study. Brain 2014; **137**(Pt 10): 2743–2758.

68. Shen T, et al. BDNF polymorphism: a review of its diagnostic and clinical relevance in neurodegenerative disorders. Aging Dis 2018; **9**(3): 523–536.

69. Aarsland D, Kramberger MG. Neuropsychiatric symptoms in Parkinson's disease. J Parkinsons Dis 2015; **5**(3): 659–667.

70. Brockmann K, et al. GBA-associated PD presents with nonmotor characteristics. Neurology 2011; **77**(3): 276–280.

71. Swan M, et al. Neuropsychiatric characteristics of GBA-associated Parkinson disease. J Neurol Sci 2016; **370**: 63–69.

72. Malek N, et al. Features of GBA-associated Parkinson's disease at presentation in the UK Tracking Parkinson's study. J Neurol Neurosurg Psychiatry 2018; **89**(7): 702–709.

73. Wang C, et al. Clinical profiles of Parkinson's disease associated with common leucine-rich repeat kinase 2 and glucocerebrosidase genetic variants in Chinese individuals. Neurobiol Aging 2014; **35**(3): 725.e1–725.e6.

74. Song J, et al. Non-motor symptoms in Parkinson's disease patients with Parkin mutations: more depression and less executive dysfunction. J Mol Neurosci 2020; **70**: 246–253.

75. Abou-Sleiman PM, et al. The role of pathogenic DJ-1 mutations in Parkinson's disease. Ann Neurol 2003; **54**(3): 283–286.

76. Ricciardi L, et al. Phenotypic variability of PINK1 expression: 12 years' clinical follow-up of two Italian families. Mov Disord 2014; **29**(12): 1561–1566.

77. Bonifati V, et al. Early-onset parkinsonism associated with PINK1 mutations: frequency, genotypes, and phenotypes. Neurology 2005; **65**(1): 87–95.

78. Ephraty L, et al. Neuropsychiatric and cognitive features in autosomal-recessive early parkinsonism due to PINK1 mutations. Mov Disord 2007; **22**(4): 566–569.

79. Thaler A, et al. Parkinson's disease phenotype is influenced by the severity of the mutations in the GBA gene. Parkinsonism Relat Disord 2018; **55**: 45–49.

80. Kasten M, Klein C. The many faces of alpha-synuclein mutations. Mov Disord 2013; **28**(6): 697–701.

81. Song J, et al. Non-motor symptoms in Parkinson's disease patients with Parkin mutations: more depression and less executive dysfunction. J Mol Neurosci 2020: p. 10.1007/s12031-019-01444-3.

82. Khan NL, et al. Parkin disease: a phenotypic study of a large case series. Brain 2003; **126**(Pt 6): 1279–1292.

83. Struhal W, et al. VPS35 Parkinson's disease phenotype resembles the sporadic disease. J Neural Transm 2014; **121**(7): 755–759.

84. D'Souza T, Rajkumar, AP. Systematic review of genetic variants associated with cognitive impairment and depressive symptoms in Parkinson's disease. Acta Neuropsychiatr 2019; **32**(1): 10–22.

85. Cagni FC, et al. Association of BDNF Val66 MET polymorphism with Parkinson's disease and depression and anxiety symptoms. J Neuropsychiatry Clin Neurosci 2017; **29**(2): 142–147.

86. Zheng J, et al. Association between gene polymorphism and depression in Parkinson's disease: a case-control study. J Neurol Sci 2017; **375**: 231–234.

87. Hua P, et al. Association of Tef polymorphism with depression in Parkinson disease. Mov Disord 2012; **27**(13): 1694–1697.

88. Barrero FJ, et al. Depression in Parkinson's disease is related to a genetic polymorphism of the cannabinoid receptor gene (CNR1). The Pharmacogenomics J 2005; **5**(2): 135–141.

89. Chang J, et al. ApoE ε4 allele is associated with incidental hallucinations and delusions in patients with AD. Neurology 2004; **63**(6): 1105–1107.

90. Lenka A, et al. Genetic substrates of psychosis in patients with Parkinson's disease: a critical review. J Neurol Sci 2016; **364**: 33–41.

91. Papapetropoulos S, et al. Phenotypic associations of tau and ApoE in Parkinson's disease. Neurosci Lett 2007; **414**(2): 141–144.

92. Cormier-Dequaire F, et al. Suggestive association between OPRM1 and impulse control disorders in Parkinson's disease. Mov Disord 2018; **33**(12): 1878–1886.

93. Ffytche DH, et al. The psychosis spectrum in Parkinson disease. Nat Rev Neurol 2017; **13**(2): 81–95.

94. Morgante F, et al. Impulsive-compulsive behaviors in parkin-associated Parkinson disease. Neurology 2016; **87**(14): 1436–1441.

95. Sharp ME, et al. The relationship between obsessive-compulsive symptoms and PARKIN genotype: the CORE-PD study. Mov Disord 2015; **30**(2): 278–283.

96. Ricciardi L, et al. Phenotypic variability of PINK1 expression: 12 years' clinical follow-up of two Italian families. Mov Disord 2014; **29**(12): 1561–1566.

97. Ephraty L, et al. Neuropsychiatric and cognitive features in autosomal-recessive early parkinsonism due to PINK1 mutations. Mov Disord 2007; **22**(4): 566–569.

98. Bhattacharjee S. Impulse control disorders in Parkinson's disease: review of pathophysiology, epidemiology, clinical features, management, and future challenges. Neurol India 2018; **66**(4): 967–975.

99. Dong J, et al. Genome-wide association analysis of the sense of smell in U.S. older adults: identification of novel risk loci in African-Americans and European-Americans. Mol Neurobiol 2017; **54**(10): 8021–8032.

100. Shu L, et al. Clinical heterogeneity among LRRK2 variants in Parkinson's disease: a meta-analysis. Front Aging Neurosci 2018; **10**: 283.

101. Wang Y, et al. Olfaction in Parkin carriers in Chinese patients with Parkinson disease. Brain Behav 2017; **7**(5): e00680.

102. Avenali M, et al. Evolution of prodromal parkinsonian features in a cohort of GBA mutation-positive individuals: a 6-year longitudinal study. J Neurol Neurosurg Psychiatry 2019; **90**(10): 1091–1097.

103. Thaler A, et al. A "dose" effect of mutations in the GBA gene on Parkinson's disease phenotype. Parkinsonism Relat Disord 2017; **36**: 47–51.

104. Kagi G, et al. Nonmotor symptoms in Parkin gene-related parkinsonism. Mov Disord 2010; **25**(9): 1279–1284.

105. Brockmann K, et al. GBA-associated PD presents with nonmotor characteristics. Neurology 2011; **77**(3): 276–280.

106. Li Y, et al. Clinicogenetic study of GBA mutations in patients with familial Parkinson's disease. Neurobiol Aging 2014; **35**(4): 935.e3–8.

107. Redenšek S, et al. Dopaminergic pathway genes influence adverse events related to dopaminergic treatment in Parkinson's disease. Front Pharmacol 2019; **10**: 8.

108. Antonini A, et al. Pain in Parkinson's disease: facts and uncertainties. Eur J Neurol 2018; **25**(7): 917-e69.

109. Ha AD, Jankovic J. Pain in Parkinson's disease. Mov Disord 2012; **27**(4): 485–491.

110. Greenbaum L, et al. Contribution of genetic variants to pain susceptibility in Parkinson disease. Eur J Pain 2012; **16**(9): 1243–1250.

111. Duan G, et al. The effect of SCN9A variation on basal pain sensitivity in the general population: an experimental study in young women. J Pain 2015; **16**(10): 971–980.

112. Lin C-H, et al. Depression and catechol-O-methyltransferase (COMT) genetic variants are associated with pain in Parkinson's disease. Sci Rep 2017; 7(1): 6306.

113. Kresojević N, et al. Presenting symptoms of GBA-related Parkinson's disease. Parkinsonism Relat Disord 2015; 21(7): 804–807.

114. Simuni T, et al. Clinical and dopamine transporter imaging characteristics of non-manifest LRRK2 and GBA mutation carriers in the Parkinson's Progression Markers Initiative (PPMI): a cross-sectional study. Lancet Neurol 2020; 19(1): 71–80.

Chapter 19

Drug-Induced Non-Motor Symptoms in Parkinson's Disease

Camila Aquino

Introduction

People with Parkinson's disease (PD) experience a variety of non-motor symptoms. Many of these non-motor symptoms can appear in the early phases, in still drug-naïve patients. Others tend to develop over time, with prolonged disease duration and exposure to higher doses of dopaminergic therapy [1]. Often, non-motor symptoms fluctuate in response to levodopa similarly to the pattern observed in motor fluctuations [2]. Complex mechanisms underlie the development of PD non-motor symptoms, therefore, the term "drug-induced" used in this chapter does not mean to "blame" the therapy for such complications. Instead, as discussed throughout this chapter, in most cases, the antiparkinsonian therapy simply worsens or triggers specific non-motor symptoms because PD increases patients' susceptibility [3]. With that in mind, a careful evaluation of patients' circumstances, including disease duration, medications, timing of symptom onset in relation to beginning of therapy, and relationship between medication doses and symptoms, is required to understand the contribution of the PD therapy to a given non-motor symptom [4].

Drug–induced non-motor symptoms can affect different domains, such as behavioral and neuropsychiatric, sleep, autonomic and others. Table 19.1 summarizes the non-motor symptoms affecting different domains, and the classes of drugs to which they have been associated. Several of these symptoms have been extensively discussed in other chapters in this book. Herein, we will focus on selected symptoms in each of these domains.

Drug-Induced Behavioral and Neuropsychiatric Symptoms

Parkinson's disease psychosis, impulse control disorders and behaviors, dopamine dysregulation syndrome, and dopamine withdrawal syndrome are the most well-known behavioral/neuropsychiatric symptoms linked to dopaminergic therapy. In this chapter we will cover PD psychosis.

Parkinson's Disease Psychosis

The reported prevalence of PD psychosis has varied according to the methodologies and definitions used [6]. With the inclusion of the less severe, i.e. minor psychotic symptoms in the spectrum of PD psychosis, the prevalence increased from approximately 40% to 60%, with nearly 45% of patients reporting at least one minor symptom, and 42% reporting at least one type of hallucination [7]. PD psychosis is one of the leading reasons for nursing home placement, caregiver burden, and is considered a predictor of mortality, thus being called a sign of poor prognosis in PD patients [8].

Phenomenology of Parkinson's Disease Psychosis

A continuum spectrum of psychotic symptoms has been documented in PD, typically starting with minor psychotic symptoms and subsequently progressing to more complex well-formed visual hallucinations and delusions [9]. In the early phases, illusions or visual misperceptions of stimuli are reported by patients, who usually describe seeing an animal or face in place of an object. Often, a stationary spot or object is noticed as a moving bug or animal. Approximately 50% of patients with PD report a "false sense of presence" of someone else in the environment. Interestingly, most patients with the "presence hallucination" experience a "vivid feeling" that someone is there, but in fact cannot describe details or recognize the person. In some cases, the "passage hallucination" phenomenon is reported, which consists of seeing a moving shadow in the periphery of the visual field [9–11].

Table 19.1 Summary of drug-induced non-motor symptoms in Parkinson's disease

Domain/symptom	Description	Classes of drugs implicated
Behavioral and Neuropsychiatric		
Impulse control disorders	Behaviors that are performed repetitively, excessively, and compulsively to an extent that interferes in major areas of life functioning.	DA, levodopa, amantadine, MAO inhibitors
Dopamine dysregulation syndrome	Addiction-like state marked by self-medication with inappropriately high doses of dopaminergic medications, particularly levodopa and high-potency, short-acting dopamine agonists.	Levodopa, apomorphine
Impulse control behaviors	Repetitive, purposeless behaviors.	DA, levodopa?
Punding Characterized by an intense preoccupation with specific items or activities (e.g. collecting, arranging, or taking apart objects).		
Hobbyism	Higher-level repetitive behaviors (e.g. excessive exercise, Internet use, reading, art work, and work on projects).	DA, levodopa
Hoarding	The acquisition of, and failure to discard, a large number of items with little or no objective value, which, in some cases, can lead to unsafe or unsanitary living conditions.	DA, levodopa
Psychosis	Refers to a spectrum of illusions, hallucinations, and delusions that occur throughout the disease course.	Levodopa, DA, amantadine, anticholinergics
Dopamine agonist withdrawal syndrome	Severe, stereotyped cluster of physical and psychological symptoms that correlate with dopamine agonist withdrawal in a dose-dependent manner, cause clinically significant distress or social/occupational dysfunction.	Withdrawal of DA
Sleep		
Excessive daytime sleepiness	Inappropriate and undesirable sleepiness during waking hours	DA, levodopa
Sleep attacks	Abrupt sleep onset, occurring without warning and non-preceded by sleepiness.	DA
Autonomic		
Orthostatic hypotension	Drop in systolic blood pressure (BP) of ≥ 20 or diastolic ≥ 10 mmHg within 3 minutes of standing.	DA, levodopa, MAO inhibitors
Nausea	Gastric discomfort with a sensation of vomiting often induced by dopaminergic drugs.	Levodopa, DA
Edema	Peripheral edema, especially pedal edema of the subcutaneous tissue, often accompanied by a red coloration of the skin in the area.	Amantadine, DA, levodopa
Cutaneous		
Livedo reticularis	Reticulated vascular pattern that appears as a lace-like purplish discoloration of the skin, most often in the legs.	Amantadine, rasagiline*
Melanoma	Patients with PD are at higher risk for melanoma and this has been one of the most common skin-related adverse events of levodopa trials.	Levodopa
Hypertensive and hyperthermia states		
Parkinsonism-Hyperpyrexia syndrome	Potentially fatal complication after reduction or cessation of levodopa, resembles neuroleptic malignant syndrome.	Withdrawal/reduction of levodopa

213

Table 19.1 (cont.)

Serotonin syndrome	A potentially life-threatening condition associated with increased serotonergic activity that manifests with abnormal level of consciousness, autonomic symptoms (diaphoresis, tachycardia, hyperthermia, hypertension), and neuromuscular hyperactivity (rigidity, myoclonus, hyperreflexia).	MAO inhibitors
Multi-domain		
Non-motor fluctuations	Fluctuations in non-motor symptoms according to dopamine levels.	Levodopa, DA

DA: dopamine agonist; MAO: monoamine oxidase. *One case report [5]

Altogether, these minor symptoms are the most common manifestations of psychosis in patients with PD [7].

Moving along the spectrum of psychotic symptoms, visual hallucinations, consisting of well-formed hallucinations in the absence of visual stimuli, are the most recognized modality of psychosis associated to PD [12]. These develop in the context of an otherwise stable condition and medication regimen, in the absence of delirium or other toxic-metabolic disorders [13]. Patients with visual hallucinations often report seeing "people" or "animals" on a regular basis. The content of such hallucinations is usually stereotyped, to the point that patients become somewhat "familiar" with them. Visual hallucinations are more frequent in the evening, during periods of dim light and silence, when external stimuli are reduced. Most patients have a good understanding that the hallucinations are unreal, at least during the first years of this problem. Over time, this insight is lost, and patients can start to act on their hallucinations. Patients with visual hallucinations with retained insight have been found to have poorer verbal fluency, although other cognitive domains might be relatively intact, whereas the lack of insight is associated with greater cognitive impairment, particularly the posterior cortical scores [14].

Some patients also develop non-visual hallucinations, such as auditory, olfactory, or tactile hallucinations. Interestingly, these tend to be associated with the visual hallucinations, for instance noises that are soundtracks for the visual component, or sensation of bugs on the skin [12]. Usually, at this stage, cognitive impairment is more frequent, but non-visual hallucinations can also occur in people with mild cognitive impairment or relatively intact cognition. Delusion is more common in later stages of PD psychosis and may or may not be associated with cognitive impairment. Studies suggest a different cognitive profile between patients with delusions and visual hallucinations. The content of delusional episodes can be quite complex and usually involves persecution, jealousy, theft, religion, grandiosity, guilt, and misidentification syndromes [9].

Diagnostic Criteria and Rating Scales

Until 2007 a working group from the National Institute of Neurological Disorders and Stroke (NINDS) and National Institute of Mental Health (NIMH) proposed the diagnostic criteria for PD psychosis, which is currently applied in clinical and research settings (Table 19.2).

A major challenge is the assessment of the severity of PD psychosis. In 2008, a task force from the Movement Disorder Society (MDS) compiled the available resources and classified them in "recommended," "suggested," and "listed" according to the level of evidence [16]. The recommended scales included: the Neuropsychiatric Inventory (NPI) [17], the Brief Psychiatric Rating Scale (BPRS), the Schedule for Assessment of Positive Symptoms (SAPS), and the Positive and Negative Syndrome Scale (PANSS) [18]. These scales are not specifically designed for assessment of PD psychosis, therefore, there are limitations to its use [16].

Table 19.2 Diagnostic criteria for Parkinson's disease psychosis [15]

Characteristic symptoms	Presence of at least one of the following symptoms: • Illusions • False sense of presence • Hallucinations • Delusions
Primary diagnosis	UK brain bank criteria for PD
Chronology of the onset of symptoms of psychosis	The symptoms occur after the onset of PD
Duration	The psychotic symptom(s) are recurrent or continuous for 1 month
Exclusion of other causes	The psychotic symptoms are not better accounted for by another cause of Parkinsonism such as dementia with Lewy bodies, psychiatric disorders such as schizophrenia, schizoaffective disorder, delusional disorder, or mood disorder with psychotic features, or a general medical condition including delirium
Associated features	With or without insight With or without dementia With or without treatment for PD (specify drug, surgical, other)

A more general assessment has been done through part I of the MDS Unified PD Rating Scale (MDS-UPDRS) [19], and the Non-Motor Symptoms Scale (NMSS) [20]. More recently, a shortened version of the SAPS has been developed and proposed as an instrument to assess psychosis in PD clinical trials [21].

Pathophysiological Mechanisms

The treatment-related nature of PD psychosis is a matter of debate with contradictory evidence. The current concept is that dopaminergic therapy has a modifier instead of causal effect on psychosis [15]. The fact that PD psychosis can occur in drug-naïve patients, and the lack of correlation between levodopa equivalent daily dose and the risk of psychosis have supported the non-causal relationship between treatment and development of psychosis [12]. On the other hand, some large cohorts have pointed towards an association between initiation of therapy, elevated levodopa or DA dose, higher levodopa equivalence, and the presence of dyskinesia as risk factors for psychosis [22–25].

The potential association between PD psychosis, particularly visual hallucinations and delusions, with distinct cognitive profile has been investigated in several studies. In general, deficits in visual perception, executive function, attention and memory have been documented in patients with visual hallucinations with either PD-MCI or intact cognition [9]. To date, there is no evidence

suggesting significant differences in overall cognitive function or a given cognitive profile in patients with minor hallucinations without dementia [10], however, these minor psychotic symptoms have been correlated with the higher levels of depressive symptoms in patients with PD [11, 26]. Visual hallucinations have been associated with REM sleep behavior disorder, vivid dreams, and mood disorders, especially depression [9].

The pathophysiology of PD psychosis likely involves multiple neurotransmitters and systems beyond the dopaminergic. Two models, the activation-input-modulation, and perception and attention deficit have been proposed. A study with functional MRI found evidence for altered cortical visual processing in PD, with greater frontal and subcortical activation and less visual cortical activation. The serotoninergic system has also been implicated and has been used as a target in drug therapy for PD psychosis. A study found increased serotonin 2A ($5-HT_{2A}$) receptor binding in the inferior temporal cortex of PD patients with visual hallucinations, suggesting enhanced $5-HT_{2A}$-mediated neurotransmission [27]. This has been supported by studies using setoperone F18, a PET ligand to serotonin receptors, in PD patients with visual hallucinations [28, 29]. Finally, it is possible that cholinergic symptoms are also involved due to degeneration of the pedunculopontine nucleus observed in PD patients with visual hallucinations [30].

Management of Parkinson's Disease Psychosis

When psychosis first manifests, it is good practice to rule out changes in health status, such as systemic infection, dehydration, and medication changes. Patients with PD are at high risk for developing psychotic symptoms when started on anticholinergic drugs (sometimes prescribed for overactive bladder), opioids, or certain antibiotics, e.g. ciprofloxacin. Patients with PD can also enter a severe psychotic state in cases of abrupt cessation or reduction of their dopaminergic therapy. In those circumstances, treatment of the underlying condition and/or removal of the triggering factors are recommended whenever possible. Considering that PD drugs are "modifiers" of PD psychosis, the evaluation of patients with PD psychosis includes a careful review of PD therapy. In some cases, discontinuation of anticholinergics or amantadine might be helpful in improving hallucinations and avoiding or postponing the introduction of drug therapy for psychosis.

Three drugs have been considered acceptable for the treatment of PD psychosis, as summarized in a recently published review [31]. In clinical practice, quetiapine has been widely used for management of PD psychosis despite limited evidence. Four limited clinical studies have evaluated the efficacy of quetiapine in comparison to placebo, all with negative results [32–35]. In a study comparing quetiapine to clozapine, both were similarly efficacious, thus the MDS evidence-based committee considered quetiapine as a "possibly useful" drug for the treatment of psychosis in PD [36]. Clozapine has been used for PD hallucinations and delusions based on the evidence from two randomized placebo-controlled trials [37, 38]. Despite the evidence, its use encounters resistance in clinical practice because of the mandatory blood monitoring required due to the risk of agranulocytosis in approximately 1% of exposed patients [39].

Pimavanserin is a selective serotonin 5-HT$_{2A}$ inverse agonist approved by the Food and Drug Administration (FDA) in the United States for treatment of PD psychosis in 2016. Pimavanserin was studied in a six-week randomized placebo-controlled trial and found to be safe and effective in PD patients with psychosis [40]. Previously the drug had been studied in a smaller trial, which suggested a trend to improvement but failed to achieve statistical significance [41]. Since pimavanserin was approved, some post-marketing concerns have been raised regarding safety of the drug, due to risk of prolonged QT interval and increased mortality [42]. However, in general, the adverse event profile appears to be more favorable than antipsychotics in terms of risk of stroke, falls, blood dyscrasia, and orthostatic hypotension [9].

To date, there is no evidence suggesting that early treatment of minor hallucinations will interfere with the course of PD psychosis, therefore, treatment has been reserved for patients who feel disturbed or threatened by the symptoms.

Drug-Induced Sleep Disorders

The sleep disturbances linked to PD have been discussed in Chapter 15. Herein, we will focus on drug-induced excessive daytime sleepiness (EDS) and sleep attacks.

Excessive Daytime Sleepiness

Excessive daytime sleepiness (EDS) is a common problem in individuals with PD and consists of an inappropriate and undesirable sleepiness during waking hours [43]. EDS is associated with negative impact on safety, quality of life, and cognition, for instance with deficits in attention, memory, and judgement. Several studies have documented that the presence of EDS is independent of sleep quality at night, and that it worsens with disease duration and severity, suggesting that intrinsic PD mechanisms predisposes to this problem [44, 45]. Approximately 50% of patients with PD report EDS, with prevalence ranging in studies from 25% to 75% according to the sample characteristics. Sudden sleep attacks are less frequent, occurring in approximately 1% of patients exposed to DA [46].

Phenomenology and Pathophysiological Mechanisms

Excessive daytime sleepiness can manifest in different forms in patients with PD. Most patients will experience gradual sleepiness and a slow drift into sleep. Others will only report excessive fatigue and lack of energy during daytime [47]. On the other hand, a group of individuals will suffer a sudden uncontrollable "sleep attack," which occurs without warning and independent of being sleepy or tired. These sleep attacks have been associated with dopamine agonist (DA) therapy, and have been linked to accidents on the road and at work [48]. Some clinicians have proposed that patients with "sudden sleep attacks" actually do experience somnolence before the attacks, however, they do not recall because of some level of amnesia related to the EDS [44].

There is a lot of debate in the literature regarding the pathophysiology of EDS, with some authors suggesting a drug-induced effect, and others suggesting that the hypodopaminergic state and the dysfunction of brainstem ascending arousal systems seen in PD are responsible for the "hypoactive" state [48]. A study from the PPMI cohort found that EDS was associated with non-tremor dominant phenotype, autonomic dysfunction, depression, anxiety and behavior disorders, but not with cognitive dysfunction or severity of motor symptoms [49].The incidence of EDS rises proportionally to the dose of dopaminergic therapy, particularly with ergoline and non-ergoline DA [50]. Studies with polysomnography also demonstrate a correlation between dopaminergic therapy dose and EDS [43]. Sleep attacks, however, have been more strongly linked to DA. It is important to take into account that individuals with PD are usually on a polypharmacy regimen, and other drugs such as antidepressants, anxiolytics, and hypnotics may contribute to EDS. Also, co-morbidities such as sleep apnea, restless legs syndrome, nocturia, and nighttime akinesia may play a role.

The neurodegenerative involvement of dopaminergic systems and ascending arousal systems located in the lower brainstem and midbrain has been proposed as a mechanism for EDS. The suprachiasmatic nucleus regulates the internal rhythm, and hypocretin, a hypothalamic peptide, may have an additional regulatory role. The number of neurons secreting hypocretin and its level was found reduced in some PD studies, however, this has not been confirmed in other studies [44]. The effects of dopamine on wakefulness have been described as biphasic, by promoting sleep via direct activation of D_2 receptors on neurons of the locus ceruleus and raphe nucleus, and then depressing their activity [51].

Assessment and Treatment of Excessive Daytime Sleepiness

The assessment of EDS has been somewhat challenging. Relying on patient information is probably one of the reasons for the under-recognition of this problem. The Epworth Sleepiness Scale (ESS), although widely used, is susceptible to recall bias, as patients with chronic sleepiness may not provide accurate information on their sleepiness state or may get used to this problem [50]. Other scales including the PD Sleep Scale (PDSS) and the Scales for Outcomes in PD-Sleep (SCOPA-S) have been validated to assess sleep disorders in PD. Additionally, tests such as the Multiple Sleep Latency Test (MSLT) and the Maintenance of Wakefulness Test (MWT) can be useful. The use of general instruments, such as the Non-Motor Symptoms Questionnaire (NMSQuest) might be a useful approach to screen for EDS in the clinic population, triaging patients for further assessment and management [52].

Management of EDS starts by a careful assessment of potential causes and contributing factors, which can be accomplished through a careful medical history and review of drugs and co-morbidities. Additional testing such as polysomnography to rule-out other sleep-related disorders can be considered for selected cases. Before intervening, removal of potential causes such as sedative drugs needs to be considered. In patients with EDS receiving DA, reduction or cessation might be necessary. To date, there is no evidence to support that a switch from one agonist to another, including from oral standard release formulations to controlled release or transdermal would be beneficial, as somnolence is considered a class effect [48]. Levodopa causes less EDS than DA, but in patients not taking DA and using higher doses of levodopa, down-titration can be attempted. In patients with sleep attacks after initiation of DA, the drug should preferably be discontinued, or in selected cases, can be maintained at minimum doses. Patients should be advised about the risk of driving and operating machines after starting DA.

Interventions for treatment of EDS were appraised and summarized by the MDS evidence-based committee. Despite the insufficient evidence due to low-quality studies, Modafinil was considered "possibly useful" for treatment of EDS in PD, supported by a meta-analysis of three trials that showed significant reduction in sleepiness measured by the ESS. Caffeine has been investigated as a potential treatment for EDS, but to date is considered an investigational approach, with insufficient evidence. In PD patients with EDS and documented breathing disorders, continuous positive airway pressure (CPAP) was found to be beneficial and therefore might be recommended [36].

Drug-Induced Autonomic Symptoms

Patients with PD often experience autonomic dysfunction, which manifests in a variety of systems, including circulatory, urinary, gastrointestinal and others [53]. The PD-related autonomic dysfunction and gastrointestinal symptoms are discussed in Chapters 12 and 13, respectively. Herein, we will briefly discuss the issues of drug-induced orthostatic hypotension and nausea.

Drug-Induced Orthostatic Hypotension

Orthostatic hypotension (OH) is defined by a drop in systolic blood pressure (BP) of ≥ 20 or diastolic ≥ 10 mmHg within three minutes of standing. This can be found in approximately 60% of patients with PD, although only 30% experience symptoms, such as lightheadedness. The detection of OH requires a high level of suspicion, as patients often only report unspecific symptoms such as blurred vision, foggy thinking, "coathanger" headache, pain in the lower back or buttocks region, or lethargy upon standing. The fact that many patients are unaware of their low blood pressure levels is concerning, as OH may increase the risk of falls, fractures, and head traumas.

Drug-Induced Nausea

Nausea is one of the most commonly reported adverse effects of dopaminergic therapy in PD, particularly in the early phases of treatment. However, nausea has also been reported in drug-naïve patients, likely due to the gastroparesis that affects the majority of PD patients [53]. It can be challenging to differentiate these two conditions, but patients with gastroparesis may also complain of early satiety, diminished appetite, bloating, abdominal distension, vomiting, and weight loss. Patients with drug-induced nausea often correlate the symptom with the introduction of a new dopaminergic agent, dose changes, or dose intakes, and rarely report vomiting [53–55]. Also, most patients tend to develop better tolerance over time, and many report improvement when levodopa or DA are taken with food.

Pathophysiology, Prevention, and Management of Drug-Induced Autonomic Symptoms

Orthostatic Hypotension

In addition to the underlying PD dysautonomia, dopaminergic therapy, either DA and/or levodopa cause OH through both peripheral and central mechanisms, causing vasodilation and decreased catecholamine release. It is therefore essential to discuss this adverse effect with patients before therapy initiation, especially with DA. Preferably, titration should begin with small doses and gradually increased. In addition, the effects of these drugs on blood pressure can be potentialized by concomitant drugs, including selegiline, COMT inhibitors, acetylcholinesterase inhibitors, and drugs taken for comorbidities, such as hypertension [53, 55, 56].

When evaluating a patient with OH, a careful review of medications in use is mandatory. Whenever possible, antihypertensive agents, alpha-1 adrenoreceptor antagonists, and tricyclic antidepressants should be reduced or discontinued. Non-pharmacological approaches should be encouraged, which include the use of compression stockings, changing positions slowly, drinking plenty of water, avoiding copious and long meals and hot baths. Unfortunately, reducing dopaminergic therapy is not an option for many patients due to the risk of motor deterioration. In such cases, active treatment of OH needs to be considered. According to the MDS evidence-based review, fludrocortisone, midodrine, and droxidopa are considered possibly useful options [57]. In countries where domperidone is available, this is often used under rigorous monitoring due to the risk of QT interval prolongation and ventricular tachyarrhythmias. Complicating the treatment of OH, patients can present supine arterial hypertension, therefore it is essential to monitor blood pressure periodically in both standing and supine positions [58].

Nausea

Nausea can be caused by levodopa and DA. Levodopa is predominantly metabolized to dopamine by peripheral decarboxylase, and the dopamine can stimulate the chemoreceptors in the area postrema of the brainstem, one of the few brain structures without a blood–brain barrier. Adding a peripheral decarboxylase inhibitor, such as carbidopa or benserazide, significantly reduces nausea, although sometimes this is not enough [59]. To prevent nausea, patients should be instructed to take their medication with food, especially at the beginning of treatment. In later stages, when motor complications develop, levodopa should be preferably taken apart from meals due to competition for absorption with amino acids from diet. Smaller, more frequent meals can be encouraged. But for those with persistent nausea an antiemetic can be prescribed, but it is critical to avoid drugs that block central dopamine receptors. Domperidone has been used as first-line therapy where available based on results of small open-label studies. Trimethobenzamide has better quality evidence, and has been recommended for treatment, as well as pre-treatment prior to initiation of apomorphine [55].

Drug-Induced Non-Motor Fluctuations

Similarly to the motor fluctuations experienced by patients with PD on long-term levodopa therapy, a variety of fluctuations in non-motor symptoms may occur according to changes in central or peripheral dopamine levels. These non-motor fluctuations have typically been divided into three groups: neuropsychiatric, autonomic, and sensory/pain (Table 19.3).

Non-Motor Fluctuation in Neuropsychiatric Symptoms

Fluctuations in mood are well documented in PD, with worsening in the off-periods and improvement in the on-periods. Anxiety, irritability, and depression tend to worsen during the off-period and to improve with transition to the on-period [56]. In more severe cases of anxiety, panic attacks can occur during off-periods. Apathy, which is a common chronic symptom in PD, may also fluctuate, being worse in off-periods. Likewise, fatigue may be exacerbated with medication wearing-off [4, 60, 61].

Some patients experience neuropsychiatric symptoms related to the on-period, for instance, elevation in mood, hyper-alertness, and euphoria. In more severe cases, patients can report psychomotor agitation, hyperactivity, increased excitability, and hypomanic state, especially in the context of levodopa overuse or double-dosing [2]. Fluctuations in cognition, with "slowing of thoughts" or bradyphrenia during on-periods has been reported, as well as impairment of selective domains, however, it is controversial if those are truly cognitive effects or related to impaired arousal [2, 60].

Table 19.3 Drug-induced non-motor fluctuations in Parkinson's disease

Non-motor symptoms	Predominantly in OFF	Predominantly in ON
Neuropsychiatric symptoms	Anxiety Depression Irritability Panic attacks Apathy Fatigue	Euphoria Agitation Hyperexcitability Hypomania Mania Psychosis
Cognitive	Executive function Attention	Bradyphrenia Delayed memory retrieval Visuospatial dysfunction
Autonomic symptoms	Sweating, facial flushing, pallor, hyperthermia Urinary disturbances Bloating, abdominal discomfort, constipation Dysphagia, sialorrhea Dyspnea	Urinary disturbances Dyspnea
Sensory symptoms	Pain Numbness, paresthesia Restless legs syndrome Akathisia	

Non-Motor Fluctuations in Autonomic Symptoms

As discussed in Chapter 12, autonomic dysfunction is a common problem in PD, however, in some cases, autonomic symptoms may fluctuate according to dopamine levels [4, 62]. For instance, some patients experience marked sweating in the off-period, whereas others complain of sweating during the on-phases, mostly in the context of levodopa-induced dyskinesias [60].

Urinary problems and urgency due to detrusor hyperreflexia and constipation can become particularly worse in the off-periods. More commonly, patients report fluctuating abdominal discomfort and bloating, due to gastroparesis occurring during off-periods [2]. Dysphagia, choking, sialorrhea, which are common in later stages of PD, can also fluctuate, being worse during off-periods [54, 56]. A sensation of dyspnea can be reported by patients with PD, and can either manifest in off-periods, or, in some cases, be secondary to respiratory dyskinesia and thus, occur within on-periods [2, 63].

Non-Motor Fluctuations in Sensory Symptoms

Parkinson's disease patients can experience fluctuations in sensory symptoms, including pain, numbness, paresthesia, and restless legs, which are often experienced or exacerbated in the off-periods, and dramatically alleviated by dopaminergic medications. Akathisia, defined as a sensation of inner restlessness and inability to sit still, may also have a fluctuating pattern, however, the exact relationship to the motor state is not consistent [60].

Pain in PD tends to manifest more frequently during off-periods, and can present as burning, aching or stabbing sensations, diffuse and poorly localized. Sometimes, pain is associated with off-related dystonia, and improves substantially with transition to the on-state. On the other hand, some rare patients may experience painful dyskinesias during the on-periods [2, 4, 56]. Fluctuating oral and genital pain have also been reported in patients with PD, sometimes responsive to dopaminergic treatment, particularly to DA [2, 64]. A more detailed discussion of sensory symptoms reported by PD patients can be found in Chapter 16.

Pathophysiology, Diagnosis, and Management of Non-Motor Fluctuations

Parkinson's disease pathology affects many different brain areas including non-dopaminergic systems in the brainstem and cortical regions. The involvement of those areas may at least in part explain some non-motor symptoms and by extension, some non-motor fluctuations. In addition, the direct stimulation of dopamine receptors by PD drugs may play a role in some symptoms, similarly to an adverse effect. Finally, the underlying dopaminergic denervation and the fluctuating dopamine levels associated with levodopa dosing, pharmacokinetics, and bioavailability is likely involved, corresponding to the mechanisms underlying the motor fluctuations [2, 63, 65].

Patients and caregivers are often unaware that the fluctuations in non-motor symptoms relate to PD, and the severity of these symptoms may not correlate to the motor severity in the wearing-off, making it hard to diagnose. In addition, to date, there is no widely accepted instrument to assess non-motor fluctuations. A non-motor fluctuation assessment (NoMoFA) instrument has been developed and is currently being evaluated in a large-scale study [66]. Other instruments, such as the wearing-off questionnaire (WOQ-32) and the modified Non-Motor Symptoms Scale (mNMSS) may also be useful to guide treatment or in clinical research [65].

Correspondingly to the motor fluctuations, addressing the fluctuations in dopamine levels aiming for a non-pulsatile dopaminergic stimulation can improve some of the non-motor fluctuations, including off-related anxiety, depression, and pain. In those cases, strategies for management of wearing-off, such as levodopa dose fragmentation, use of long-acting levodopa formulations or DA, and introduction of COMT inhibitors or MAO inhibitors might be beneficial [67]. Recent findings on clinical trials with safinamide for management of motor complications points towards improvement of depression, which suggests the drug might become a potential strategy for management of non-motor fluctuations [67]. For some non-motor off symptoms, it is unclear if a more general approach to fluctuations would work, therefore a symptom-oriented approach may be necessary, for instance, for overactive bladder, constipation, and cognitive deficits [65].

Advanced therapies, such as apomorphine infusions, levodopa gel intestinal infusion, and deep brain stimulation (DBS) have documented benefits for treatment of specific non-motor symptoms and therefore can be considered for selected cases of non-motor fluctuations. A study found that DBS improved non-motor fluctuations by 58%, with the pain/sensory fluctuations showing the greatest reduction, and the neuropsychiatric fluctuations the smallest. Apomorphine infusion is highly effective in reducing motor fluctuations, although there is little evidence regarding non-motor symptoms and non-motor fluctuations. Similarly, levodopa intestinal gel has strong evidence for improvement of motor fluctuations, but only low-quality evidence for non-motor symptoms [67].

Considering the large number of different non-motor fluctuations and their enigmatic pathophysiology, it is unlikely that a single strategy will satisfactorily accommodate all various therapeutic needs, therefore a tailored approach is recommended [65].

References

1. Titova N, Chaudhuri KR. Non-motor Parkinson disease: new concepts and personalised management. Med J Aust 2018; **208**: 404–409.

2. Fox SH, Lang AE. Motor and non-motor fluctuations. Handb Clin Neurol 2007; **84**: 157–184.

3. Schaeffer E, Berg D. Dopaminergic therapies for non-motor symptoms in Parkinson's disease. CNS Drugs 2017; **31**: 551–570.

4. Chaudhuri KR, Schapira AHV. Non-motor symptoms of Parkinson's disease: dopaminergic pathophysiology and treatment. Lancet Neurol 2009; **8**: 464–474.

5. Strowd LC, Lee AD, Yosipovitch G. Livedo reticularis associated with rasagiline (azilect). J Drugs Dermatol 2012; **11**: 764–765.

6. Fénelon G, Alves G. Epidemiology of psychosis in Parkinson's disease. J Neurol Sci 2010; **289**: 12–17.

7. Fénelon G, Soulas T, Zenasni F, et al. The changing face of Parkinson's disease-associated psychosis: a cross-sectional study based on the new NINDS-NIMH criteria. Mov Disord 2010; **25**: 763–766.

8. Goetz CG, Fan W, Leurgans S, et al. The malignant course of "benign hallucinations" in Parkinson disease. Arch Neurol 2006; **63**: 713–716.

9. Ffytche DH, Creese B, Politis M, et al. The psychosis spectrum in Parkinson disease. Nat Rev Neurol 2017; **13**: 81–95.

10. Lenka A, Pagonabarraga J, Pal PK, et al. Minor hallucinations in Parkinson disease. Neurology 2019; **93**: 259–266.

11. Fenelon G, Mahieux F, Huon R, et al. Hallucinations in Parkinson's disease: prevalence, phenomenology and risk factors. Brain 2000; **123**: 733–745.

12. Goetz CG, Stebbins GT, Ouyang B. Visual plus nonvisual hallucinations in Parkinson's disease: development and evolution over 10 years. Mov Disord 2011; **26**: 2196–2200.

13. Diederich NJ, Fénelon G, Stebbins G, et al. Hallucinations in Parkinson disease. Nature Rev Neurol 2009; **5**: 331–342.

14. Llebaria G, Pagonabarraga J, Martínez-Corral M, et al. Neuropsychological correlates of mild to severe hallucinations in Parkinson's disease. Mov Disord 2010; **25**: 2785–2791.

15. Ravina B, Marder K, Fernandez HH, et al. Diagnostic criteria for psychosis in Parkinson's disease: report of an NINDS, NIMH work group. Mov Disord 2007; **22**: 1061–1068.

16. Fernandez HH, Aarsland D, Fénelon G, et al. Scales to assess psychosis in Parkinson's disease: critique and recommendations. Mov Disord 2008; **23**: 484–500.

17. Cummings JL, Mega M, Gray K, et al. The Neuropsychiatric Inventory: comprehensive assessment of psychopathology in dementia. Neurology 1994; **44**: 2308–2314.

18. Kay SR, Opler LA, Lindenmayer J-P. The Positive and Negative Syndrome Scale (PANSS): rationale and standardisation. Br J Psychiatry 1989; **155**: 59–65.

19. Goetz CG, Tilley BC, Shaftman SR, et al. Movement Disorder Society-sponsored revision of the Unified Parkinson's Disease Rating Scale (MDS-UPDRS): Scale presentation and clinimetric testing results. Mov Disord 2008; **23**: 2129–2170.

20. Chaudhuri KR, Martinez-Martin P, Brown RG, et al. The metric properties of a novel non-motor symptoms scale for Parkinson's disease: results from an international pilot study. Mov Disord 2007; **22**: 1901–1911.

21. Voss T, Bahr D, Cummings J, et al. Performance of a shortened Scale for Assessment of Positive Symptoms for Parkinson's disease psychosis. Parkinsonism Relat Disord 2013; **19**: 295–299.

22. Zhu K, van Hilten JJ, Putter H, et al. Risk factors for hallucinations in Parkinson's disease: results

from a large prospective cohort study. Mov Disord 2013; **28**: 755.

23. la Riva de P, Smith K, Xie SX, et al. Course of psychiatric symptoms and global cognition in early Parkinson disease. Neurology 2014; **83**: 1096–1103.

24. Forsaa EB, Larsen JP, Wentzel-Larsen T, et al. A 12-year population-based study of psychosis in Parkinson disease. Arch Neurol 2010; **67**: 996–1001.

25. Morgante L, Colosimo C, Antonini A, et al. Psychosis associated to Parkinson's disease in the early stages: relevance of cognitive decline and depression. J Neurol Neurosurg Psychiatry 2011; **83**: 76–82.

26. Mack J, Rabins P, Anderson K, et al. Prevalence of psychotic symptoms in a community-based Parkinson disease sample. Am J Geriatr Psychiatry 2012; **20**: 123–132.

27. Huot P, Johnston TH, Darr T, et al. Increased 5-HT2A receptors in the temporal cortex of parkinsonian patients with visual hallucinations. Mov Disord 2010; **25**: 1399–1408.

28. Cho SS, Strafella AP, Duff-Canning S, et al. The relationship between serotonin-2A receptor and cognitive functions in nondemented Parkinson's disease patients with visual hallucinations. Mov Disord Clin Pract 2017; **4**: 698–709.

29. Ballanger B, Strafella AP, van Eimeren T, et al. Serotonin 2A receptors and visual hallucinations in Parkinson disease. Arch Neurol 2010; **67**: 416–421.

30. Janzen J, t' Ent D, Lemstra AW, et al. The pedunculopontine nucleus is related to visual hallucinations in Parkinson's disease: preliminary results of a voxel-based morphometry study. J Neurol 2011; **259**: 147–154.

31. Wilby KJ, Johnson EG, Johnson HE, et al. Evidence-based review of pharmacotherapy used for Parkinson's disease psychosis. Ann Pharmacother 2017; **51**: 682–695.

32. Fernandez HH, Okun MS, Rodriguez RL, et al. Quetiapine improves visual hallucinations in Parkinson disease but not through normalization of sleep architecture: results from a double-blind clinical-polysomnography study. Int J Neurosci 2009; **119**: 2196–2205.

33. Shotbolt P, Samuel M, Fox C, et al. A randomized controlled trial of quetiapine for psychosis in Parkinson's disease. Neuropsychiatr Dis Treat 2009; **5**: 327–332.

34. Ondo WG, Tintner R, Voung KD, et al. Double-blind, placebo-controlled, unforced titration parallel trial of quetiapine for dopaminergic-

induced hallucinations in Parkinson's disease. Mov Disord 2005; **20**: 958–963.

35. Rabey JM, Prokhorov T, Miniovitz A, et al. Effect of quetiapine in psychotic Parkinson's disease patients: a double-blind labeled study of 3 months' duration. Mov Disord 2007; **22**: 313–318.

36. Seppi K, K. Ray Chaudhuri, Coelho M, et al. Update on treatments for nonmotor symptoms of Parkinson's disease – an evidence-based medicine review. Mov Disord 2019; **34**: 180–198.

37. Parkinson Study Group. Low-dose clozapine for the treatment of drug-induced psychosis in Parkinson's disease. N Engl J Med 1999; **340**: 757–763.

38. Pollak P, Tison F, Rascol O, et al. Clozapine in drug-induced psychosis in Parkinson's disease: a randomised, placebo-controlled study with open follow up. J Neurol Neurosurg Psychiatry 2004; **75**: 689–695.

39. Alvir JMJ, Lieberman JA, Safferman AZ, et al. Clozapine-induced agranulocytosis – incidence and risk factors in the United States. N Eng J Med 2010; **329**: 162–167.

40. Cummings J, Isaacson S, Mills R, et al. Pimavanserin for patients with Parkinson's disease psychosis: a randomised, placebo-controlled phase 3 trial. Lancet 2014; **383**: 533–540.

41. Meltzer HY, Mills R, Revell S, et al. Pimavanserin, a serotonin2A receptor inverse agonist, for the treatment of Parkinson's disease psychosis. Neuropsychopharmacol 2009; **35**: 881–892.

42. The Lancet Neurology. Difficult choices in treating Parkinson's disease psychosis. Lancet Neurol 2018; **17**: 569.

43. Verbaan D, van Rooden SM, Visser M, et al. Nighttime sleep problems and daytime sleepiness in Parkinson's disease. Mov Disord 2008; **23**: 35–41.

44. Knie B, Mitra MT, Logishetty K, et al. Excessive daytime sleepiness in patients with Parkinson's disease. CNS Drugs 2011; **25**: 203–212.

45. Shpirer I, Miniovitz A, Klein C, et al. Excessive daytime sleepiness in patients with Parkinson's disease: a polysomnography study. Mov Disord 2006; **21**: 1432–1438.

46. Paus S, Brecht HM, Köster J, et al. Sleep attacks, daytime sleepiness, and dopamine agonists in Parkinson's disease. Mov Disord 2003; **18**: 659–667.

47. Gros P, Videnovic A. Overview of sleep and circadian rhythm disorders in Parkinson disease. Clin Geriatr Med 2020; **36**: 119–130.

48. Chaudhuri KR, Pal S, Brefel-Courbon C. 'Sleep attacks' or 'unintended sleep episodes' occur with

dopamine agonists. Drug-Safety 2002; **25**: 473–483.

49. Amara AW, Chahine LM, Caspell-Garcia C, et al. Longitudinal assessment of excessive daytime sleepiness in early Parkinson's disease. J Neurol Neurosurg Psychiatry 2017; **88**: 653–662.

50. Razmy A, Lang AE, Shapiro CM. Predictors of impaired daytime sleep and wakefulness in patients with Parkinson disease treated with older (ergot) vs newer (nonergot) dopamine agonists. Arch Neurol 2004; **61**: 97–102.

51. Silkis IG. Search for approaches to correction of daytime sleepiness induced by dopaminergic drugs during treatment of Parkinson's disease: neurochemical aspects. Neurochem J 2009; **3**: 221–231.

52. Chaudhuri KR, Martin PM, Schapira AHV, et al. International multicenter pilot study of the first comprehensive self-completed nonmotor symptoms questionnaire for Parkinson's disease: The NMSQuest study. Mov Disord 2006; **21**: 916–923.

53. Pfeiffer RF. Non-motor symptoms in Parkinson's disease. Parkinsonism Relat Disord 2016; **22**: S119–122.

54. Pfeiffer RF. Gastrointestinal dysfunction in Parkinson's disease. Parkinsonism Relat Disord 2011; **17**: 10–15.

55. Wood LD. Clinical review and treatment of select adverse effects of dopamine receptor agonists in Parkinson's disease. Drugs Aging 2010; **27**: 295–310.

56. Schapira AHV, Chaudhuri KR, Jenner P. Non-motor features of Parkinson disease. Nat Rev Neurosci 2017; **18**: 435–450.

57. Seppi K, K. Ray Chaudhuri, Coelho M, et al. Update on treatments for nonmotor symptoms of Parkinson's disease – an evidence-based medicine review. Mov Disord 2019; **34**: 180–198.

58. Quarracino C, Otero-Losada M, Capani F, et al. State-of-the-art pharmacotherapy for autonomic dysfunction in Parkinson's disease. Expert Opin Pharmacother 2020; **21**: 445–457.

59. Chou KL. Adverse events from the treatment of Parkinson's disease. Neurol Clin 2008; **26**: 65–83.

60. Witjas T, Kaphan E, Azulay JP, et al. Nonmotor fluctuations in Parkinson's disease frequent and disabling. Neurology 2002; **59**: 408–413.

61. Kummer A, Scalzo P, Cardoso F, et al. Evaluation of fatigue in Parkinson's disease using the Brazilian version of Parkinson's Fatigue Scale. Acta Neurol Scand 2011; **123**: 130–136.

62. Todorova A, Jenner P, K. Ray Chaudhuri Non-motor Parkinson's: integral to motor Parkinson's, yet often neglected. Prac Neurol 2014; **14**(5): 310.

63 Aquino CC, Fox SH. Clinical spectrum of levodopa-induced complications. Mov Disord 2015; **30**: 80–89.

64. Aquino CC, Mestre T, Lang AE. Restless genital syndrome in Parkinson disease. JAMA Neurol 2014; **71**: 1559–1561.

65. Classen J, Koschel J, Oehlwein C, et al. Nonmotor fluctuations: phenotypes, pathophysiology, management, and open issues. J Neural Transm 2017; **124**: 1029–1036.

66. Kleiner-Fisman G, Martine R, Lang AE, et al. Development of a non-motor fluctuation assessment instrument for Parkinson disease. Parkinsons Dis 2011; **2011**: 1–13. DOI:10.4061/2011/292719

67. Fernández RM, Schmitt E, Martin PM, et al. The hidden sister of motor fluctuations in Parkinson's disease: a review on nonmotor fluctuations. Mov Disord 2016; **31**: 1080–1094.

Chapter 20

Impulse Control Disorders and the Dopamine Dysregulation Syndrome

Atbin Djamshidian, Guillaume Pagnier, Michael J. Frank, Joseph H. Friedman

History

The syndromes subsumed under the general umbrella term of impulse control disorders (ICDs), punding, compulsive disorders, and the dopamine dysregulation syndrome (DDS), all share the common theme of an overwhelming need to perform some activity. The actions are generally closer in nature to addictive disorders, being ego syntonic, and less like true impulsive disorders which patients may try to resist [1]. Punding represents a need to perform senseless activities repeatedly, such as folding and refolding clothes in a drawer for hours at a time, polishing pennies, or pulling weeds from a lawn or threads from a rug. The more common ICDs include gambling disorder, compulsive sexual disorder, consumerism, and hobbyism, but may include strikingly unusual activities that are extraordinarily narrow in their focus. The DDS seems to be a form of drug addictive behavior, similar to that of the usual addictive drugs. Although they are labelled as impulsive disorders, implying an inability to resist a sudden impulse to perform an activity that is ill considered and likely counterproductive, the activities we will discuss are generally ones the patients want to do all the time, and are not impulses that arise out of the blue. In addition, they are typically not sorry that they "gave in" to their desires, but rather, like many addicted people, minimize the negative effects.

While ICDs were first recognized to affect PD patients in 1994 [2], the role of levodopa in sexual behavior was discussed in the 1960s with the drug's introduction [3–6]. It was the subject of several reports. In contemporary lectures on PD, speakers often show old newspaper headlines reporting the purported aphrodisiac powers of levodopa. However, the publications of that time do not bear this out. In 1969 Barbeau [3] reported on 80 patients with PD or post-encephalitic parkinsonism (PEP), mean age 59.7, treated with a mean dose of 4.3 grams/day. Sexual issues did not rise to the level of even being included in the table of side effects. He noted that "a behavioral pattern with frontal lobe overtones was evident in some patients, especially in the sexual sphere. A clear-cut, visually evident increase in libido occurred in at least four male patients." The author suspected that this occurred in the women as well but did not have evidence. This was a retrospective study and the methods of determining sexual changes were not discussed. A large multicenter prospective study on levodopa, with centers chosen around the United States to reflect the American population, followed 485 parkinsonian patients, of whom about 88% had PD, for an average of 10 months. They reported in 1970 that "hypersexuality or increased libido occurred quite often but was rarely looked on as an adverse effect" [5]. Another prospective but single site study of 19 patients with PD duration between 3 and 15 months, 45–80 years old, of whom 12 were men, found that levodopa improved sexual function but not necessarily libido. Seven of 19 reported an increased "activation of sexual behavior," but no patient reported an increase of more than one point on a five-point self-report scale of sexual behavior. The authors concluded that "levodopa appears to cause a transient specific stimulation of sexual drive in only a small percentage of patients; it is therefore probably inaccurate to describe it as an aphrodisiac" [4].

A remarkably insightful review of levodopa therapy in 1974 noted no cases of hypersexuality occurring among 93 patients, 71 with idiopathic PD, rather than post-encephalitic parkinsonism, all of whom had been followed for over five years [7]. A single case report described a 76-year-old man started on levodopa 5 gm/d whose mobility improved significantly but who developed hyper-sexual behavior, making amorous advances to nurses and exposing himself [6]. Six weeks later he was seen as an outpatient, severely immobile, having stopped the levodopa voluntarily because of the discomfort of the sexual change. A retrospective study by a team of neurologists and psychiatrists, looking only at mental effects of levodopa, found that four of 12 males and none of eight women reported increased libido. This was listed in a table of mental changes only, without description. Six men reported improvement in erectile function [8]. In a summary of all reports up to the time of his writing, Goodwin summar-ized the literature on over 800 patients (including patients from an unpublished study) with regard to the effect of levodopa on sexual interest as follows. "Restoration of sexual interest has occurred frequently in patients on levodopa as a result that would seem to be consistent with the dramatic improvement in functional motor capacity. In a few cases this . . . has gone beyond the norm and has involved inappropriately exces-sive sexual drives and behavior." Rather than a specific aphrodisiac effect, Goodwin [9] thought it more likely "that the sexual behavior is part of a more general hypomanic syndrome," and typi-cally occurred with symptoms of hypomania such as euphoria, hyperactivity, grandiosity, and poor judgment." From our review of this literature, we believe this to be the case, as well, and believe, especially with the five decades of further experi-ence with levodopa, that hypersexuality is rare when levodopa is taken alone.

Definition of Impulse Control Disorders

Impulse control disorders are excessively and repeatedly performed behaviors with a lack of forethought despite potential negative conse-quences to the individual or others [1] and lead to an impairment of social and occupational func-tioning. These addictive behaviors are often non-goal-orientated, stereotyped, and compulsive. Therefore, ICDs are often labelled as impulsive compulsive behaviors (ICBs) to acknowledge both components [10–12].

The four most common ICDs in PD include compulsive sexual behavior, compulsive shop-ping, binge eating, and gambling disorder [1]. Other addictive behaviors include punding, the

dopamine dysregulation syndrome, hoarding, and excessive hobbyism [1].

Impulse control disorders are described as behavioral addictions, because of the striking similarities regarding their risk factors for other addictive disorders [13].

The prevalence of ICDs in PD patients with dopamine agonists varies and lies between 14% and 30% [14, 15] but may be even higher in patients with younger disease onset [16]. Multiple ICDs occur in approximately one-quarter of patients [14]. However, the cumulative prevalence of ICDs in PD is likely declining as doctors are more aware and have changed their prescribing practices [13].

Compulsive Sexual Behavior

Compulsive sexual behavior ranges from increased sex drive to intense urges or behaviors involving non-normative sexual interests, often termed paraphilias [17, 18]. Compulsive sexual disorders are more common in male PD patients. Initially it was reported that compul-sive sexual behavior occurs in about 3.5% [14]. More recent studies show, however, that com-pulsive sexual behavior is underdiagnosed and the actual prevalence rate may be much higher (9–14%) [15]. In one study among PD patients with ICDs, compulsive sexual behavior was the most common disorder and occurred in almost 50%. Patients with compulsive sexual behavior had a higher levodopa equivalent dose, had mul-tiple ICDs, and were younger than PD patients with other ICDs [19]. Changes in sexual beha-vior and zoophilia are less commonly observed [18, 20].

Gambling Disorder

Gambling disorder is one of the most frequently described addictions in PD. DSM-V criteria for gambling disorder in the general population is defined as an inappropriate, persistent, and mala-daptive gambling behavior. In treated PD patients, prevalence rates vary between 5% and 8% depending on culture and access to gambling venues [14, 15]. PD patients usually prefer gam-bling that needs little cognitive activity such as scratch cards and slot machines where loss peri-ods are short and can be instantly re-gambled. These gambles also offer "near misses" which further increase the addiction. Often patients use "lucky charms" in order to improve their winning chances [21].

Compulsive Shopping

Compulsive shopping is defined as a maladaptive preoccupation with buying, manifest as impulses that are irresistible, intrusive, or senseless and result in spending more than can be afforded or purchasing items that are not needed [22]. In PD patients treated with dopaminergic therapy (a combination of levodopa and dopamine agonists) compulsive buying has been reported between 3.4% [23] and 5.7% [14]. Often the item itself is not expensive and patients frequently report that they had an urge to buy a bargain. It has been hypothesized that the repetitive negative emotional state that emerges when patients cannot go shopping as well as the loss of control over spending resembles craving in patients with illicit drug abuse [24].

Binge Eating

Binge eating usually occurs at night. PD patients describe a lack of control over eating and often consume large portions of either carbon-rich meals or sweets. These episodes occur at least once in a week over three months and differ significantly from previous eating patterns. It was reported in 4.3% of US-PD patients treated with dopamine agonists [14].

Dopamine Dysregulation Syndrome

Dopamine dysregulation syndrome (DDS) was first described by Giovannoni in 2000 and is defined as the compulsive overuse of dopaminergic medication [25]. Typically, patients and their families report dysphoria in the "off state" and disabling dyskinesias during the "on state." Self-medicating and self-escalation of dopaminergic drugs (mostly fast-acting levodopa or apomorphine pen injections) are characteristic. In contrast to compulsive sexual behavior, gambling disorder, and compulsive shopping, DDS is associated with the use of levodopa. It is more frequently seen in men with a younger onset of disease. Motor complications, including motor fluctuations and dyskinesias, as well as neuropsychiatric comorbidities such as anxiety, aggression, depression, and panic attacks are common [26]. Patients typically describe avoidance of "off"

periods as the reason for self-escalation of their dopaminergic medication [27]. Some patients also acknowledge a subjective "high" or mood benefit after taking levodopa [25]. PD patients frequently describe debilitating withdrawal symptoms during "off" times [28].

Punding

The first ICD associated with PD was punding [2]. Punding was a term used by amphetamine addicts, a shortened form of "pund-huvud," [29] meaning "block head." The term generally refers to behaving "stupidly or foolishly." Among addicts the term means "aimless, stereotyped, repetitive behaviors" that present during the "run" and sometimes during the "crash" [29]. The first known reference to punding in any context was made by Rylander in 1971 in a book chapter on stimulant abuse [30] before appearing in the general literature [31].

The first two publications reporting punding in PD attributed the behavior to levodopa, and not agonists [2, 32]. The first paper was a letter describing a non-demented PD patient who began shuffling papers and tallying the same numbers repeatedly, humming, and telling inappropriate jokes, despite knowing they were inappropriate, within days of an increase in levodopa from 400 to 900 mg/day [2]. He was also taking selegiline, but no dopamine agonist. Within four days of a reduction to 500 mg/day of levodopa his behaviors returned to baseline. The letter suggested that once looked for, this syndrome was probably going to be found considerably more common than a single case report would indicate. In the second paper, all three patients were taking both levodopa and pergolide, a dopamine agonist.

Punding attracted a great deal of attention when two review papers appeared in 2004 [33, 34] discussing the problem of compulsive behaviors in PD. As predicted, the publication record on punding increased dramatically afterward, but more importantly, punding was put into the context of compulsive disorders and became associated with dopamine agonists, rather than levodopa.

Punding is idiosyncratic depending on the individual interests. The prevalence of punding in PD probably increases with disease duration and varies between 0.34% to 14% [35].

Miscellaneous Impulsive Behaviors

Reckless generosity [36], excessive hoarding [37], compulsive smoking [38], reckless driving [39], aggression and walkabouts [25], drug addiction [40], compulsive pet killing [41], and criminal behavior [42] are other, albeit rarer, addictive behaviors seen in PD.

Obsessive Compulsive Disorders

Obsessive compulsive disorders (OCDs) differ from impulsive behavior, usually being perservative and non-goal-orientated. However, there is a clear overlap between impulsive and compulsive disorders. Furthermore, habit formation, (where a stimulus triggers an action, in contrast to goal-orientated behavior) in combination with stress and anxiety likely contributes to the development of compulsive behavior [43].

Neuropsychological tests reveal motor disinhibition and an impaired ability to stop a sequence in both impulsive and compulsive patients [44]. Moreover, fMRI and volumetric data have revealed hypoactivation of the prefrontal cortex, orbitofrontal cortex, and striatal volumetric changes as well as cortico-striatal dysfunction in patients with ICDs and OCDs. Dysfunction of glutamate, serotonin, and particularly opioids, which in turn have a modulatory effect on dopamine and serotonin levels, have been also hypothesized to trigger both OCDs and ICDs [45]. However, no study has yet confirmed this hypothesis.

Obsessive compulsive disorders are excessive, intrusive, irresistible thoughts that can impair the patients' and their families' quality of life. Typical clinical symptoms include, but are not limited to, excessive washing, persistent checking (e.g. whether doors are locked), hoarding, ordering and rearranging of items. As in patients with ICDs, insight can be low. Over time it has been postulated that impulsivity and rash processes increase in patients with OCDs [45]. The prevalence of OCDs is about 2.5–3% in the general population [46]. Age of onset is bimodal and there are differences in severity in comorbidity. Early-onset OCD (mean age 11) tends to be more severe, responds less well to medication, and is more frequently associated with tics than late-onset OCD (mean age 23) [47]. The diagnosis is made clinically on the presence of symptoms that last more than 1 hour per day, are distressing and impair daily function, and are not a result of substance abuse or illness. In the new DSM-V criteria anxiety was removed as it is not a "core criterion" for OCD [48].

Risk Factors for Binge Eating, Gambling Disorder, Compulsive Sexual Disorder, and Compulsive Shopping

The most important risk factor for the following three ICDs (compulsive sexual behavior, compulsive shopping, and gambling disorder) in PD is the use of dopamine agonist therapy. For example, gambling disorder almost exclusively evolves under dopamine agonist therapy and has been only rarely reported with levodopa monotherapy [21]. Although craving for sweets is common in PD, particularly in those who have ICDs [49], the association of binge eating and dopamine agonist therapy is less clear. While previous studies have linked dopamine agonist use and binge eating [14], a more recent, but smaller, cross-sectional study identified deep brain stimulation (DBS) as the only predictor for overeating [50].

On the other hand, untreated PD is not associated with ICDs. This has been confirmed in a case control study in drug-naïve PD patients [51]. There have been conflicting reports whether ICDs correlate with dopamine agonist dose. It seems, however, that the combination of a dopamine agonist with levodopa increases the risk further [12, 14, 52–54]. A longitudinal study conducted in 411 patients showed that the maximum lifetime dopamine agonist dose as well as the duration of treatment were associated with ICDs [55].

The most commonly used dopamine agonists are highly selective for the dopamine D3 receptor, which are mainly expressed in the mesolimbic system. This has led to the hypothesis that D3 receptor stimulation of the limbic system may play a crucial role in reward processing in susceptible patients and may be responsible for causing ICDs in PD [56]. There may be, however, differences in triggering ICDs between the dopamine agonists. ICDs were less frequently associated with the transdermal dopamine agonist rotigotine than pramipexole or ropinirole [57]. Other addictive behaviors, such as punding, DDS, hobbyism, walkabouts, and hoarding occur more commonly with "pulsatile" (short-acting) dopaminergic therapy, such as levodopa and apomorphine.

Impulse control disorders have rarely been described with other dopaminergic and non-dopaminergic drugs such as rasagiline and amantadine [1]. In 2016 the US Food and Drug Administration (FDA) issued a safety warning of a possible association of aripiprazol and ICDs, which was later confirmed [58, 59]. Indeed, aripiprazol acts as a dopamine D3 receptor agonist which further strengthens the link between dopamine D3 stimulation and addictions [58].

Patients with early-onset PD, who are single and have more motor complications such as unpredictable motor fluctuations as well as non-motor symptoms such as depression are also at higher risk [60–63]. Dyskinesias are seen frequently in PD patients with ICDs. In one recent study more than 50% of patients with dyskinesias had ICDs, of which 36% were clinically significant [64]. In the Parkinson Progression Markers Initiative (PPMI) cohort, drug-naïve PD patients who went on to develop ICDs had higher anxiety scores as well as worse autonomic and global cognitive function at baseline [65]. There are also gender differences. While compulsive sexual behavior has been more frequently reported in men, compulsive shopping and binge eating has been more frequently observed in female PD patients [14, 17]. The relationship between sleep and ICDs is incompletely understood. While ICDs can often lead to sleep restriction and sleep fragmentation (e.g. nocturnal punding or excessive Internet use) [66], REM sleep behavior abnormalities have been proposed as a risk factor in some [67] but not all studies [68].

Depression is a frequent concomitant problem in patients with ICDs. In one recent study using the data of the PPMI, depression at baseline was associated with ICDs at follow-up after four years. This risk increased even further when patients were treated with dopamine agonists [69].

Risk Factors for Dopamine Dysregulation Syndrome and Punding

As mentioned earlier, DDS as well as punding are mainly triggered by dopamine D1 receptor stimulation. It has been hypothesized that DDS is an addiction that could arise in individuals who are also susceptible to developing substance abuse. Some authors have argued that a previous history of substance abuse, higher past history of alcohol intake, and higher novelty seeking personality traits are found in those who are more prone to developing DDS [70]. More motor complications such as dyskinesias, unpredictable motor fluctuations, but also non-motor problems such as depression, panic attacks, as well as male gender, a younger onset of PD, and the use of a large amount of rapid-release levodopa or apomorphine injections are other proposed risk factors [26, 28, 62]. Furthermore, other ICDs, as well as psychosis, are frequently seen in patients with DDS [26].

Similarly, punding has been associated with male gender, younger onset of PD, young age, depression, dyskinesias, more advanced PD, and a history of alcohol abuse [71, 72]. Furthermore, punding frequently co-occurs in patients with DDS [71]. There are isolated case reports of punding associated with non-dopaminergic drugs, including the dopamine receptor blocking drug, quetiapine [73].

Psychiatric Comorbidities

Psychiatric comorbidities are common in PD patients with ICDs. A personal or family history of alcohol addiction, illicit drug abuse in the past, and high novelty seeking personality traits are common in patients with ICDs [24, 60, 67, 74]. Higher aggressiveness, irritability, disinhibition [75], and impairment on various neuropsychological tests have been also described [10]. Alexithymia, difficulty identifying emotions, has been also linked with increased impulsivity in drug-naïve PD patients [76] and has been proposed as a risk factor for ICDs [76, 77]. Othello syndrome, a delusion of infidelity, has been associated with dopamine-agonist use and ICDs [78, 79]. In line with this a large cross-sectional study has found a significant association between psychosis and ICDs [62].

Apathy, a reduction in emotions, interests, and motivation is common in PD. These patients may describe fatigue but usually it is their family who report a lack of spontaneous initiation. Along with other hypodopaminergic behaviors, such as depression and anxiety, apathy lies on the opposite spectrum of hyperdopaminergic behaviors [80]. However, studies have shown that apathy is common among patients with ICDs [68] and thus, may share a common behavioral spectrum [81].

As mentioned above, depression is common among PD patients with ICDs and has even been identified as a risk factor [63]. Patients with ICDs exhibit higher scores for anxiety. Interestingly, anxiety seems to occur particularly in patients with gambling disorder [60]. Moreover, young-onset PD patients have significantly more frequent psychiatric co-morbidities such as depression, substance abuse, and psychosocial dysfunction relative to age-, sex- and gender-matched disabled patients [82].

The Genetics of Impulse Control Disorders

It is still unclear why some PD patients develop ICDs, while others do not. For many years, it was speculated that certain genes may predispose to addiction. Twin studies in the non-PD population have shown that genetic factors account for between 33–54% of the risk of developing pathological gambling [83]. The DOMINON study, involving over 3000 subjects, reported that ICDs in PD are more common in those who have a family history of gambling addiction [14].

In a recent prospective study, 276 drug-naïve PD patients without ICDs were followed for three years. Of the 238 patients who received dopaminergic therapy, 40% were treated with dopamine agonists. In this study a total of 19% of all patients developed ICDs at follow-up. Whole exome sequencing using 12 candidate variants (*DRD2, DRD3, DAT1, COMT, DDC, GRIN2B, ADRA2C, SERT, TPH2, HTR2A, OPRK1*, and *OPRM1* genes) increased ICD predictability up to 87% in a given patient, which was significantly better than using clinical data alone (71%). Of these 12 variants the strongest associations were found with the *OPRK1, HTR2A* and *DDC* gene. These three genes are of particular interest as they encode for opioid (*OPRK1*), serotonin (*HTR2A*), and dopamine (*DDC*) receptors [84].

Another study found no difference in the frequency of ICDs in PD patients with Parkin mutations compared to those without. However, PD patients with ICDs had a younger disease onset, were more likely smokers, and had more severe ICDs than PD controls with ICDs [85].

Clinical Measures of Impulse Control Disorders

A thorough clinical assessment is still likely the best way to screen for ICDs [86]. Until 2009, no standardized questionnaire to assess ICDs in PD existed. The Questionnaire for Impulsive Compulsive Disorders in Parkinson's disease (QUIP) [87] and the QUIP- rating scale [11] are the most commonly used tools to screen for and measure addictions in PD. While the QUIP is widely used, it does not assess ICD severity. This has been supplemented with the QUIP- rating scale. However, the QUIP- rating scale is not recommended to screen for DDS [86]. A detailed list of screening scales for ICDs are listed in Table 20.1.

Pathomechanism

Structural Magnetic Resonance Imaging

Higher cortical thickness in the anterior cingulate as well as the orbitofrontal cortex have been found in some [88, 89] but not all structural MRI studies of PD patients with an ICD [90]. Moreover, a prospective study failed to show a difference on cortical thickness in drug-naïve PD patients who developed ICDs after dopaminergic medication during follow-up and those who remained ICD unaffected [65]. Therefore, the role of structural imaging to measure cortical thickness in PD patients with ICDs is still inconclusive.

Functional Magnetic Resonance Imaging

Several fMRI studies have shown decreased activation of the prefrontal cortex and the bilateral striatum [91, 92]. In addition, decreased connectivity from the caudate to the superior parietal cortex and an increased connectivity from the caudate to the insula area have been reported [91].

Lower blood oxygenation levels as well as a reduction in cerebral blood flow were found in the ventral striatum in PD patients with ICDs compared to those without ICDs during risk-taking tasks [93]. At resting state, the presence of ICDs was associated with a functional disconnection between the anterior putamen and the inferior temporal and anterior cingulate gyrii [90]. In contrast, an elevated connectivity in the mesocorticolimbic network has been observed, more specifically between the ventral striatum and its

Table 20.1 Impulse Control Disorder Screening scales in Parkinson's disease

	In use by other investigators	Classification for diagnostic screening	Classification for severity rating
Questionnaire for Impulsive-Compulsive Disorders in Parkinson's Disease (QUIP)	+	Recommended	–
QUIP-Rating Scale (QUIP-RS)	+	Recommended	Recommended
Self-Assessment Scale for Dopamine Dependent Behaviors in Parkinson's Disease (Ardouin short screen)	+	–	Recommended
Scales for Outcomes in Parkinson's Disease–Psychiatric Complications (SCOPA-PC)	+	–	Recommended for compulsive sexual disorder, compulsive shopping, and gambling disorder
Minnesota Impulsive Disorders Interview (MIDI)	+	Suggested	–
The Parkinson's Impulse Control Scale (PICS)	–	Suggested	Suggested
Scale for Evaluation of Neuropsychiatric Disorders in Parkinson's Disease (SEND-PD)	–	–	Suggested
Parkinson's Disease Dopamine Dysregulation Syndrome-Patient and Caregiver Inventory (DDS-PC)	–	–	Suggested

Table adapted from Evans et al. [86]. The terms "suggested" and "recommended" are defined within the article, as defined by the Movement Disorders Society.

connectivity to the anterior cingulate gyrus, orbitofrontal cortex, insula, putamen, globus pallidus, and thalamus [92].

In summary, fMRI data show altered connectivity between and within dopaminergic neuronal circuits involving mesocorticolimbic regions in PD patients with ICDs [94].

Positron Emission Tomography

A significant dopamine agonist-induced reduction of activity (measured by changes in regional cerebral blood flow assessed with ^{15}O-H_2O PET) in brain areas that are important for impulse control and response inhibition (lateral orbitofrontal cortex, rostral cingulate zone, amygdala, external pallidum) was found in PD patients with ICDs compared to those who were ICD free [95].

Although the mesocorticolimbic system is thought to play a crucial role in ICDs in PD, a cerebral 18 F-fluorodeoxyglucose PET study showed that a much larger network, also involving the caudate, the parahippocampus, and the prefrontal cortex, are dysfunctional in PD

patients with ICDs [96]. It has been therefore hypothesized that ICDs in PD are associated with an increased metabolism in the fronto-insular network with reduced dopamine agonist-induced inhibition [94].

A [11 C] raclopride PET study measured striatal dopamine D2/D3 receptor binding and release of dopamine in PD patients with gambling disorder. A greater decrease in post-synaptic [11 C] raclopride binding in the ventral striatum and thus greater striatal dopamine release was found in the ICD group [97]. Furthermore, an increased ventral striatal dopamine release was found in another PET study in PD patients with a variety of ICDs compared to PD controls following a reward-related cue [98]. In line with this, a [11 C] raclopride PET study in patients with DDS who were off medication showed enhanced ventral striatal dopamine release compared to PD controls following administration of levodopa [99]. This increased striatal dopamine release seen in DDS patients as well as in PD patients with ICDs (during gambling, following reward-related images, or following levodopa administration) may be due to neuroplastic changes, leading to sensitization of the ventral striatum.

Multimodal Imaging

Three factors associated with severity of ICDs in PD have been identified combining MRI with PET data. Patients with more severe ICDs had lower dopamine synthesis in the nucleus accumbens and a reduced connectivity between the accumbens and rostral cingulate cortex. On the other hand, a positive correlation with cortical thickness of the subgenual rostral anterior cingulate cortex and ICD severity was found [100].

Basic Science

To consider the basic mechanisms underlying ICD, we focus on the anatomical and functional characteristic of the basal ganglia (BG) and its innervation by dopamine. In PD, the neurons affecting motor function that degenerate are the dopaminergic neurons projecting from the substantia nigra pars compacta (SNC) to the striatum, resulting in diminished levels of striatal dopamine [101].

Theoretical models suggest that the frontal cortex "proposes" candidate motor action plans, which are then evaluated and dynamically gated by the BG and its innervation of the thalamus [102–104]. More specifically, the striatum, the main input region of the BG, contains two distinct major cellular populations of medium-sized spiny neurons (MSNs): MSNs that contain the dopamine D1 receptor and MSNs that contain the dopamine D2 receptor. These distinct populations project to different downstream targets of the basal ganglia: MSNs containing the D1 receptor project directly to the internal portion of the internal globus pallidus (GPi) while the MSNs with the D2 receptor project to the external globus pallidus (GPe). The D1 MSNs are part of the "direct pathway" (because they directly project to the GPi) while the D2 MSNs project to the "indirect pathway." In the following section, we will describe how ICDs and DDS can be attributed to atypical direct and indirect pathway activity. Critically, there are distinct and dissociable types of impulsivity that can emerge following atypical direct and indirect pathway function.

For instance, boosting dopamine in the striatum (perhaps due to dopamine replacement therapy) increases one type of impulsive behavior. This impulsive behavior can be characterized as a strengthening of impulses and is a result of two distinct dopamine-related phenomena: 1) dopamine modulating action selection (choice) and 2) dopamine modulating learning.

Extensive work in animals and humans in the past few decades has clarified dopamine's role in action selection (i.e. choice behavior). High levels of striatal dopamine activate D1-containing MSNs (and thus, the direct pathway) while simultaneously inhibiting D2-containing MSNs (and silencing the indirect pathway). Conversely, low levels of striatal dopamine are associated with reduced activation of D1-containing MSNs but enhanced activation of D2-containing MSNs. Therefore, the amount of striatal dopamine differentially activates the direct and indirect pathways. Classically, direct pathway activation is commonly thought to promote movement via thalamic disinhibition while indirect activation canonically suppresses movement [105]. This model accounts for how dopamine-depleted PD patients regain movement after dopamine replacement therapy. More modern theoretical models refine this notion to propose that the striatal dopamine levels amplify the effective subjective value of actions, rather than promoting movement per se, specifically by reweighting the prospective benefits of alternative actions (encoded in D1 direct pathway neurons) versus the costs of these actions (via D2 indirect activation) [103, 106]. This more nuanced account explains why high striatal dopamine not only increases motor response [103, 107, 108] but also promotes risky behavior in both humans and rodents [109, 110] when the potential gain is large – similar to what ICD patients experience. Zalocusky and colleagues showed that D2 MSN activity is elevated following negative outcomes resulting from risky choice [111]. Using targeted optogenetic stimulation, they further demonstrated that D2 activity during the choice period does not inhibit movement altogether, but instead causally shifts an animal's active choice from risk-seeking to risk-avoiding, whereas D2 inhibition has the opposite effect. In humans, Cools and colleagues demonstrated that PD patients on levodopa bet higher amounts compared to unmedicated PD patients and healthy controls [112].

The effects of dopamine medication on impulsivity may also be emphasized in PD patients because of disease pathology. In PD, nigrostriatal neurons are primarily the ones that degenerate as opposed to mesolimbic neurons which are relatively unaffected [101]. Therefore, the nucleus accumbens (involved in reward processing) may still be relatively normal in PD but the extra dopamine medication potentially causes a local dopamine overdose [113].

The reconceptualization of the D1/D2 dichotomy in terms of valuation rather than motor output per se raises the question: how do the D1- and D2-containing MSNs come to represent the costs and benefits of an action? The answer rests on the finding that in addition to striatal dopamine affecting choice behavior, striatal dopamine also modulates the learning process. Indeed, striatal dopamine has long been linked to learning how rewarding an action is [114]. After an action is taken, the positive or negative outcome is translated into a reward prediction error (RPE; an outcome that is better or worse than expected) that is used to organize future behavior. RPEs in humans and animals are quantified by the increase or decrease of dopamine-releasing cellular activity. Specifically, positive RPEs increase dopaminergic cell activity while negative RPEs reduce dopaminergic cell activity. The resultant transient increases and decreases in dopamine differentially activate the direct and indirect pathways to induce activity-dependent plasticity, make suggested actions more or less likely and thus, instigate learning. As such, with cumulative experience, D1 MSNs come to represent the prospective benefits of actions that lead to positive RPEs, whereas D2 MSNs come to represent their costs. Indeed, striatal dopamine has been experimentally shown to modulate learning of positive and negative outcomes in animals and humans and consequently to drive adaptive behavior [103, 115–118]. An important implication from this work is that high levels of striatal dopamine induces better learning from positive outcomes while low levels of striatal dopamine induces better learning from negative outcomes [103, 106]. As a result, unmedicated PD patients exhibit enhanced learning from negative feedback while medicated PD patients learn better from positive feedback [119–122]. This is believed to be a function of direct and indirect basal ganglia activity influencing the actual learning of reward. Indeed, in rodents, optogenetic stimulation of the direct pathway induced persistent reinforcement while stimulation of the indirect pathway was aversive [123], regardless of whether the reinforced action increased or decreased movement [124].

This logic can account for why medicated patients sometimes develop ICDs: dopaminergic medication may produce better than expected feedback signals that mask the negative consequences of impulsive actions [103, 121, 125]. This also results in a positive feedback loop as D1 neurons, being consistently active, will experience long-term potentiation (LTP), promoting activity in the future while underactive D2 neurons will experience long-term depression (LTD). If boosted levels of dopamine lead to impulsiveness, then reduced levels of dopamine (i.e. unmedicated PD patients) will result in the opposite effect: LTP in the indirect D2 pathway and LTD in the direct D1 pathway. Indeed, empirical animal data finds that blocking D2 receptors (and thus stimulating the indirect pathway) triggers LTP in the indirect pathway [126]. Moreover, animals who are dopamine depleted (analogous to unmedicated PD patients) are cataleptic for progressively longer periods [127]. Under the framework that direct pathway activation represents the benefits of an action and the indirect pathway represents the costs, these dopamine-depleted animals emphasize the costs of any action and become cataleptic as they unconsciously "learn" that actions are too costly [128, 129].

In summary, a type of impulsivity that ICD patients exhibit is most likely due to increased striatal dopamine that changes patients' learning and choice behavior. However, it is important to note that increased dopamine alone does not trigger ICD. The extra dopamine most likely interacts with pre-existing vulnerabilities to result in varying degrees of ICD behavior that differ extensively between patients [130, 131]. It is possible that ICD patients exhibit emphasized striatal impulses (as a function of a dopamine "overdose") as well as diminished ability to control response threshold (perhaps due to DBS or individual differences).

Pathology

One recent post-mortem immunohistochemistry study assessed α-synuclein load and tyrosine hydroxylase activity in the ventral and dorsal striatum of 31 PD patients with ICDs and 29 PD cases without ICDs matched for age, sex, disease duration, and onset of PD. In addition, dopamine D2 and D3 receptors were measured in the frontal cortex, the dorsal and ventral striatum via western blotting. Both α-synuclein load as well as dopamine D3 receptors were reduced in the nucleus accumbens of PD patients with ICDs compared to those without addictive behaviors [132]. These findings dovetail with the previous pathological studies in PD patients without ICDs which showed a relatively less affected ventral compared to the dorsal striatum [101]. Therefore, and according to the "overdose hypothesis," dopaminergic drugs that are necessary to restore the depleted dorsal striatal dopamine levels overstimulate the ventral striatum in some PD patients [133] who may be later more prone to develop ICDs [132]. The lower dopamine D3 receptors found in the ICD group are either a consequence of downregulation, as these patients also had a higher levodopa equivalent dose, or a premorbid trait which may make them more susceptible to develop ICDs [132].

Clinical Vignettes

Case 1: Dopamine Dysregulation Syndrome

A 56-year-old man with PD developed compulsive sexual disorder soon after starting pramipexole. His medication was switched to levodopa monotherapy but soon afterwards, he reported the feeling of being "high" each time after taking levodopa. He started taking levodopa excessively ("like smarties") and demanded multiple levodopa prescriptions from outpatient clinics and his GPs. Eventually he was treated with apomorphine via a continuous pump system with partial improvement of his addictive behavior.

Case 2: Collecting

A 72-year-old man with mild PD started collecting uranium glass a year after starting pramipexole. Neither he nor his wife view this as a problem, although he notes that in retirement he spends a lot of his free time driving to flea markets to find specimens. He reports having over 200 pieces, and likes them because they glow in the dark and have a nice green color [we checked and confirmed that these are harmless and pose no health risks].

Case 3: Compulsive Clothing Change

A 61-year-old woman with mild PD, taking only ropinirole for about three years, reported that she had noticed a change in her behavior. She stated that at every visit she was asked about compulsive behaviors and had never had any, but she had recently started to change her clothes two or three times before she left for work. She found this a puzzling change, as she had never been particularly finicky about dressing and could not explain to herself why she was doing it. After stopping the ropinirole and starting levodopa, this behavior stopped.

Case 4: Hobbyism

A 58-year-old man with a 12-year history of PD, taking both levodopa and pramipexole, reported no problems with compulsive behavior, although he always came to appointments alone. He had always been an avid fisherman, and spent holidays visiting friends who lived near interesting places to fish. Two years after his last visit, having had DBS and reduced his dopaminergic medications, including his dopamine agonist, he reported that although he was still an avid fisherman, his "need" to fish had markedly decreased and he was no longer fishing off the rocks on the ocean during the winter, or in other unsafe situations.

Case 5: Compulsive Behaviors

A 68-year-old woman with PD for ten years started spending hours on making various different lists after starting pramipexole. She also had the compulsion to keep stockings within reach wherever she was in the house in case her feet got cold.

Treatment

Given the lack of specific treatment options, prevention of ICDs is extremely important. All patients and their families as well as caregivers should be informed of the potential risk of developing addictive behaviors after the initiation of dopaminergic therapy, especially dopamine agonists. Doctors should be especially vigilant in male patients, those with depression, young-onset PD, and those with a personal or family history of addictive behaviors. In these patients it may be better to avoid dopamine agonist therapy. Moreover, ICDs evolve slowly over time and therefore patients as well as their families should watch out for subtle personality changes as well as insomnia and sleep fragmentation [10, 134]. In line with this, a recent study has shown that 24% of patients with subsyndromal ICDs (defined as behaviors without reaching the formal diagnostic criteria for ICD) developed full symptoms of an ICD at follow-up after 1 year [68]. It is likely that an individual critical dose of dopamine agonists is necessary before an ICD develops.

When an ICD is noticed, general measures such as limitation of Internet use, credit cards, or bank accounts are advised. Spouses or other caregivers should be involved. General practitioners should be informed to avoid multiple prescriptions. In general, the prognosis is better if treatment starts as soon as possible, however, in rare cases the addictive behavior may not need any specific management and can be monitored (e.g. if the patient is mentally or physically too disabled to engage excessively with the addictive behavior).

Among other non-pharmacological approaches, cognitive behavioral therapy may be useful. A recent evidence-based review considered cognitive behavioral therapy for ICDs as likely efficacious. However, all cognitive behavioral therapy studies bear the risk of bias, as a double blinding study design is not possible [135].

The specific therapy of ICDs in PD relies mostly in reducing and weaning off dopamine agonists in those who have gambling disorder, compulsive sexual disorder, and compulsive shopping disorder. A recent study provides class IV evidence that switching from a dopamine agonist to levodopa improves ICDs and patients' activities of daily living at follow-up after three months. However, in about 16%, this switch was impossible due to side effects such as worsening of motor or non-motor symptoms [136]. Furthermore, withdrawal symptoms such as anxiety, depression, irritability as well as craving, known as the dopamine agonist withdrawal syndrome (DAWS) are frequently seen [137] and may require hospital admission.

In those with DDS a reduction of levodopa or the fast-acting apomorphine injections are necessary. Usually attempts to reduce the total levodopa dose (or apomorphine injections) are met with great resistance and therefore relapses are frequent. In our opinion patients with DDS and those with compulsive sexual disorders have the lowest insight and the poorest prognosis.

Punding usually improves after reducing the levodopa dose but may induce worsening of

motor symptoms. In those cases the use of entacapone, an MAO-B inhibitor, or amantadine can be considered [138]. In addition, physiotherapy may be particularly important for these patients, as a recent study has reported higher postural deformities in PD patients with punding compared to PD controls [72].

Previous studies have linked dyskinesias with ICDs in PD [61]. In fact, oscillatory activity in the subthalamic nucleus has been recorded within the theta–delta band in patients with dyskinesias as well as ICDs albeit with different topography [139]. Therefore, it is not surprising that a reduction of dyskinesias by tapering off the dopamine agonists will often lead to improvement of ICDs and DDS in PD. This has been shown in small uncontrolled studies, which have provided preliminary evidence that continuous delivery of levodopa/carbidopa or apomorphine via a pump system can improve addictive behaviors [140, 141]. The role of DBS targeting the subthalamic nucleus to improve ICDs and DDS is still controversial with conflicting reports [142] but may be considered in carefully selected patients. This procedure presumably is helpful because it allows a major reduction in medication for PD motor problems.

Sleep fragmentation is prevalent in PD particularly in those with ICDs. Although the relationship between sleep deprivation and impulsivity is complex, an improvement of nocturnal sleep is important. Amitriptyline may be useful in selected patients but side effects such as cognitive impairment and dry mouth are limitations. Preferred alternative antidepressants include trazodone and the alpha 2 adrenoreceptor antagonist mirtazapine [66]. The evidence for neuroleptic medication such as quetiapine and clozapine is limited. There are reports that clozapine can improve ICDs [143], but the potential risk of agranulocytosis and the regular blood tests limit its use. However, neuroleptic drugs may be useful to treat concomitant psychosis.

Outcome

Long-term follow-up studies (1–8 years) have shown remission of addictive behaviors in about 40–80% of patients. Reduction and ideally stoppage of dopamine agonist therapy was associated with better outcome [55, 144–146]. The variable outcome may be due to different ICD-severity and the continued use of dopamine agonists due to withdrawal symptoms in some studies [144]. Other factors such as better working memory capacities have also been linked with better long-term outcome of addictive behaviors in PD [147].

References

1. Gatto EM, Aldinio V. Impulse control disorders in Parkinson's disease. A brief and comprehensive review. Front Neurol 2019; **10**: 351.

2. Friedman JH. Punding on levodopa. Biol Psychiatry 1994; **36**(5): 350–351.

3. Barbeau A. L-dopa therapy in Parkinson's disease: a critical review of nine years' experience. Can Med Assoc J 1969; **101**(13): 59–68.

4. Bowers MB Jr, Van Woert M, Davis L. Sexual behavior during L-dopa treatment for Parkinsonism. Am J Psychiatry 1971; **127**(12): 1691–1693.

5. Keenan RE. The Eaton collaborative study of levodopa therapy in parkinsonism: a summary. Neurology 1970; **20**(12): 46–65.

6. Shapiro SK. Hypersexual behavior complicating levodopa (I-dopa) therapy. Minn Med 1973; **56**(1): 58–59.

7. Markham CH, Treciokas LJ, Diamond SG. Parkinson's disease and levodopa. A five-year follow-up and review. West J Med 1974; **121**(3): 188–206.

8. O'Brien CP, et al. Mental effects of high-dosage levodopa. Arch Gen Psychiatry 1971; **24**(1): 61–64.

9. Goodwin FK. Behavioral effects of L-dopa in man. Semin Psychiatry 1971; **3**(4):477–492.

10. Averbeck BB, O'Sullivan SS, Djamshidian A. Impulsive and compulsive behaviors in Parkinson's disease. Annu Rev Clin Psychol 2014; **10**: 553–580.

11. Weintraub D, et al. Questionnaire for Impulsive-Compulsive Disorders in Parkinson's Disease-Rating Scale. Mov Disord 2012; **27**(2): 242–247.

12. Evans AH, et al. Impulsive and compulsive behaviors in Parkinson's disease. Mov Disord 2009; **24**(11): 1561–1570.

13. Weintraub D. Impulse control disorders in Parkinson's disease: a 20-year odyssey. Mov Disord 2019; **34**(4): 447–452.

14. Weintraub D, et al. Impulse control disorders in Parkinson disease: a cross-sectional study of 3090 patients. Arch Neurol 2010; **67**(5): 589–595.

15. Antonini A, et al. ICARUS study: prevalence and clinical features of impulse control disorders in Parkinson's disease. J Neurol Neurosurg Psychiatry 2017; **88**(4): 317–324.

16. Vela L, et al. The high prevalence of impulse control behaviors in patients with early-onset Parkinson's disease: a cross-sectional multicenter study. J Neurol Sci 2016; **368**: 150–154.

17. Voon V, et al. Prevalence of repetitive and reward-seeking behaviors in Parkinson disease. Neurology 2006; **67**(7): 1254–1257.

18. Solla P, et al. Paraphilias and paraphilic disorders in Parkinson's disease: a systematic review of the literature. Mov Disord 2015; **30**(5): 604–613.

19. Barbosa PM, et al. Compulsive sexual behaviour in Parkinson's disease is associated with higher doses of levodopa. J Neurol Neurosurg Psychiatry 2018; **89**(10): 1121–1123.

20. Almeida KJ, et al. Zoophilia and Parkinson's disease. Parkinsonism Relat Disord 2013; **19**(12): 1167–1168.

21. Djamshidian A, et al. Pathological gambling in Parkinson's disease–a review of the literature. Mov Disord 2011; **26**(11): 1976–1984.

22. McElroy SL, et al. Compulsive buying: a report of 20 cases. J Clin Psychiatry 1994; **55**(6): 242–248.

23. Lee JY, et al. Association between the dose of dopaminergic medication and the behavioral disturbances in Parkinson disease. Parkinsonism Relat Disord 2009; **16**(3): 202–207.

24. Cossu G, Rinaldi R, Colosimo C. The rise and fall of impulse control behavior disorders. Parkinsonism Relat Disord 2018; **46**(Suppl 1): S24–S29.

25. Giovannoni G, et al. Hedonistic homeostatic dysregulation in patients with Parkinson's disease on dopamine replacement therapies. J Neurol Neurosurg Psychiatry 2000; **68**(4): 423–428.

26. Warren N, et al. Dopamine dysregulation syndrome in Parkinson's disease: a systematic review of published cases. J Neurol Neurosurg Psychiatry 2017; **88**(12): 1060–1064.

27. Bearn J, et al. Recognition of a dopamine replacement therapy dependence syndrome in Parkinson's disease: a pilot study. Drug Alcohol Depend 2004; **76**(3): 305–310.

28. O'Sullivan SS, Evans AH, Lees AJ. Dopamine dysregulation syndrome: an overview of its epidemiology, mechanisms and management. CNS Drugs 2009; **23**(2): 157–170.

29. Schiorring E. Psychopathology induced by "speed drugs." Pharmacol Biochem Behav 1981; **14**(Suppl 1): 109–122.

30. Rylander G. Stereotype behavior in man following amphetamine abuse. In: SB DeC Baker (ed.). *The*

Correlation of Adverse Effects in Man with Observations in Animals. International Congress Series no. 230, vol. **12**. Excerpta Medica; 1971, 28–31.

31. Rylander G. Psychoses and the punding and choreiform syndromes in addiction to central stimulant drugs. Psychiatr Neurol Neurochir 1972; **75**(3): 203–212.

32. Fernandez HH, Friedman JH. Punding on L-dopa. Mov Disord 1999; **14**(5): 836–838.

33. Evans AH, et al. Punding in Parkinson's disease: its relation to the dopamine dysregulation syndrome. Mov Disord 2004; **19**(4): 397–405.

34. Voon V. Repetition, repetition, and repetition: compulsive and punding behaviors in Parkinson's disease. Mov Disord 2004; **19**(4): 367–370.

35. Spencer AH, et al. The prevalence and clinical characteristics of punding in Parkinson's disease. Mov Disord 2011; **26**(4): 578–586.

36. O'Sullivan SS, et al. Reckless generosity in Parkinson's disease. Mov Disord 2010; **25**(2): 221–223.

37. O'Sullivan SS, et al. Excessive hoarding in Parkinson's disease. Mov Disord 2010; **25**(8): 1026–1033.

38. Bienfait KL, et al. Impulsive smoking in a patient with Parkinson's disease treated with dopamine agonists. J Clin Neurosci 2010; **17**(4): 539–540.

39. Avanzi M, et al. The thrill of reckless driving in patients with Parkinson's disease: an additional behavioural phenomenon in dopamine dysregulation syndrome? Parkinsonism Relat Disord 2008; **14**(3): 257–258.

40. Friedman JH, Chang V. Crack cocaine use due to dopamine agonist therapy in Parkinson disease. Neurology 2013; **80**(24): 2269–2270.

41. Micheli F, et al. Pet killing as a manifestation of impulse control disorder secondary to pramipexol. Clin Neuropharmacol 2015; **38**(2): 55–56.

42. Santens P, et al. Crime and Parkinson's: the jury is out. Mov Disord 2018; **33**(7): 1092–1094.

43. Gillan CM, et al. The role of habit in compulsivity. Eur Neuropsychopharmacol 2016; **26**(5): 828–840.

44. Robbins TW, et al. Neurocognitive endophenotypes of impulsivity and compulsivity: towards dimensional psychiatry. Trends Cogn Sci 2012; **16**(1): 81–91.

45. Fontenelle LF, et al. Obsessive-compulsive disorder, impulse control disorders and drug addiction: common features and potential treatments. Drugs 2011; **71**(7): 827–840.

46. Robbins TW, Vaghi MM, Banca P. Obsessive-compulsive disorder: puzzles and prospects. Neuron 2019; **102**(1): 27–47.

47. Taylor S. Early versus late onset obsessive-compulsive disorder: evidence for distinct subtypes. Clin Psychol Rev 2011; **31**(7): 1083–1100.

48. Hirschtritt ME, Bloch MH, Mathews CA. Obsessive-Compulsive Disorder: Advances in Diagnosis and Treatment. JAMA 2017; **317**(13): 1358–1367.

49. de Chazeron I, et al. Compulsive eating behaviors in Parkinson's disease. Eat Weight Disord 2019; **24**(3): 421–429.

50. Zahodne LB, et al. Binge eating in Parkinson's disease: prevalence, correlates and the contribution of deep brain stimulation. J Neuropsychiatry Clin Neurosci 2011; **23**(1): 56–62.

51. Weintraub D, et al. Screening for impulse control symptoms in patients with de novo Parkinson disease: a case-control study. Neurology 2013; **80**(2): 176–180.

52. Bharmal A, et al. Outcomes of patients with Parkinson disease and pathological gambling. Can J Neurol Sci 2010; **37**(4): 473–477.

53. Gallagher DA, et al. Pathological gambling in Parkinson's disease: risk factors and differences from dopamine dysregulation. An analysis of published case series. Mov Disord 2007; **22**(12): 1757–1763.

54. Hassan A, et al. Dopamine agonist-triggered pathological behaviors: surveillance in the PD clinic reveals high frequencies. Parkinsonism Relat Disord 2011; **17**(4): 260–264.

55. Corvol JC, et al. Longitudinal analysis of impulse control disorders in Parkinson disease. Neurology 2018; **91**(3): e189–e201.

56. Grall-Bronnec M, et al. Dopamine agonists and impulse control disorders: a complex association. Drug Saf 2018; **41**(1): 19–75.

57. Garcia-Ruiz PJ, et al. Impulse control disorder in patients with Parkinson's disease under dopamine agonist therapy: a multicentre study. J Neurol Neurosurg Psychiatry 2014; **85**(8): 840–844.

58. Etminan M, et al. Risk of gambling disorder and impulse control disorder with aripiprazole, pramipexole, and ropinirole: a pharmacoepidemiologic study. J Clin Psychopharmacol 2017; **37**(1): 102–104.

59. Lertxundi U, et al. Aripiprazole and impulse control disorders: higher risk with the intramuscular depot formulation? Int Clin Psychopharmacol 2018; **33**(1): 56–58.

60. Voon V, et al. Impulse control disorders in Parkinson disease: a multicenter case–control study. Ann Neurol 2011; **69**(6): 986–996.

61. Voon V, et al. Impulse control disorders and levodopa-induced dyskinesias in Parkinson's disease: an update. Lancet Neurol 2017; **16**(3): 238–250.

62. Hinkle JT, et al. Markers of impaired motor and cognitive volition in Parkinson's disease: correlates of dopamine dysregulation syndrome, impulse control disorder, and dyskinesias. Parkinsonism Relat Disord 2018; **47**: 50–56.

63. Marin-Lahoz J, et al. Depression as a risk factor for impulse control disorders in Parkinson disease. Ann Neurol 2019; **86**(5): 762–769.

64. Biundo R, et al. Impulse control disorders in advanced Parkinson's disease with dyskinesia: the ALTHEA study. Mov Disord 2017; **32**(11): 1557–1565.

65. Ricciardi L, et al. Can we predict development of impulsive-compulsive behaviours in Parkinson's disease? J Neurol Neurosurg Psychiatry 2018; **89**(5): 476–481.

66. Djamshidian A, Poewe W, Hogl B. Impact of impulse control disorders on sleep-wake regulation in Parkinson's disease. Parkinsons Dis 2015; **2015**: 970862.

67. Fantini ML, et al. Increased risk of impulse control symptoms in Parkinson's disease with REM sleep behaviour disorder. J Neurol Neurosurg Psychiatry 2015; **86**(2): 174–179.

68. Baig F, et al. Impulse control disorders in Parkinson disease and RBD: a longitudinal study of severity. Neurology 2019; **93**(7):. e675–e687.

69. Marin-Lahoz J, et al. Depression as a risk factor for impulse control disorders in Parkinson disease. Ann Neurol 2019; **86**(5): 762–769.

70. Evans AH, et al. Factors influencing susceptibility to compulsive dopaminergic drug use in Parkinson disease. Neurology 2005; **65**(10): 1570–1574.

71. Fasano A, Petrovic I. Insights into pathophysiology of punding reveal possible treatment strategies. Mol Psychiatry 2010; **15**(6): 560–573.

72. Aoki R, et al. Deterioration of postural deformity in Parkinson's disease patients with punding and hobbyism. J Clin Neurosci 2019; **69**: 179–183.

73. Miwa H, et al. Stereotyped behaviors or punding after quetiapine administration in Parkinson's disease. Parkinsonism Relat Disord 2004; **10**(3): 177–180.

74. Djamshidian A, et al. Novelty seeking behaviour in Parkinson's disease. Neuropsychologia 2011; **49**(9): 2483–2488.

75. Latella D, et al. Impulse control disorders in Parkinson's disease: a systematic review on risk factors and pathophysiology. J Neurol Sci 2019; **398**: 101–106.

76. Poletti M, et al. Alexithymia is associated with impulsivity in newly diagnosed, drug-naive patients with Parkinson's disease: an affective risk factor for the development of impulse-control disorders? J Neuropsychiatry Clin Neurosci 2012; **24**(4): E36–37.

77. Goerlich-Dobre KS, et al. Alexithymia: an independent risk factor for impulsive-compulsive disorders in Parkinson's disease. Mov Disord 2014; **29**(2): 214–220.

78. Graff-Radford J, et al. Dopamine agonists and Othello's syndrome. Parkinsonism Relat Disord 2010; **16**(10): 680–682.

79. Kataoka H, Sugie K. Delusional jealousy (Othello syndrome) in 67 patients with Parkinson's disease. Front Neurol 2018; **9**: 129.

80. Sierra M, et al. Apathy and impulse control disorders: yin and yang of dopamine-dependent behaviors. J Parkinsons Dis 2015; **5**(3): 625–636.

81. Leroi I, et al. Apathy and impulse control disorders in Parkinson's disease: a direct comparison. Parkinsonism Relat Disord 2012; **18**(2): 198–203.

82. Willis AW, et al. Epidemiology and neuropsychiatric manifestations of young onset Parkinson's disease in the United States. Parkinsonism Relat Disord 2013; **19**(2): 202–206.

83. Eisen SA, et al. Familial influences on gambling behavior: an analysis of 3359 twin pairs. Addiction 1998; **93**(9): 1375–1384.

84. Kraemmer J, et al. Clinical-genetic model predicts incident impulse control disorders in Parkinson's disease. J Neurol Neurosurg Psychiatry 2016; **87**(10): 1106–1111.

85. Morgante F, et al. Impulsive-compulsive behaviors in parkin-associated Parkinson disease. Neurology 2016; **87**(14): 1436–1441.

86. Evans AH, et al. Scales to assess impulsive and compulsive behaviors in Parkinson's disease: critique and recommendations. Mov Disord 2019; **34**(6): 791–798.

87. Weintraub D, et al. Validation of the questionnaire for impulsive-compulsive disorders in Parkinson's disease. Mov Disord 2009; **24**(10): 1461–1467.

88. Tessitore A, et al. Cortical thickness changes in patients with Parkinson's disease and impulse

control disorders. Parkinsonism Relat Disord 2016; **24**: 119–125.

89. Pellicano C, et al. Morphometric changes in the reward system of Parkinson's disease patients with impulse control disorders. J Neurol 2015; **262**(12): 2653–2661.

90. Carriere N, et al. Impaired corticostriatal connectivity in impulse control disorders in Parkinson disease. Neurology 2015; **84**(21): 2116–2123.

91. Filip P, et al. Disruption of multiple distinctive neural networks associated with impulse control disorder in Parkinson's disease. Front Hum Neurosci 2018; **12**: 462.

92. Petersen K, et al. Ventral striatal network connectivity reflects reward learning and behavior in patients with Parkinson's disease. Hum Brain Mapp 2018; **39**(1): 509–521.

93. Rao H, et al. Decreased ventral striatal activity with impulse control disorders in Parkinson's disease. Mov Disord 2010; **25** (11): 1660–1669.

94. Roussakis AA, Lao-Kaim NP, Piccini P. Brain imaging and impulse control disorders in Parkinson's disease. Curr Neurol Neurosci Rep 2019; **19**(9): 67.

95. van Eimeren T, et al. Drug-induced deactivation of inhibitory networks predicts pathological gambling in PD. Neurology 2010; **75**(19): 1711–1716.

96. Verger A, et al. Brain PET substrate of impulse control disorders in Parkinson's disease: a metabolic connectivity study. Hum Brain Mapp 2018; **39**(8): 3178–3186.

97. Steeves TD, et al. Increased striatal dopamine release in Parkinsonian patients with pathological gambling: a [11 C] raclopride PET study. Brain 2009; **132**(Pt 5): 1376–1385.

98. O'Sullivan SS, et al. Cue-induced striatal dopamine release in Parkinson's disease-associated impulsive-compulsive behaviours. Brain 2011; **134**(Pt 4): 969–978.

99. Evans AH, et al. Compulsive drug use linked to sensitized ventral striatal dopamine transmission. Ann Neurol 2006; **59**(5): 852–858.

100. Hammes J, et al. Dopamine metabolism of the nucleus accumbens and fronto-striatal connectivity modulate impulse control. Brain 2019; **142**(3): 733–743.

101. Kish SJ, Shannak K, Hornykiewicz O. Uneven pattern of dopamine loss in the striatum of patients with idiopathic Parkinson's disease. Pathophysiologic and clinical implications. N Engl J Med 1988; **318**(14): 876–880.

102. Mink JW. The basal ganglia: focused selection and inhibition of competing motor programs. Prog Neurobiol 1996; **50**(4): 381–425.

103. Frank MJ. Dynamic dopamine modulation in the basal ganglia: a neurocomputational account of cognitive deficits in medicated and nonmedicated Parkinsonism. J Cog Neurosci 2005; **17**(1): 51–72.

104. Frank MJ. Hold your horses: a dynamic computational role for the subthalamic nucleus in decision making. Neural Netw 2006; **19**(8): 1120–1136.

105. Albin RL, Young AB, Penney JB. The functional anatomy of basal ganglia disorders. Trend Neurosci 1989; **12**(10): 366–375.

106. Collins AG, Frank MJ. Opponent actor learning (OpAL): modeling interactive effects of striatal dopamine on reinforcement learning and choice incentive. Psychol Rev 2014; **121**(3): 337.

107. Zénon A, et al. The human subthalamic nucleus encodes the subjective value of reward and the cost of effort during decision-making. Brain 2016; **139**(6): 1830–1843.

108. Beierholm U, et al. Dopamine modulates reward-related vigor. Neuropsychopharmacol 2013; **38**(8): 1495.

109. Rigoli F, et al. Dopamine increases a value-independent gambling propensity. Neuropsychopharmacol 2016; **41**(11): 2658.

110. St. Onge JR, Floresco SB. Prefrontal cortical contribution to risk-based decision making. Cereb Cortex 2009; **20**(8): 1816–1828.

111. Zalocusky KA, et al. Nucleus accumbens D2 R cells signal prior outcomes and control risky decision-making. Nature 2016; **531**(7596): 642.

112. Cools R, et al. L-Dopa medication remediates cognitive inflexibility, but increases impulsivity in patients with Parkinson's disease. Neuropsychologia 2003; **41**(11): 1431–1441.

113. Cools R, et al. Enhanced or impaired cognitive function in Parkinson's disease as a function of dopaminergic medication and task demands. Cereb Cortex 2001; **11**(12): 1136–1143.

114. Schultz W. Predictive reward signal of dopamine neurons. J Neurophysiol 1998; **80**(1): 1–27.

115. de Boer L, et al. Dorsal striatal dopamine D1 receptor availability predicts an instrumental bias in action learning. Proc Nat Acad Sci 2019; **116** (1): 261–270.

116. Cools R, Clark L, Robbins TW. Differential responses in human striatum and prefrontal cortex to changes in object and rule relevance. J Neurosci 2004; **24**(5): 1129–1135.

117. Pessiglione M, et al. Dopamine-dependent prediction errors underpin reward-seeking behaviour in humans. Nature 2006; **442**(7106): 1042.

118. Schönberg T, et al. Reinforcement learning signals in the human striatum distinguish learners from nonlearners during reward-based decision making. J Neurosci 2007; **27**(47): 12860–12867.

119. Frank MJ, Seeberger LC, O'Reilly RC. By carrot or by stick: cognitive reinforcement learning in parkinsonism. Science 2004; **306**(5703): 1940–1943.

120. Bódi N, et al. Reward-learning and the novelty-seeking personality: a between- and within-subjects study of the effects of dopamine agonists on young Parkinson's patients. Brain 2009; **132** (9): 2385–2395.

121. Voon V, et al. Impulsive choice and response in dopamine agonist-related impulse control behaviors. Psychopharmacol 2010; **207**(4): 645–659.

122. Cools R, et al. Top–down attentional control in Parkinson's disease: salient considerations. J Cog Neurosci 2010; **22**(5): 848–859.

123. Kravitz AV, Tye LD, Kreitzer AC. Distinct roles for direct and indirect pathway striatal neurons in reinforcement. Nat Neurosci 2012; **15**(6): 816.

124. Yttri EA, Dudman JT. Opponent and bidirectional control of movement velocity in the basal ganglia. Nature 2016; **533**(7603): 402.

125. McCoy B, et al. Dopaminergic medication reduces striatal sensitivity to negative outcomes in Parkinson's disease. Brain 2019; **142**(11): 3605–3620.

126. Centonze D, et al. Chronic haloperidol promotes corticostriatal long-term potentiation by targeting dopamine D2 L receptors. J Neurosci 2004; **24**(38): 8214–8222.

127. Klein A, Schmidt WJ. Catalepsy intensifies context-dependently irrespective of whether it is induced by intermittent or chronic dopamine deficiency. Behav Pharmacol 2003; **14**(1): 49–53.

128. Beeler JA, Frazier CR, Zhuang X. Putting desire on a budget: dopamine and energy expenditure, reconciling reward and resources. Front Integr Neurosci 2012; **6**: 49.

129. Wiecki TV, Frank MJ. Neurocomputational models of motor and cognitive deficits in Parkinson's disease. Prog Brain Res 2010; **183**: 275–297.

130. Weintraub D, et al. Questionnaire for impulsive-compulsive disorders in Parkinson's disease–rating scale. Mov Disord 2012; **27**(2): 242–247.

131. Voon V, Mehta AR, Hallett M. Impulse control disorders in Parkinson's disease: recent advances. Curr Opin Neurol 2011; **24**(4): 324.

132. Barbosa P, et al. Lower nucleus accumbens alpha-synuclein load and D3 receptor levels in Parkinson's disease with impulsive compulsive behaviours. Brain 2019; **142**(11): 3580–3591.

133. Vaillancourt DE, et al. Dopamine overdose hypothesis: evidence and clinical implications. Mov Disord 2013; **28**(14): 1920–1929.

134. O'Sullivan SS, et al. Sleep disturbance and impulsive-compulsive behaviours in Parkinson's disease. J Neurol Neurosurg Psychiatry 2011; **82** (6): 620–622.

135. Seppi K, et al. Update on treatments for nonmotor symptoms of Parkinson's disease-an evidence-based medicine review. Mov Disord 2019; **34**(2): 180–198.

136. Lee JY, et al. Behavioural and trait changes in parkinsonian patients with impulse control disorder after switching from dopamine agonist to levodopa therapy: results of REIN-PD trial. J Neurol Neurosurg Psychiatry 2019; **90**(1): 30–37.

137. Rabinak CA, Nirenberg MJ. Dopamine agonist withdrawal syndrome in Parkinson disease. Arch Neurol 2010; **67**(1): 58–63.

138. Fasano A, et al. Management of punding in Parkinson's disease: an open-label prospective study. J Neurol 2011; **258**(4): 656–660.

139. Rodriguez-Oroz MC, et al. Involvement of the subthalamic nucleus in impulse control disorders associated with Parkinson's disease. Brain 2011; **134**(Pt 1): 36–49.

140. Barbosa P, et al. A retrospective evaluation of the frequency of impulsive compulsive behaviors in Parkinson's disease patients treated with continuous waking day apomorphine pumps. Mov Disord Clin Pract 2017; **4**(3): 323–328.

141. Todorova A, et al. Infusion therapies and development of impulse control disorders in advanced Parkinson disease: clinical experience after 3 years' follow-up. Clin Neuropharmacol 2015; **38**(4): 132–134.

142. Eisinger RS, et al. Medications, deep brain stimulation, and other factors influencing

impulse control disorders in Parkinson's disease. Front Neurol 2019; **10**: 86.

143. Rotondo A, et al. Clozapine for medication-related pathological gambling in Parkinson disease. Mov Disord 2010; **25**(12): 1994–1995.

144. Barbosa PM, et al. The long-term outcome of impulsive compulsive behaviours in Parkinson's disease. J Neurol Neurosurg Psychiatry 2019; **90**(11): 1288–1289.

145. Sohtaoglu M, et al. Long-term follow-up of Parkinson's disease patients with impulse control disorders. Parkinsonism Relat Disord 2010; **16** (5): 334–337.

146. Mamikonyan E, et al. Long-term follow-up of impulse control disorders in Parkinson's disease. Mov Disord 2008; **23**(1): 75–80.

147. Siri C, et al. Long-term cognitive follow-up of Parkinson's disease patients with impulse control disorders. Mov Disord 2015; **30**(5): 696–704.

Chapter 21

Serotonin Syndrome and Drug Interactions, Hypertensive Complications, and, Adverse Effects of Monoamine Oxidase Inhibitors in Patients with Parkinson's Disease

Eoin Mulroy, Kailash P. Bhatia

The Role of Monoamine Oxidase in Dopamine and Serotonin Metabolism

Monoamine oxidase (MAO), located in the outer mitochondrial membrane, is a critical enzyme in the metabolism of a number of neurotransmitters. Two isoforms of the enzyme exist, MAO-A and MAO-B [1]. These differ both in their tissue distribution and substrate selectivity. MAO-A is predominantly located in the periphery (including the gut) and preferentially catalyses the oxidation of 5-hydroxytyptamine (5-HT, serotonin) and norepinephrine [1]. MAO-B selectively metabolizes beta-phenylethylamine, while tyramine and dopamine are substrates for both types [1]. MAO inhibition, either non-specific or selective, increases the synaptic concentrations of the usually metabolized neurochemicals, providing symptomatic benefit in a variety of neurological and psychiatric disorders.

A Brief History of Monoamine Oxidase Inhibition in Parkinson's Disease

The first published reports detailing the use of MAOIs in Parkinson's disease (PD) began emerging in the mid-twentieth century. These involved the administration of non-selective monoamine oxidase inhibitors (MAOIs), either alone or in combination with levodopa, to small numbers of patients with PD [2]. In 1968, Johnston discovered the two different forms of monoamine oxidase (MAO), MAO-A and MAO-B [3]. Selegiline (initially termed L-deprenyl) was the first MAO-B

inhibitor to be synthesized. Initially patented as an antidepressant in the mid-1960s, its potential as a treatment of motor and non-motor features of PD would only become recognized a decade later [2].

Monoamine oxidase inhibitors can be classified into three types according to which form of the enzyme they inhibit:

1. Irreversible non-selective inhibitors. These are predominantly older medications such as phenelzine and tranylcypromine.
2. Selective, irreversible MAO-B inhibitors such as selegiline, rasagiline, and safinamide.
3. Reversible, selective MAO-A inhibitors such as moclobemide.

The utility and side-effect profiles vary depending on individual medication types. Classical non-selective MAOIs and selective MAO-A inhibitors are primarily useful in the treatment of mood disorders, likely because of their ability to influence serotonergic and noradrenergic signaling. Conversely, selective MAO-B inhibitors are the class of drugs which are used to target the motor features of PD, owing to both their influence on the dopaminergic system and the absence of MAO-A inhibition-related adverse effects.

Evidence Base for Monoamine Oxidase Inhibitors Use in the Treatment of Parkinson's Disease

Motor Symptoms

Selegiline was the first MAOI to be approved by the FDA for the treatment of PD. It is used both as monotherapy and as an adjunctive treatment for PD [4]. Unequivocal demonstration of its safety and efficacy in PD patients came through the landmark DATATOP trial. This demonstrated that patients with early PD receiving selegiline had a longer time to disability requiring levodopa therapy than those receiving placebo (or vitamin E) [5]. Note was made of some cardiac arrhythmias in the selegiline group, likely as a result of the amphetamine metabolites of this drug [5]. Further clinical trials demonstrated that the addition of selegiline permitted a 30% to 40% sparing in levodopa dose, though functional disability was not affected (albeit that patients without selegiline required higher doses of levodopa) [6, 7]. There were also some signals of increased motor fluctuations, dyskinesia, or even increased mortality in the selegiline arms [6, 7].

The TEMPO and ADAGIO studies, both randomized, double-blind, placebo-controlled trials, demonstrated the safety and efficacy of rasagiline monotherapy in patients with PD [8]. The former demonstrated the efficacy of rasagiline at 1 mg and 2 mg doses above placebo in reducing mean total Unified Parkinson's Disease Rating Scale (UPDRS) scores at 26-week follow-up [9]. A further one-year extension of this trial showed benefit to early initiation of treatment, a finding which was replicated in the ADAGIO trial at the 1 mg but not the 2 mg dose, making conclusions about its disease-modifying effects difficult [10]. The PRESTO trial demonstrated the efficacy of rasagiline in improving motor fluctuations in patients already optimized to levodopa therapy, while in the LARGO study, rasagiline reduced mean daily off time to a degree similar to entacapone [11, 12].

Safinamide has recently been approved by both the European Commission and the US Food and Drug Administration (FDA) as an add-on therapy to levodopa/carbidopa in the treatment of PD. It works through multiple mechanisms, including reversible, selective MAO-B inhibition and modulation of glutamate release [13]. In addition, it is purported to have an anti-dyskinetic effect, though this has not been conclusively demonstrated in human studies.

Non-Motor Symptoms

Theoretically at least, the main non-motor symptom of PD which would be targeted by the administration of MAOIs is depression. This however requires either the use of older non-selective drugs such as tranylcypromine, MAO-A inhibitors such as moclobemide, or the administration of high doses of MAO-B inhibitors such that they produce non-selective MAO effects [2]. While studies have demonstrated the efficacy of these drugs in depression, especially atypical depression, MAOIs are rarely employed to treat mood disorders in PD, and their use in the psychiatric realm is declining [14]. This is both due to the dietary restrictions required (in order to avoid tyramine reactions) and to the potential for drug–drug interaction, in particular leading to serotonin syndrome, which is a particular concern in patients with PD.

Selegiline is occasionally employed as a treatment for another common non-motor symptom in PD, fatigue [15]. Its mechanism of action in this instance is thought to result from its metabolism into the stimulant compounds, L-amphetamine and L-methamphetamine. Such metabolites are not produced from metabolism of rasagiline, safinamide, or indeed new sublingual delivery systems of selegiline, which are designed to avoid such first-pass metabolism [16].

In the PRESTO study [11], rates of depression were significantly lower in patients taking rasagiline 0.5 mg daily as compared to placebo (p = 0.04). A meta-analysis of 11 controlled clinical trials of major depressive disorder in PD showed that rasagiline was effective, but especially at the 2 mg dose, which is above the recommended dose of 1 mg daily used in the treatment of motor Parkinsonism [17].

Disease-Modifying Effect

The potential disease-modifying effect of MAOIs has proven a vexed subject, with abundant arguments for and against the motion. A disease-modifying effect of both selegiline and rasagiline has been suggested in in-vitro and animal models.

The interest in potential disease-modifying effects of MAO-B inhibitors began with the observation that MAO-B was required for the conversion of MPTP to the active and toxic MPP+ [18]. This also suggested a possible mechanism through which MAO-B inhibition may limit neurodegeneration, namely through modulation of the mitochondrial oxidative stress pathway [18]. Since these early studies, other possible neuroprotective mechanisms including increased neurotrophin production or upregulation of anti-apoptotic factors have been suggested [19–21]. Notably however, despite promising in-vitro and animal models, a true disease-modifying effect of MAO-B inhibitors has not been conclusively proven in the controlled trial setting.

Adverse Effects of Monoamine Oxidase Inhibition

Serotonin Syndrome

Serotonin syndrome, probably the most publicized and feared complication of MAOI use, is a life-threatening condition resulting from excess central and peripheral serotonergic agonism. First reported in 1960 following the co-administration of L-tryptophan with a MAOI [22], the disorder comprises three cardinal manifestations: altered mental status, autonomic dysfunction, and neuromuscular effects. Its true prevalence is unknown, and it is likely than many mild cases remain unrecognized or unreported. Occurring exclusively as a complication of medication administration, the vast majority of cases result from intentional drug overdose, with the remainder mainly ensuing from inadvertent drug–drug interactions [23].

Serotonergic innervation of the central nervous system stems from neurons in the midline Raphe nuclei of the brainstem [24]. These project both rostrally (contributing to the regulation of wakefulness, thermoregulation, mood, and behavior) and caudally to spinal regions where they influence spinal tone and nociception [24]. Peripherally, serotonin is involved in the regulation of vascular tone, gastrointestinal motility, and platelet function.

Serotonergic neurotransmission involves release of pre-synaptic vesicles containing serotonin into the synaptic cleft. Here they exert an effect both on post-synaptic receptors, effecting neurotransmission, and on pre-synaptic receptors which suppress the further release of serotonin [24]. Serotonergic signalling is primarily terminated by re-uptake of serotonin into pre-synaptic neurons, a process mainly regulated by serotonin reuptake transporter protein (SERT) [24]. Once re-uptake is complete, serotonin is metabolized, predominantly by MAO-A, to 5-hydroxyindoleacetic acid (5-HIAA).

Serotonin syndrome results from excess stimulation of post-synaptic 5-HT receptors, particularly the 5-HT_{1A} and 5-HT_{2A} subtypes, with the former likely mediating some of the milder and the latter (requiring higher concentrations of serotonin to be activated) some of the more severe symptoms of serotonin toxicity [24]. This likely explains why severe SS is generally only encountered with particular combinations of drugs which act in concert to significantly increase serotonergic receptor activation. Indeed, while SS has occasionally been reported following exposure to a single drug (either in overdose or after dose escalation in susceptible individuals), severe SS is usually encountered only following administration of at least two drugs, with the combination of MAOIs alongside other serotonergic drugs being particularly dangerous. Furthermore, attention must be paid not only to drugs with obvious serotonergic properties, but also to those which may inhibit drug metabolism (particularly through the CYP450 pathway) as well as medications which are not commonly recognized to influence serotonin metabolism or serotonergic neurotransmission (see Table 21.1).

Serotonin Syndrome in Parkinson's Disease

Significant depression is encountered in up to 50% of patients with Parkinson's disease, making this one of the most common neuropsychiatric manifestations of this disorder [25]. Nigral dopaminergic neuronal loss producing dopamine deficiency in mesolimbic circuits as well as degenerative neuropathology extending to serotonergic and noradrenergic neurons likely accounts for this high prevalence [26]. Untreated, depressive symptoms in PD negatively impact quality of life and caregiver burden but also result in greater physical disability, cognitive deterioration, and increased mortality [27–29]. Many patients with PD require pharmacologic treatment for their mood symptoms, often with selective serotonin reuptake inhibitors (SSRIs), serotonin norepinephrine reuptake inhibitors (SNRIs), or tricyclic antidepressants, often in combination with MAO-B inhibitors. Such a polypharmaceutic milieu could theoretically predispose PD patients to SS.

Clinical Manifestations of Serotonin Syndrome

The manifestations of serotonin syndrome are protean and exist along a spectrum ranging from mild clinical symptoms and signs which could be

Table 21.1 Examples of drugs implicated in serotonin syndrome

Mechanism	Specific agents
Reduced serotonin metabolism	*MAO-inhibitors* **Antidepressants:** phenylzine, pargyline, clorgyline, tranylcypromine, moclobemide **Anti-Parkinsonian medications:** selegiline, rasagiline **Antibiotics:** linezolid, isoniazid **Others:** methylene blue, procarbazine, Syrian rue
Reduced serotonin reuptake	**SSRIs:** fluoxetine, paroxetine, citalopram, sertraline, escitalopram, fluvoxamine, trazodone **SNRIs:** venlafaxine, duloxetine **TCAs:** imipramine, clomipramine **Opioids:** meperidine, buprenorphine, tramadol, dextromethorphan, pethidine, methadone, fentanyl **Antiepileptics:** valproate, carbamazepine **Antiemetics:** ondansetron, granisetron, metoclopramide **Others:** St. John's Wort
Increased serotonin release	**Drugs of abuse:** cocaine, MDMA **Amphetamine and its derivatives:** phentermine, fenfluramine, and dexfenfluramine **Others:** dextromethorphan
5-HT receptor agonists	**Triptans** e.g. rizatriptan, sumatriptan, zolmitriptan, frovatriptan, naratriptan **Ergots and ergot derivatives:** dihydroergotamine **Opiates:** fentanyl, meperidine **Drugs of abuse:** LSD **Antiepileptics:** sodium valproate, carbamazepine
CYP2D6 and CYP3A4 inhibitors	**Antibiotics:** ciprofloxacin, erythromycin **Antifungals:** fluconazole **Antivirals:** ritonavir

easily overlooked through to shock, multi-organ failure, and death. In mild cases, neuromuscular symptoms may include tremor, myoclonus, and hyperreflexia, progressing to frank rigidity and spontaneous clonus in more severe instances. Interestingly, reflexes and tone are often considerably more exaggerated in the lower limbs compared to the upper limbs [30]. Autonomic dysfunction manifests as tachycardia, hypertension, diaphoresis, shivering, mydriasis, and variable degrees of temperature elevation. In mild cases, mental state examination may reveal hypervigilance and enhanced startle, which progresses to agitated delirium and obtundation with increasing severity. Bowel sounds are generally hyperactive, and patients may have diarrhea. Ocular clonus may be seen [30]. In more severe cases, metabolic acidosis, significant hyperthermia, elevated serum creatine kinase, disseminated intravascular coagulation, and cardiovascular collapse may occur.

Especially in its milder forms, the syndrome may be difficult to differentiate from other causes of worsening of PD. Indeed, the callow physician may inappropriately attribute an increase in rigidity, altered mental status, and autonomic dysfunction to urinary or respiratory tract infections rather than considering the possibility of offending medications.

The symptomatic overlap between the clinical features of SS and another medication-related syndrome occasionally encountered in PD,

neuroleptic malignant syndrome (NMS), can make differentiating between these difficult. NMS results from the administration of dopamine antagonists, or abrupt reduction or cessation of dopaminergic stimulation e.g. of levodopa or dopamine agonists in PD. As such, a thorough medication history is often the most helpful differentiator. Shivering, hyperreflexia, myoclonus, and diarrhea, all common symptoms in SS, are unusual in NMS [30]. Timeline of symptom onset is also purported to help, with SS generally occurring within 6 hours of drug ingestion or dose escalation, while NMS generally develops over days (see Table 21.2). Things are often however not so clear cut, and delayed-onset SS commonly occurs, depending on the pharmacokinetics of the ingested medications. In this regard, the SSRI fluoxetine can be particularly misleading, owing to its metabolism to the serotonergic metabolite norfluoxetine, whose serum half-life is considerably longer than its parent compound [30].

Diagnosis of Serotonin Syndrome

A number of criteria have been designed in order to aid with the diagnosis of serotonin syndrome. These include the Sternbach, Radomski, and Hunter criteria (see Table 21.3) [31–33]. All of these come with their own set of pros and cons. The Sternbach criteria have historically been most frequently employed, though their strict application may overlook mild cases [31]. The Hunter criteria on the other hand may be more accurate,

Table 21.2 Clinical features which aid in the differentiation of serotonin syndrome from neuroleptic malignant syndrome

	Medication history	Usual time to onset of symptoms	Muscle tone	Reflexes	Pupils	Bowels	Shivering	Clonus (including ocular)	Myoclonus	Mental status
Serotonin syndrome	Recent addition or increase of serotonergic agent	< 12 hours	Increased (lower > upper limbs)	Increased	Dilated	Hyperactive, diarrhea frequent	Common	Common	Common	Agitation, confusion, coma
Neuroleptic Malignant Syndrome	Recent addition or increase in dopamine antagonist Recent withdrawal of dopamine receptor agonist of levodopa	1–3 days	Increased (lead-pipe)	Normal/ decreased	Normal	Normal	Rare	Rare	Rare	Stupor, bradyphrenia, coma

Table 21.3 Diagnostic criteria for serotonin syndrome

Sternbach	Radomski		Hunter
Recent addition or increase in a known serotonergic agent, PLUS at least three of the following features:	Recent initiation of increase in a known serotonergic agent PLUS four minor OR three major and two minor symptoms:		In the presence of a serotonergic agent, the presence of ONE of the following clinical features:
	Major	**Minor**	
Mental status changes (confusion, hypermania)	Mental		• Spontaneous clonus
Agitation	• Impaired consciousness	• Restlessness	• Inducible clonus AND agitation OR diaphoresis
Myoclonus	• Elevated mood	• Insomnia	• Ocular clonus AND agitation OR diaphoresis
Hyperreflexia	• Semicoma/coma		• Tremor AND hyperreflexia
Diaphoresis			• Hypertonic AND temperature > 38 °C AND ocular clonus OR inducible clonus
Shivering	Neurological		
Tremor	• Myoclonus	• Incoordination	
Diarrhea	• Tremor	• Dilated pupils	
Incoordination	• Shivering	• Akathisia	
Fever	• Rigidity		
	• Hyperreflexia		
AND	Vegetative		
	• Fever	• Tachycardia	
• Other etiologies (e.g. infectious, metabolic, or endocrine, substance abuse or withdrawal) have been ruled out.	• Sweating	• Tachypnea/ dyspnea	
		• Diarrhea	
		• Hyper/ hypotension	
• A neuroleptic drug had not been started or increased in dosage prior to the onset of the signs and symptoms listed above.	AND		
	• Clinical features not an integral part of the underlying psychiatric disorder prior to commencing the serotonergic agent.		
	• Other etiologies (e.g. infectious, metabolic or endocrine, substance abuse or withdrawal) have been ruled out.		
	• A neuroleptic drug has not been started or increased in dosage prior to the onset of the signs and symptoms listed above.		

but were specifically designed for patients with SSRI overdose, rather than serotonin syndrome [33].

Treatment of Serotonin Syndrome

A high index of suspicion combined with early treatment including withdrawal of the offending agent(s), supportive care, and active management of hyperthermia and autonomic instability offers the best chances of improvement. The degree of active management required depends on syndrome severity. Mild cases can often be managed with medication withdrawal, supportive care, and administration of benzodiazepines to help with rigidity and hyperkinesia. More severe cases may require additional sedation, intubation, and neuromuscular paralysis. The $5-HT_{2A}$ antagonist, cyproheptadine, is recommended in severe cases, though its effectiveness has not been rigorously established [30].

Specific Issues Relating to Monoamine Oxidase B Inhibition in Parkinson's Disease

The observation that both non-selective MAOIs and MAO-A inhibitors were frequently implicated in cases of severe serotonin syndrome understandably caused some concern surrounding an increased risk for the development of serotonin toxicity in patients with PD treated with MAO-B inhibitors. This was especially so due to the frequent co-administration of serotonergic compounds for treatment of co-existent mood and anxiety disorders in this population. While theoretically, the selective inhibition of MAO-B would render this risk low (most serotonin being metabolized by MAO-A), it is recognized that both selegiline and rasagiline lose their selectivity for MAO-B at high doses, whereupon they also begin to inhibit MAO-A [34]; safinamide is vastly more selective for MAO-B than either selegiline or rasagiline.

The potential for induction of serotonin syndrome by MAO-B use has been examined in a number of trials. A 1997 survey of the Parkinson Study Group of an estimated 4568 patients treated with the combination of selegiline and an SSRI found 11 patients (0.24%) who had symptoms possibly related to serotonin excess [35]. In only two patients (0.04%) was this considered to be serious. A 2014 large multicenter retrospective cohort study of 1504 patients with PD found no cases of serotonin syndrome in 471 patients co-prescribed rasagiline and antidepressants (most commonly SSRIs) [36]. A post-hoc analysis of the ADAGIO study examining 191 patients on rasagiline and antidepressant therapy found no evidence of serotonin syndrome [37].

Pragmatically therefore, there is little concrete evidence to substantiate an increased risk of serotonin syndrome in PD patients treated with combinations of MAO-B inhibitors and either SSRIs or SNRIs, as long as recommended doses are not exceeded [35, 37].

In practice however, reports of serotonin syndrome in patients receiving MAO-B inhibitors along with other serotonergic medications have surfaced. Hébant et al. reported a case of serotonin syndrome in a patient with PD beginning three weeks after the addition of paroxetine to pre-existing rasagiline therapy [38]. Single cases also describe SS resulting from co-administration of escitalopram [39, 40], fluoxetine [41], sertraline [42], nortriptyline [43], and linezolid [44] with MAO-B inhibitors. In addition, a case of serotonin syndrome resulting from rasagiline overdose, without concurrent administration of other serotonergic drugs, has been described [45]. Concurrent administration of MAO-B inhibitors with certain analgesics (meperidine, tramadol, methadone, and propoxyphene) and the antitussive dextromethorphan remains contraindicated. Official FDA guidance also suggests that it is prudent to avoid administering MAO-B inhibitors alongside SSRIs, SNRIs, and tricyclic antidepressants, and suggests a 14-day washout period (five weeks for fluoxetine), though in practice, co-administration is common. Some degree of vigilance must therefore continue to be observed when patients are co-prescribed these medications.

Identifying patients who have heightened risk of developing serotonin syndrome remains difficult. An individual's genetic makeup likely plays a part however. SSRIs are metabolized by the cytochrome P450 family of enzymes, particularly CYP2D6 and CYP3A4. Genetic polymorphisms in these enzymes, causing a hypometabolic state, could theoretically predispose an individual to SS following SSRI administration [46]. Furthermore, individuals with the T102C single nucleotide polymorphisms in the $5-HT_{2A}$ receptor gene may be at heightened risk of SS, as may those with polymorphisms in the SERT gene [46]. Testing for such polymorphisms however remains outside the scope of routine clinical practice.

Cardiovascular Complications

The "Cheese Reaction"

Cheese, especially aged cheese, is the classic food associated with hypertensive reactions in patients undergoing MAO inhibition, hence the common description of the syndrome as the "cheese reaction." Though noted by some individuals to have a relationship with hypertensive crises (a British pharmacist for example noted that his wife, who was on an MAOI, would experience severe headaches whenever she consumed cheese), it was not until 1965 that the causative dietary compound was identified as tyramine [47].

Dietary tyramine is metabolized by MAO-A in the gut lining. In the setting of MAO-A inhibition, tyramine is absorbed and taken up by pre-synaptic noradrenergic nerve terminals where it acts as a false substrate. Tyramine displaces noradrenaline from pre-synaptic vesicles, the release of which can produce a hypertensive crisis.

Theoretically, this complication should only be encountered with MAO-A inhibition, and as such, should not occur with selective MAO-B inhibitors, unless these are taken at above recommended dosages (thereby producing off-target effects). No dietary restriction is therefore necessary in PD patients prescribed MAO-B inhibitors. The incidence of this adverse effect has declined steeply in recent years, in line with the trend towards falling prescription rates of non-selective MAOIs and MAO-A inhibitors.

Again however, as with the serotonin syndrome, theory does not always translate into clinical practice. There have been reported cases of selegiline taken at recommended doses inducing hypertensive crises either alone [48] or following SSRI or tyramine administration [49]. There are also cases of hypertension following co-administration with ephedrine, a sympathomimetic, as well as exaggerated pressor responses e.g. following dopamine infusion, likely due to impaired drug metabolism [50].

Orthostatic Hypotension

Orthostatic hypotension is one of the most frequent side effects of MAOI use in patients with PD. This can be particularly problematic, given that this patient group is pre-disposed to this phenomenon, both due to dysfunctional pressor responses from synucleinopathy and levodopa administration.

Gradual displacement of adrenaline from peripheral nerve terminals by amines which, in the absence of MAO inhibition would be metabolized in the gut, is the proposed mechanism for the generation of postural hypotension [51]. In clinical practice, the occurrence of blood pressure alterations with MAO-B inhibitors is seen most commonly with selegiline [6, 52, 53], and probably to a lesser extent with rasagiline and safinamide [54, 55].

Cardiovascular Mortality

United Kingdom PD study group research found a significant increase in mortality in patients taking selegiline as add-on therapy to levodopa [6]. This was explained to be due to increased incidence of orthostatic hypotension in those prescribed selegiline, attributed to its amphetamine metabolites. Such an increase in mortality in patients taking selegiline was however not observed in further clinical trials [56]. No such concerns have been raised with either rasagiline or safinamide.

Other Adverse Effects

Other adverse effects variably reported during the studies of MAO-B inhibitors included anorexia, nausea, vomiting, infection, headache, dizziness, and asthenia [9, 11]. A number of skin cancers, in particular melanomas, were also observed, though the incidence of melanoma is increased in PD per se, and there is no clear evidence that this is further increased by MAOI administration.

Confusion, hallucinations, and insomnia have been observed as side effects of selegiline, possibly due to its amphetamine metabolites [57, 58]. Avoiding administration late in the day may mitigate this to some extent. Rasagiline appears to have less neurobehavioral side effects, with no significant increase in confusion or hallucinations detected during post-hoc analyses of the PRESTO and TEMPO trials, even when a sub-analysis for patients over 70 years of age was performed.

Conclusion

There are two main indications for the use of MAOIs in patients with PD. By far the most common is the administration of selective MAO-B inhibitors, either as monotherapy or in combination with levodopa in order to ease the motor symptoms of PD. By and large, these drugs are safe when administered in recommended doses.

Certain characteristics of patients with PD however make them prone to potential drug interactions. The first is the high rate of depressive illness in this population, often requiring pharmacotherapy, frequently in the form of an SSRI. While this is generally safe, occasional reports of serotonin syndrome resulting from drug–drug interactions in the PD population reinforces that this potentially life-threatening condition must be kept in mind as a cause of deterioration in motor function and cognition in patients with PD, especially when accompanied by other clinical signs such as autonomic changes and mental state alterations. Moreover, the clinical presentation of serotonin syndrome can be mistaken for other common causes of deterioration in the PD population, such as infection.

The use of MAOIs as treatments for depression have become unpopular in recent years, particularly due to the imposed dietary restrictions on consumption of tyramine-rich foods in order to avoid hypertensive events. Such tyramine-related hypertensive "cheese reactions" are rarely encountered with MAO-B inhibitors.

Theoretical risks have been raised about increased cardiovascular mortality in patients prescribed selegiline, though this has not been conclusively reproduced across studies. Postural hypotension is however a common and recognized side effect of MAO-B inhibitors, which can be particularly problematic in PD patients, in whom such events decrease quality of life but may also accelerate cognitive decline [59].

In summary, MAO-B inhibition represents a useful adjunct to the treatment of motor and non-motor manifestations in PD. These medications have a relatively benign side-effect profile. Serious side effects, mainly relating to drug–drug interactions, are possible, and though exceedingly rare, merit careful consideration in the appropriate clinical setting.

References

1. Kalgutkar AS, Dalvie DK, Castagnoli N Jr, Taylor TJ. Interactions of nitrogen-containing xenobiotics with monoamine oxidase (MAO) isozymes A and B: SAR studies on MAO substrates and inhibitors. Chem Res Toxicol 2001; **14**(9): 1139–1162.

2. Riederer P, Laux G. MAO-inhibitors in Parkinson's Disease. Exp Neurobiol 2011; **20**(1): 1–17.

3. Johnston JP. Some observations upon a new inhibitor of monoamine oxidase in brain tissue. Biochem Pharmacol 1968; **17**(7): 1285–1297.

4. Robakis D, Fahn S. Defining the role of the monoamine oxidase-B inhibitors for Parkinson's disease. CNS Drugs 2015; **29**(6): 433–441.

5. Parkinson Study Group. Effects of tocopherol and deprenyl on the progression of disability in early Parkinson's disease. N Engl J Med 1993; **328**(3): 176–183.

6. Lees AJ. Comparison of therapeutic effects and mortality data of levodopa and levodopa combined with selegiline in patients with early, mild Parkinson's disease. Parkinson's Disease Research Group of the United Kingdom. Br Med J. 1995; **311**(7020): 1602–1607.

7. Myllylä VV, Sotaniemi KA, Hakulinen P, Mäki-Ikola O, Heinonen EH. Selegiline as the primary treatment of Parkinson's disease–a long-term double-blind study. Acta Neurol Scand 1997; **95**(4): 211–218.

8. Nayak L, Henchcliffe C. Rasagiline in treatment of Parkinson's disease. Neuropsychiatr Dis Treat 2008; **4**(1): 23–32.

9. Parkinson Study Group. A controlled trial of rasagiline in early Parkinson disease: the TEMPO Study. Arch Neurol 2002; **59**(12): 1937–1943.

10. Olanow CW, Rascol O, Hauser R, et al. A double-blind, delayed-start trial of rasagiline in Parkinson's disease. N Engl J Med 2009; **361**(13): 1268–1278.

11. Parkinson Study Group. A randomized placebo-controlled trial of rasagiline in levodopa-treated patients with Parkinson disease and motor fluctuations: the PRESTO study. Arch Neurol 2005; **62**: 241–248.

12. Rascol O, Brooks DJ, Melamed E, et al. Rasagiline as an adjunct to levodopa in patients with Parkinson's disease and motor fluctuations (LARGO, Lasting effect in Adjunct therapy with Rasagiline Given Once daily, study): a randomised, double-blind, parallel-group trial. Lancet 2005; **365**: 947–954.

13. Bette S, Shpiner DS, Singer C, Moore H. Safinamide in the management of patients with Parkinson's disease not stabilized on levodopa: a review of the current clinical evidence. Ther Clin Risk Manag 2018; **14**: 1737–1745.

14. Shulman KI, Fischer HD, Herrmann N, et al. Current prescription patterns and safety profile of irreversible monoamine oxidase inhibitors: a population-based cohort study of older adults. J Clin Psychiatry. 2009; **70**(12): 1681–1686.

15. Karlsen K, Larsen JP, Tandberg E, Jørgensen K. Fatigue in patients with Parkinson's disease. Mov Disord 1999; **14**: 237–241.

16. Clarke A, Brewer F, Johnson ES, et al. A new formulation of selegiline: improved bioavailability and selectivity for MAO-B inhibition. J Neural Transm 2003; **110**(11): 1241–1255.

17. Sandoval-Rincón M, Sáenz-Farret M, Miguel-Puga A, Micheli F, Arias-Carrión O. Rational pharmacological approaches for cognitive dysfunction and depression in Parkinson's disease. Front Neurol 2015; **6**: 71.

18. Schapira AH. Monoamine oxidase B inhibitors for the treatment of Parkinson's disease: a review of symptomatic and potential disease-modifying effects. CNS Drugs 2011; **25**(12): 1061–1071.

19. Boll MC, Alcaraz-Zubeldia M, Rios C. Medical management of Parkinson's disease: focus on neuroprotection. Curr Neuropharmacol 2011; **9** (2): 350–359.

20. Tatton W, Chalmers-Redman R, Tatton N. Neuroprotection by deprenyl and other propargylamines: glyceraldehyde-3-phosphate dehydrogenase rather than monoamine oxidase B. J Neural Transm 2003; **110**(5): 509–515.

21. Wu RM, Chen RC, Chiueh CC. Effect of MAO-B inhibitors on MPP? toxicity in vivo. Ann N Y Acad Sci 2000; **899**: 255–261.

22. Oates JA, Sjoerdsma A. Neurologic effects of tryptophan in patients receiving a monoamine oxidase inhibitor. Neurology 1960; **10**: 1076–1078.

23. Moss MJ, Hendrickson RG. Toxicology Investigators Consortium (ToxIC). Serotonin toxicity: associated agents and clinical characteristics. J Clin Psychopharmacol 2019; **39** (6): 628–633.

24. Scotton WJ, Hill LJ, Williams AC, Barnes NM. Serotonin syndrome: pathophysiology, clinical features, management, and potential future directions. Int J Tryptophan Res 2019; **12**: 1178646919873925.

25. Reijnders JS, Ehrt U, Weber WE, Aarsland D, Leentjens AF. A systematic review of prevalence studies of depression in Parkinson's disease. Mov Disord 2008; **23**(2): 183–189; quiz 313.

26. Aarsland D, Påhlhagen S, Ballard CG, Ehrt U, Svenningsson P. Depression in Parkinson disease–epidemiology, mechanisms and management. Nat Rev Neurol 2011; **8**(1): 35–47.

27. Starkstein SE, Mayberg HS, Leiguarda R, et al. A prospective longitudinal study of depression, cognitive decline, and physical impairments in patients with Parkinson's disease. J Neurol Neurosurg Psychiatry 1992; **55**: 377–382.

28. Müller B, Assmus J, Herlofson K, Larsen JP, Tysnes OB. Importance of motor vs. non-motor symptoms for health-related quality of life in early Parkinson's disease. Parkinsonism Relat Disord 2013; **19**(11): 1027–1032.

29. Hughes TA, Ross HF, Mindham RH, Spokes EG. Mortality in Parkinson's disease and its association with dementia and depression. Acta Neurol Scand 2004; **110**: 118–123.

30. Boyer EW, Shannon M. The serotonin syndrome. N Engl J Med 2005; **352**(11): 1112–1120.

31. Sternbach H. The serotonin syndrome. Am J Psychiatry 1991; **148**: 705–713.

32. Radomski JW, Dursun SM, Reveley MA, Kutcher SP. An exploratory approach to the serotonin syndrome: an update of clinical phenomenology and revised diagnostic criteria. Med Hypotheses 2000; **55**(3): 218–224.

33. Dunkley EJ, Isbister GK, Sibbritt D, Dawson AH, Whyte IM. The Hunter Serotonin Toxicity Criteria: simple and accurate diagnostic decision rules for serotonin toxicity. QJM 2003; **96**(9): 635–642.

34. Youdim MB, Gross A, Finberg JP. Rasagiline [N-propargyl-1 R(+)-aminoindan], a selective and potent inhibitor of mitochondrial monoamine oxidase B. Br J Pharmacol 2001; **132**(2): 500–506.

35. Richard IH, Kurlan R, Tanner C, et al. Serotonin syndrome and the combined use of deprenyl and an antidepressant in Parkinson's disease. Parkinson Study Group. Neurology 1997; **48**(4): 1070–1077.

36. Panisset M, Chen JJ, Rhyee SH, Conner J, Mathena J. STACCATO study investigators. Serotonin toxicity association with concomitant antidepressants and rasagiline treatment: retrospective study (STACCATO). Pharmacotherapy 2014; **34**(12): 1250–1258.

37. Smith KM, Eyal E, Weintraub D, ADAGIO Investigators. Combined rasagiline and antidepressant use in Parkinson disease in the ADAGIO study: effects on nonmotor symptoms and tolerability. JAMA Neurol 2015; **72**(1): 88–95.

38. Hébant B, Guillaume M, Desbordes M, et al. Combination of paroxetine and rasagiline induces serotonin syndrome in a parkinsonian patient. Rev Neurol 2016; **172**(12): 788–789.

39. Sanyal D, Chakraborty S, Bhattacharyya R. An interesting case of serotonin syndrome precipitated by escitalopram. Indian J Pharmacol 2010; **42**(6): 418–419.

40. Suphanklang J, Santimaleeworagun W, Supasyndh O. Combination of escitalopram and rasagiline induced serotonin syndrome: a case report and review literature. J Med Assoc Thai 2015; **98**(12): 1254–1257.

41. Bilbao Garay J, Mesa Plaza N, Castilla Castellano V, Dhimes Tejada P. Serotonin syndrome: report of a fatal case and review of the literature. Rev Clin Esp 2002; **202**(4): 209–211.

42. Duval F, Flabeau O, Razafimahefa J, Spampinato U, Tison F. Encephalopathy associated with rasagiline and sertraline in Parkinson's disease: possible serotonin syndrome. Mov Disord 2013; **28**(10): 1464.

43. Hinds NP, Hillier CE, Wiles CM. Possible serotonin syndrome arising from an interaction between nortriptyline and selegiline in a lady with parkinsonism. J Neurol 2000; **247**(10): 811.

44. Hisham M, Sivakumar MN, Nandakumar V, Lakshmikanthcharan S. Linezolid and rasagiline – a culprit for serotonin syndrome. Indian J Pharmacol 2016; **48**(1): 91–92.

45. Fernandes C, Reddy P, Kessel B. Rasagiline-induced serotonin syndrome. Mov Disord 2011; **26**(4): 766–767.

46. Francescangeli J, Karamchandani K, Powell M, Bonavia A. The serotonin syndrome: from molecular mechanisms to clinical practice. Int J Mol Sci 2019; **20**(9): E2288.

47. Blackwell B, Mabbitt LA. Tyramine in cheese related to hypertensive crises after monoamine oxidase inhibition. Lancet 1965; **1**: 938–940.

48. Ito D, Amano T, Sato H, Fukuuchi Y. Paroxysmal hypertensive crises induced by selegiline in a patient with Parkinson's disease. J Neurol 2001; **248**(6): 533–534.

49. Montastruc JL, Chamontin B, Senard JM, et al. Pseudophaeochromocytoma in parkinsonian patients treated with fluoxetine plus selegiline. Lancet 1993; **341**(8844): 555.

50. Rose LM, Ohlinger MJ, Mauro VF. A hypertensive reaction induced by concurrent use of selegiline and dopamine. Ann Pharmacother 2000; **34**(9): 1020–1024.

51. Cockhill LA, Remick RA. Blood pressure effects of monoamine oxidase inhibitors–the highs and lows. Can J Psychiatry 1987; **32**(9): 803–808.

52. Pursiainen V, Korpelainen TJ, Haapaniemi HT, et al. Selegiline and blood pressure in patients with Parkinson's disease. Acta Neurol Scand 2007; **115**: 104–108.

53. Shoulson I, Oakes D, Fahn S, et al. Impact of sustained deprenyl (selegiline) in levodopa-treated PD: a randomized placebo-controlled extension of the deprenyl and tocopherol antioxidant therapy of parkinsonism trial. Ann Neurol 2002; **51**: 604–612.

54. Abassi ZA, Binah O, Youdim MB. Cardiovascular activity of rasagiline, a selective and potent inhibitor of mitochondrial monoamine oxidase B: comparison with selegiline. Br J Pharmacol 2004; **143**(3): 371–378.

55. Minguez-Minguez S, Solis-Garcia del Pozo J, Jordan J. Rasagiline in Parkinson's disease: a review based on meta-analysis of clinical data. Pharmacol Res 2013; **74**: 78–86.

56. Dezsi L, Vecsei L. Monoamine oxidase B inhibitors in Parkinson's disease. CNS Neurol Disord Drug Targets 2017; **16**(4): 425–439.

57. Montastruc JL, Chaumerliac C, Desboeuf K, et al. Adverse drug reactions to selegiline: a review of the French pharmacovigilance database. Clin Neuropharmacol 2000; **23**(5): 271–275.

58. Kamakura K, Mochizuki H, Kaida K, et al. Therapeutic factors causing hallucination in Parkinson's disease patients, especially those given selegiline. Parkinsonism Relat Disord 2004; **10**(4): 235–242.

59. Centi J, Freeman R, Gibbons CH, et al. Effects of orthostatic hypotension on cognition in Parkinson disease. Neurology 2017; **88**(1): 17–24.

Chapter 22

Parkinson's Disease and Pregnancy

Shira McMahan, Ramon Lugo-Sanchez, Nestor Galvez-Jimenez

Parkinson's disease (PD) in pregnancy is a rare occurrence. PD presents before the age of 40 in only 5% of cases and less than 400 women less than 50 years of age are diagnosed with PD each year in the United States [1]. However, as the average maternal age is increasing, it may become more common. Incidence of pregnancy in PD is unknown and knowledge is limited to case reports.

Animal models suggest estrogen has a neuroprotective effect on dopaminergic neurons by influencing anti-oxidative, anti-inflammatory, and anti-apoptotic pathways with studies showing cell death can be significantly decreased by administration of estrogen [2]. Other animal studies showed estrogen has dopaminergic effect by inhibiting catechol-O-methyltransferase (COMT) and striatal dopamine transporter activity as well as enhancing tyrosine hydroxylase [3, 4]. Incidence of PD is less in women, yet after menopause risk of PD increases [5]. Women tend to have less severe disease but more dyskinesia [6, 7]. When estrogen levels drop during the week prior to menses, one study showed 50% to 60% of women reported worsening PD symptoms [8]. Exogenous estrogen use has been associated with reduced symptom severity in postmenopausal women with both early PD as well as women with motor fluctuations [9, 10]. There are also population studies describing no link between lifetime estrogen exposure and the development of PD [8, 11, 12]. Even some data suggests that exposure to exogenous estrogens is related to an increased risk of PD and an earlier menopause reduces PD risk [13]. There have also been numerous reports of worsening PD symptoms throughout duration of pregnancy when estrogen levels are high [14] so there is much conflicting data on this topic.

Reports in English literature from 1985–2016 reviewed 79 cases of pregnancy and PD from 28 articles with 75 live births. A total of 41% of women experienced worsening of PD symptoms and 44% showed no change or improvement in symptoms [1]. A case report involving a 33-year-old woman on sinemet while pregnant highlighted increased motor dysfunction during pregnancy despite dose increases and adding mirapex. She didn't return to baseline postpartum [15].

During pregnancy, women's plasma volume, volume of distribution, and metabolic states are altered thus resulting in modified pharmacokinetics and possible subtherapeutic dosing of anti-parkinsonian medications. Pregnancy also causes physical and psychological stress which may also cause worsening PD.

Anti-parkinsonian medication use in literature includes levodopa, ergot-derived dopamine agonists, catecholamine-O-methyltransferase (COMT) inhibitors, monoamine oxidase-B (MAO-B) inhibitors, amantadine, and anticholinergics.

Levodopa is most commonly used and relatively safe in pregnancy. Levodopa is transferred through the placenta resulting in fetal exposure. Levodopa is metabolized by the fetus but carbidopa does not cross the placental barrier [16]. Articles of patients on 100–2500 mg reported eight complications including seizure, pre-eclampsia (on amantadine as well), osteomalacia, ventral septal defects (VSDs), placental abruption, and transient hypotonia. All babies developed normally. Overall levodopa is not associated with an increased rate of spontaneous abortion, birth complications, or teratogenicity and available data supports its use as first-line treatment in pregnant women [17].

Regarding dopamine agonists, ergot-derived agonists have traditionally been used in women with hyperprolactinemia. No associated complications were reported in 650 cabergoline- and 1410 bromocriptine-exposed pregnancies but doses are much smaller than those used in PD.

A French study involved 183 women receiving at least one dopamine agonist during pregnancy, but only four of them had PD. Bromocriptine was the most frequently prescribed drug and is approved for PD in France. None of them took levodopa. Eighty-six percent of exposed women gave birth to healthy term babies but risks of pregnancy loss and preterm birth were significantly increased [18]. A case report of a 42-year-old woman who became pregnant at 41 years of age was treated with pramipexole 4.5 and refused to stop it while pregnant. She had worsening motor disability and had to have a Caesarean section due to motor impairment. The baby was healthy and showed normal development [19]. Despite this, no issues with fertility, conception, or birthing process were noted in women with idiopathic PD and diagnosis alone does not increase the risk of birth complications and should not directly dictate delivery method [1].

Regarding selegiline and rasagiline, ventral septal defects (VSDs) were noted in selegiline exposure but patients were also on levodopa and entacapone [6]. No adverse effects were reported on the fetus of a patient who continued taking levodopa and selegiline throughout her pregnancy [20]. Selegiline administered as monotherapy for rabbits caused an increase in resorption and decrease in the number of live fetuses, with similar results noted in rat studies. Based on animal studies, use may be contraindicated during pregnancy [21].

Amantadine has been reported to be embryotoxic and teratogenic in animal studies and its use is widely discouraged during pregnancy [17].

Regarding the outcomes of deep brain stimulation (DBS) in pregnancy, women with PD could reduce their medications and it also reduced motor fluctuations and dopamine dysregulation symptoms, allowing for pregnancy to occur post-DBS. Women tolerated DBS adjustments well [22].

With regards to breastfeeding, dopamine agonists and levodopa will suppress prolactin release and reduce/inhibit lactation. Data is limited on the degree that medications are secreted into breast milk and have effects on infants, but it is likely babies are exposed to low levels. It is typically not advised to breastfeed while taking anti-PD medications [17].

References

1. Seier M, Hiller A. Parkinson's disease and pregnancy: an updated review. Parkinsonism Relat Disord 2017; **40**: 11–17.

2. Gatto NM, Deapen D, Stoyanoff S, et al. Lifetime exposure to estrogens and Parkinson's disease in California teachers. Parkinsonism Relat Disord 2014; **20**: 1149–1156.

3. Nageshwaran S, Smith M, Bordelon YM. Movement disorders and pregnancy. In: Klien A, O'Neal MA, Scifres C, (eds.). *Neurological Illness in Pregnancy: Principles and Practice*, 1st ed. Wiley-Blackwell; 2016, 179–190.

4. Disshon KA, Boja JW, Dluzen DE. Inhibition of striatal dopamine transporter activity by 17B-estradiol. Eur J Pharmacol 1998; **345**: 207–211.

5. Bendetti MD, Maraganore DM, Bower JH, et al. Hysterectomy, menopause and estrogen use preceding Parkinson's disease: an exploratory case control study. Mov Disord 2001; **16**: 830–837.

6. Lyons KE, Hubble JP, Troster AI, et al. Gender differences in Parkinson's disease. Clin Neuropharmacol 1998; **21**: 118–121.

7. Picillo M, Nocioletti A, Fetoni V, et al. The relevance of gender in Parkinson's disease: a review. J Neurol 2017; **9**: 1–25.

8. Rubin SM. Parkinson's disease in women. Dis Mon 2007; **53**: 206–213.

9. Saunders-Pullman R, Gordon-Elliot J, Parides M, et al. The effect of estrogen replacement on early Parkinson's disease. Neurology 1999; **52**: 141.

10. Tsang K, Ho S, Lo S. Estrogen improves motor disability in parkinsonian postmenopausal women with motor fluctuations. Neurology 2000; **54**: 2292–2298.

11. Liu R, Baird D, Park Y, et al. Female reproductive factors, menopausal hormone use and Parkinson's disease. Mov Disord 2014; **29**: 889–896.

12. Shulman LM. Is there a connection between estrogen and Parkinson's disease? Parkinsonism Relat Disord 2002; **8**: 289–295.

13. Wang P, Li J, Qiu S, Wen H, Du J. Hormone replacement therapy and Parkinson's disease risk in women: a meta-analysis of 14 observational studies. Neuropsychiatr Dis Treat 2015; **11**: 59–66.

14. Popat R, Van Den Eeden S, Tanner C, et al. Effect of reproductive factors and postmenopausal hormone use on the risk of Parkinson. Neurology 2005; **65**: 383–390.

15. Shulman LM, Minagar A, Weiner WJ. The effect of pregnancy in Parkinson's disease. Mov Disord 2000; **15**: 132–135.

16. Merchant CA, Cohen G, Mytilineous C, et al. Human transplacental transmission of carbidopa/levodopa. Neurology 1994; **44**(Suppl 2): A247–248.

17. Tufekcioglu Z, Hanagasi H, Yalcin Cakmakli G, et al. Use of anti-Parkinson medication during pregnancy: a case series, J Neurol 2018; **265**(8): 1922–1929.

18. Hurault-Delarue C, Montastruc JL, Beau AB, Lacriox I, Damase-Michel C. Pregnancy outcome in women exposed to dopamine agonists during pregnancy: a pharmacoepidemiology study in EFEMERIS database. Arch Gyencol Obstet 2014; **290**: 263–270.

19. Mucchiut M, Belgrado E, Cutuli D, Antonini A, Bergonzi P. Pramipexole-treated Parkinson's disease during pregnancy. Mov Disord 2004; **19**: 1114–1115.

20. Kupsch A, Oertel WH. Selegiline, pregnancy and Parkinson's disease. Mov Disord 1998; **13**: 175–176.

21. Eldepryl (selegiline) [product information]. Tampa (FL): Somerset Pharmaceutical; 1996.

22. Kranick SM, Mowry EM, Colcher A, Horn S, Golbe LI. Movement disorders and pregnancy: a review of the literature. Mov Disord 2010; **25**: 665–671.

Index